CANCER GENES

Functional Aspects

PEZCOLLER FOUNDATION SYMPOSIA

SERIES EDITOR:
Enrico Mihich, *Roswell Park Cancer Institute, Buffalo, New York*

STANDING PEZCOLLER SYMPOSIA COMMITTEE:
Enrico Mihich (Chairman), *Roswell Park Cancer Institute, Buffalo, New York*
David M. Livingston (Vice-Chairman), *Dana–Farber Cancer Institute, Boston, Massachusetts*
Giuseppe Bernardi, *Pezcoller Foundation, Trento, Italy*
Carlo M. Croce, *Jefferson Medical College, Philadelphia, Pennsylvania*
Giuseppe Della Porta, *European Institute of Oncology, Milan, Italy*
Vincent T. DeVita, *Yale Comprehensive Cancer Center, New Haven, Connecticut*
Giorgio Lenaz, *University of Bologna, Bologna, Italy*
Paolo Schlechter, *Pezcoller Foundation, Trento, Italy*
Ellen Solomon, *Imperial Cancer Research Fund, London, England*
Tadatsugu Taniguchi, *University of Tokyo, Tokyo, Japan*
Fulvio Zuelli, *University of Trento, Trento, Italy*

PROGRAM COMMITTEE:
Enrico Mihich (Chair), *Roswell Park Cancer Institute, Buffalo, New York*
David Housman (Co-Chair), *MIT Center for Cancer Research, Cambridge, Massachusetts*
Jane Azizkhan, *Roswell Park Cancer Institute, Buffalo, New York*
Paolo Comoglio, *University of Turin, Turin, Italy*
Giulio Draetta, *European Institute of Oncology, Milan, Italy*
David M. Livingston, *Dana–Farber Cancer Institute, Boston, Massachusetts*
Alex Matter, *Ciba-Geigy Ltd., Basel, Switzerland*

Recent volumes published by Plenum Press:

A Continuation Order Plan is available for this series. A continuation order will bring delivery of each new volume immediately upon publication. Volumes are billed only upon actual shipment. For further information please contact the publisher.

CANCER GENES

Functional Aspects

Edited by

Enrico Mihich
Roswell Park Cancer Institute
Buffalo, New York

and

David Housman
MIT Center for Cancer Research
Cambridge, Massachusetts

SPRINGER SCIENCE+BUSINESS MEDIA, LLC

Library of Congress Cataloging-in-Publication Data

Cancer genes : functional aspects / edited by Enrico Mihich and David
  Housman.
        p.   cm. -- (Pezcoller Foundation symposia ; v. 7)
    "Proceedings of the Seventh Pezcoller Symposium on Cancer Genes:
  Functional Aspects, held June 14-16, 1995, in Trento, Italy"--T.p.
  verso.
    Includes bibliographical references and index.
    ISBN 978-0-306-45482-0   ISBN 978-1-4615-5895-8 (eBook)
    DOI 10.1007/978-1-4615-5895-8
    1. Oncogenes--Congresses. 2. Antioncogenes--Congresses.
  I. Mihich, Enrico. II. Housman, David E. III. Pezcoller Symposium
  on Cancer Genes: Functional Aspects (1995 : Trento, Italy)
  IV. Series: Pezcoller Foundation symposia ; 7.
    [DNLM: 1. Oncogenes--physiology--congresses. 2. Neoplasms-
  -genetics--congresses. 3. Gene Expression Regulation, Neoplastic-
  -physiology--congresses. 4. Gene Therapy--methods--congresses.   W1
  PE995 v.7 1996 / QZ 202 C21527 1996]
  RC268.42.C36   1996
  616.99'4042--dc20
  DNLM/DLC
  for Library of Congress   96-41755
                                                             CIP

Proceedings of the Seventh Pezcoller Symposium on Cancer Genes: Functional Aspects,
held June 14–16, 1995, in Trento, Italy

ISBN 978-0-306-45482-0

©1996 Springer Science+Business Media New York
Originally published by Plenum Press, New York in 1996

10 9 8 7 6 5 4 3 2 1

THE PEZCOLLER FOUNDATION

The Pezcoller Foundation was created in 1979 by Professor Alessio Pezcoller (1896–1993) who was the chief surgeon of the S. Chiara Hospital in Trento from 1937 to 1966 and who gave a substantial portion of his estate to support its activities; the Foundation also benefits from the cooperation of the Savings Bank Cassa di Risparmio di Trento e Rovereto.

The main goal of this non-profit foundation is to provide and recognize scientific progress on life-threatening diseases, currently focusing on cancer. Towards this goal, the Pezcoller Foundation awards, every two years, the Pezcoller Prize, recognizing highly meritorious contributions to medical research; it also sponsors a series of annual symposia promoting interactions among scientists working at the cutting edge of basic oncological sciences.

The award selection process is managed by the European School of Oncology in Milan, Italy, with the aid of an international committee of experts chaired by Professor U. Veronesi.

The symposia are held in the Trentino Region of Northern Italy and their scientific focus is selected by Enrico Mihich with the collaboration of an international Standing Symposia Committee. A Program Committee determines the content of each symposium.

The first symposium focused on *Drug Resistance: Mechanisms and Reversal* (E. Mihich, Chairman, 1989); the second on *The Therapeutic Implications of the Molecular Biology of Breast Cancer* (M.E. Lippman and E. Mihich, Co-Chairmen, 1990); the third on *Tumor Suppressor Genes* (D.M. Livingston and E. Mihich, Co-Chairmen, 1991), the fourth on *Cell Adhesion Molecules: Cellular Recognition Mechanisms* (M.E. Hemler and E. Mihich, Co-Chairmen, 1992), the fifth on *Apoptosis* (E. Mihich and R.T. Schimke, Co-Chairmen, 1993), the sixth on *Normal and Malignant Hematopoiesis: New Advances* (E. Mihich and D. Metcalf, Co-Chairmen, 1994). The eighth symposium (1996) was focused on Genomic Instability and Immortality in Cancer (E. Mihich, L. Hartwell and C. Greider, Co-Chairmen).

PREFACE

The seventh Annual Pezcoller Symposium entitled, Cancer Genes: Functional Aspects, was held in Trento, Italy, June 14–16, 1995 and was focused on oncogenes function, tumor suppressor gene function, transcription regulation, cell cycle progression regulation and apoptosis, and the clinical implications of oncogene function and regulation for prevention and therapy of cancer. With presentations at the cutting edge of progress and stimulating discussions, this Symposium addressed issues related to the mechanisms of control of cell growth and death by certain genes such as c-myc, src, fyns, bcl2, the function of cdk inhibitors, the functions of p53 and WTI, the mechanisms of transcriptional activation of specific oncogenes, the genetic characterization of certain hematological malignancies, the interference with specific sites along signal transduction and the genetic alterations of tumor immunity.

We wish to thank the participants in the Symposium for their substantial contributions and their participation in the spirited discussions which followed. We would also like to thank Drs. Jane Azizkhan, Paolo Comoglio, Giulio Draetta, David M. Livingston and Alex Matter for their essential input as members of the Program Committee, and Ms. A. Toscani for her invaluable assistance. The aid of the Bank Cassa di Risparmio di Trento and Rovereto, and the Municipal, Provincial and Regional Administrations in supporting this Symposium through the Pezcoller Foundation are also acknowledged with deep appreciation. Finally, we wish to thank the staff of Plenum Publishing Corporation for their efficient cooperation in the production of these Proceedings.

Enrico Mihich
David Housman

CONTENTS

THE INTEGRATED CONTROL OF CELL PROLIFERATION AND CELL VIABILITY

Gerard I. Evan, Elizabeth H. Harrington, Nicola J. McCarthy, Trevor D. Littlewood and David C. Hancock

Imperial Cancer Research Fund Laboratories
44, Lincolns Inn Fields
London WC2A 3PX, United Kingdom

THE NEOPLASIA PROBLEM

One of the major problems faced by multicellular organisms is the continuous suppression of outgrowth of somatic cells that acquire a growth advantage through mutation. In principle, any somatic cell that acquires a growth advantage should spontaneously outgrow its siblings, spread, invade and so form a tumour. Moreover, clonal expansion of the mutant cell necessarily increases number of targets for additional carcinogenic mutations that would foster tumour progression. Thus, cancer appears to be an inevitable consequence of natural selection within the soma—given enough mutations. In man, this "neoplasia problem" is further exacerbated by three factors: our substantial physical size, our longevity, and the self-renewing (i.e. proliferating) nature of many of our tissues. The larger an organism is, the greater the number of potential cellular targets for neoplastic mutations. Likewise, the longer an organism lives, the greater the chances of neoplasia occurring at some point in its life. Finally, many of our tissues (notably epithelial and haematopoietic) exhibit substantial proliferation throughout our lives so cells within them sustain a risk of *de novo* mutation throughout life.

Nonetheless, cancer affects only 1 in 3 individuals. As cancer is a clonal disease that arises through expansion of a single affected cell, this implies that the cancer cell also arises only in 1 in 3 persons, out of some 10^{14}–10^{15} somatic cells and some 10^{18} cell divisions. The cancer cell is, therefore, extremely rare. Such rarity implies the existence of powerful mechanisms that suppress neoplasia.

Metazoans thus face a deep conundrum. To generate their tissues and maintain their integrity, massive cell proliferation must occur both during development and (in larger organisms like vertebrates) throughout life. However, at the same time, any faster growing clonal variants must be specifically and tightly removed or suppressed. Recently, an important clue has emerged as to the answer of how organisms such as man maintain high levels of somatic cell proliferation (with its consequent obligate accumulation of carcino-

Cancer Genes, edited by Mihich and Housman
Plenum Press, New York, 1996

genic mutations) whilst at the same time suppressing neoplastic outgrowth. Dominant on-cogenes appear to be potent triggers of programmed cell death (apoptosis), suggesting that the processes of cell proliferation and cell suicide are intimately entwined.

COUPLING OF PROLIFERATION AND CELL DEATH PATHWAYS: c-*myc* AS A PARADIGM

Proto-oncogenes are well established in their role as genes encoding essential com-ponents of signal transduction pathways regulating cell proliferation and whose inappro-priate activation promotes cellular transformation. Surprisingly, several dominant oncogenes have recently been shown to possess an unexpected biological prop-erty—namely, the ability to trigger programmed cell death. This has been most graphi-cally demonstrated in the case of the proto-oncogene c-*myc*. Expression of c-*myc* is necessary and, in some cases appears sufficient, for cell proliferation [reviewed in (Evan and Littlewood., 1993)]. Deregulated c-*myc* expression is virtually ubiquitous in all tu-mour cells (Spencer and Groudine., 1991) and is associated with inability to withdraw from the cell cycle (Amati et al., 1994; Eilers et al., 1991; Evan et al., 1992) and suppres-sion of differentiation (Coppola and Cole., 1986; Denis et al., 1987; Dmitrovsky et al., 1986; Freytag., 1988; Freytag et al., 1990). c-*myc* encodes a short-lived sequence-specific DNA-binding phosphoprotein possessing an N-terminal domain transcriptional activating domain and a C-terminal DNA-binding/dimerisation bHLH-LZ domain akin to that pre-sent in several known transcription factors (Amati et al., 1993; Amati et al., 1992; Amati et al., 1994; Kato et al., 1990; Kretzner et al., 1992). Mutagenesis studies show that c-Myc function is dependent upon the integrity of all of these domains, strongly suggesting that c-Myc promotes cell proliferation through its action as a transcription factor. However, with very few exceptions (Bello et al., 1993; Benvenisty et al., 1992; Eilers et al., 1991), target genes regulated by c-Myc have remained elusive.

Paradoxically, c-*myc* is not only a potent inducer of cell proliferation but also a powerful trigger of cell death by apoptosis. Transgenic animals whose lymphocytes ex-press deregulated c-*myc* exhibit massive apoptosis within lymphoid organs (Dyall and Cory., 1988; Langdon et al., 1988; Neiman et al., 1991). Moreover, substantial oncogenic synergy is apparent between c-*myc* and the anti-apoptotic gene *bcl*-2 (Bissonnette et al., 1992; Fanidi et al., 1992; Wagner et al., 1993), implying that cell death is a major limita-tion in the oncogenic progression of proto-tumours driven by c-*myc* alone. Recent *in vitro* studies of the induction of cell death by c-Myc have demonstrated that death occurs by the active process of apoptosis (Figures 1 and 2). Serum-deprived fibroblasts expressing a conditional Myc allele, in which the c-Myc protein is fused to the hormone binding do-main of the human oestrogen receptor (MycER) to render it functionally dependent upon oestrogen, die only when Myc is activated by addition of ß-oestradiol to the culture me-dium (Evan et al., 1992). This demonstrates that the apoptosis observed in these cells is specifically triggered by c-Myc. Moreover, the higher the level of c-Myc expressed in cells, the easier it becomes to trigger apoptosis. Fibroblasts expressing low levels of c-Myc found in normal cells (i.e. about 2,000 molecules of c-Myc protein per cell) die rap-idly only if serum is completely removed. In contrast, cells expressing the high levels of c-Myc found in many tumour cells (i.e. 20,000 molecules per cell observed in many colo-nic carcinomas) exhibit some apoptosis even in 10% serum, and die rapidly if serum level is dropped to 2% (Figure 3). Thus, cells with elevated c-Myc replicate more rapidly than their normal counterparts but are also more prone to undergo apoptosis (Evan et al., 1992).

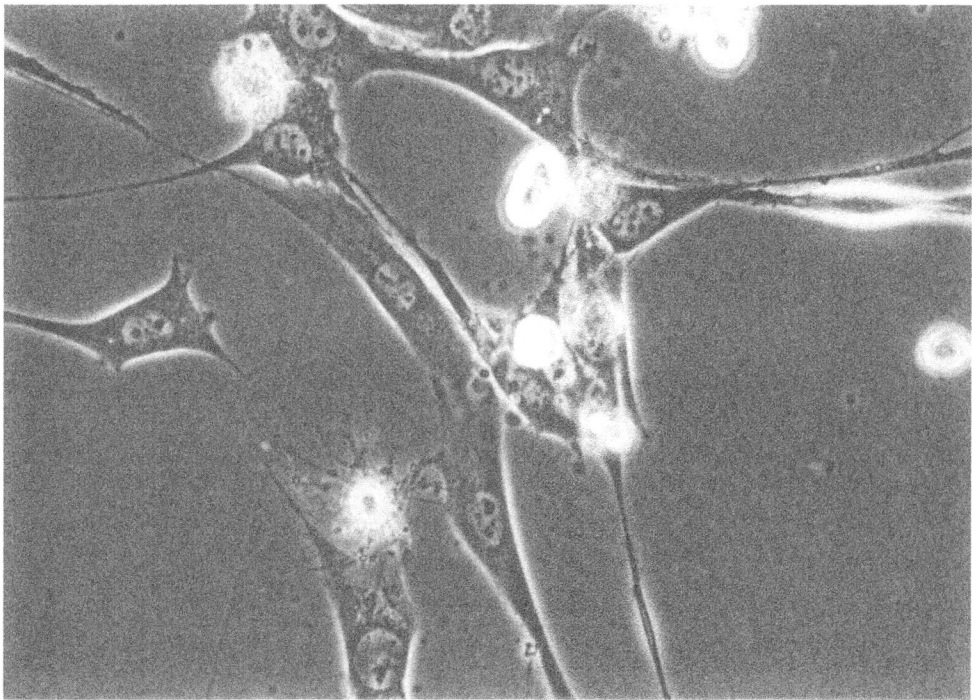

Figure 1. Induction of apoptosis in rodent fibroblasts by c-Myc. Rat-1 fibroblasts transfected with the conditional c-Myc allele c-MycER™ were cultured in medium containing 10% foetal calf serum. Foetal calf serum was then removed and the cells cultured for a further 24 hours. Apoptotic cells appear as refractile and rounded bodies. Unaffected cells appear normal.

Nonetheless, even "normal" levels of c-Myc are sufficient to induce programmed cell death.

The cytotoxic attribute of c-Myc is genetically indissociable from its mitogenic property. Identical regions of the c-Myc protein are required for both growth promotion and induction of apoptosis. Both the N-terminal *trans*-activation domain and the C-terminal DNA-binding and dimerisation bHLH-LZ domain (Evan et al., 1992); mediating inter-

Table 1. Comparisons of properties of c-Myc mutants

Mutant	Attribute	Co-Transforming?	Mitogenic?	Induces Apoptosis?
wt		Yes	Yes	Yes
Δ7-93	trans-activation	No	No	No
Δ41-53	1st Myc Box phosphoryation site	Super	Yes	Super
Δ106-143	trans-activation	No	No	No
Δ141-262	none known	Yes	Yes	Yes
Δ265-317	none known	Yes	Yes	Yes
Δ371-413	delete helix-loop-helix	No	No	No
D414-433	delete leucine zipper	No	No	No
360 N → P	corrupt DNA binding	No	No	No
364/6/7 R→ A	corrupt DNA binding	No	No	No
In 414	disrupt leucine zipper	No	No	No

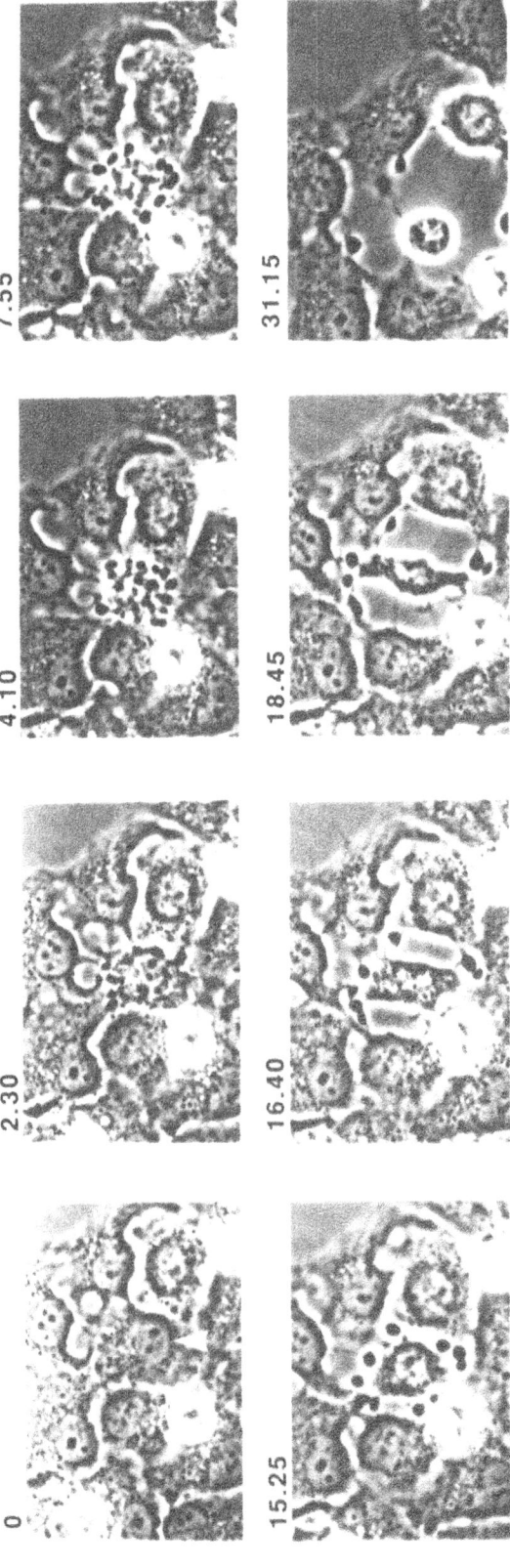

Figure 2. Time course of Myc-induced apoptosis. Rat-1 fibroblasts transfected with the conditional c-Myc allele c-MycER™ were cultured in medium containing 10% foetal calf serum. Foetal calf serum was then removed and cells observed by time-lapse video microscopy at a rate of one frame every 10 seconds. The series shows selected time points (in minutes) of one fibroblast undergoing Myc-induced apoptosis.

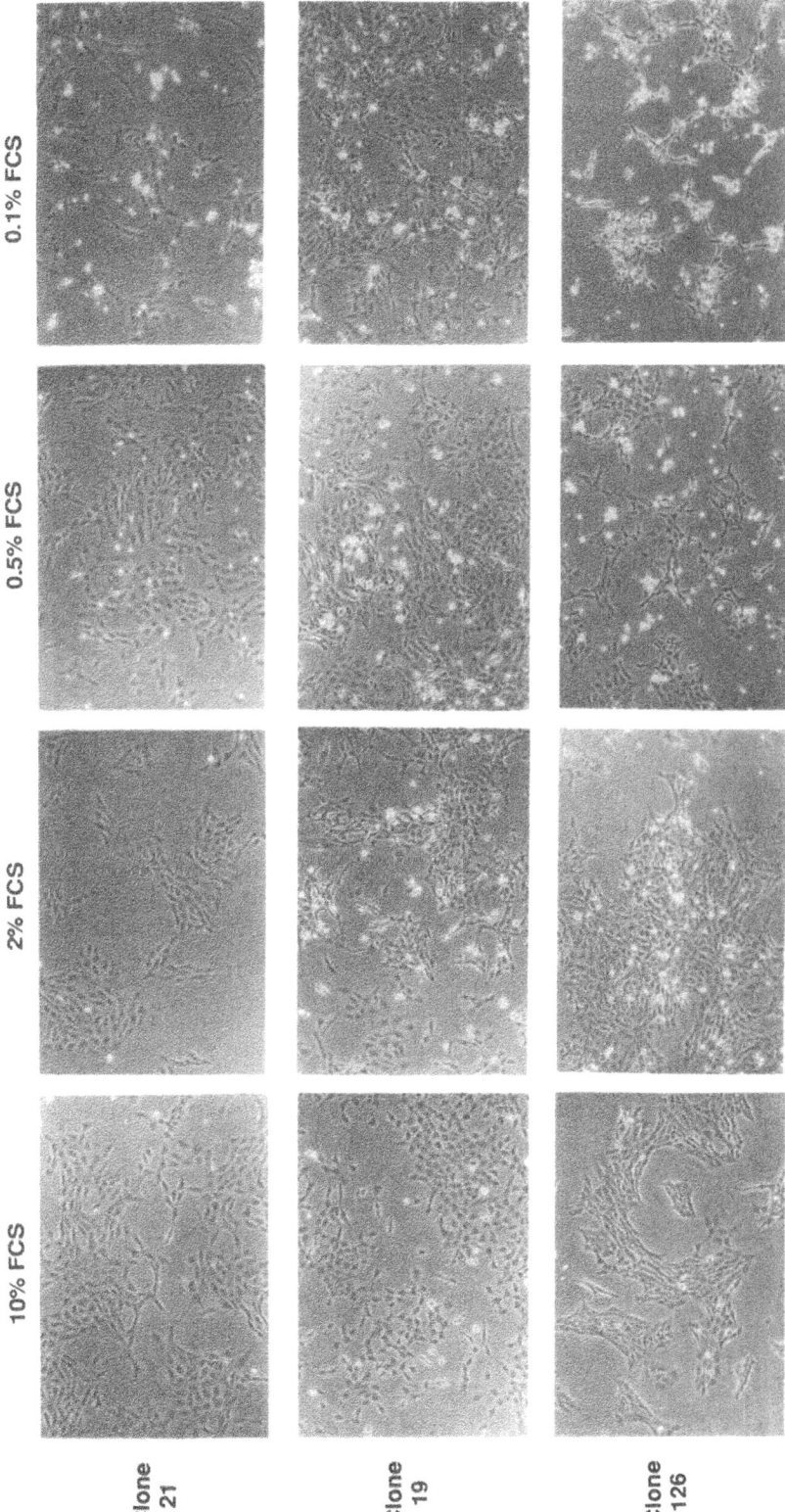

Figure 3. Induction of apoptosis by c-Myc is dependent upon level of expression and level of serum in the culture medium. Three clones of Rat-1 fibroblasts constitutively express-ing differing level of c-Myc protein were incubated for 24 hours in media containing the specified concentrations of foetal calf serum. Clone 21 cells express about 4,000 molecules c-Myc per cell (equivalent to the level of c-Myc in normal proliferating fibroblasts); clone 19 expresses about 9,000 molecules/cell (the level usually expressed in Burkitt's lym-phoma cells) and clone 26 about 22,000 (the level expressed in many colon carcinomas).

action with the heterologous partner protein Max (Amati et al., 1993) are necessary for both transforming and apoptotic functions of c-Myc (Table 1). Moreover, physical interaction with Max is absolutely required for induction of both proliferation and apoptosis (Amati et al., 1994). These observations all strongly suggest that c-Myc induces apoptosis via a transcriptional mechanism—presumably through the modulation of appropriate target genes.

Thus, c-Myc can drive two completely contradictory processes within a cell: proliferation and death. This is clearly a paradoxical state of affairs: every proliferating cell expresses one or other member of the *myc* gene family, usually c-*myc*. It is therefore obvious that not every cell that replicates undergoes apoptosis—somehow a decision is made whether the cell will replicate or commit suicide. How could such a critical decision be manifest?

DUAL SIGNAL MODEL FOR c-Myc ACTION

Recently, we demonstrated that the reason fibroblasts expressing c-Myc in high serum do not die is that serum contains certain cytokines whose action is to suppress apoptosis—specifically PDGF and IGF-I (Harrington et al., 1994a). The anti-apoptotic effects of IGF-I and PDGF are not linked to either cytokine's mitogenic properties. Both cytokines block apoptosis in cells arrested with cytostatic agents, under which conditions neither factor can promote cell proliferation. Moreover, both IGF-I and PDGF also block apoptosis in post-commitment S/G2 cells, which do not require any mitogens for cell cycle progression (Harrington et al., 1994a). Thus, IGF-I and PDGF activate specific signalling pathways in mesenchymal cells that regulate cell viability, and these signalling pathways are discrete from those that mediate mitogenesis. Further evidence that the IGF-I survival signalling pathway is discrete from the mitogenic one arises from the demonstration that IGF-I can block cell death even in cells blocked in macromolecular synthesis. Fibroblasts treated with the protein synthesis inhibitor cycloheximide and/or the RNA synthesis inhibitor actinomycin D exhibit delayed apoptosis in the presence of IGF-I—even if the IGF-I is added after the drugs (Harrington et al., 1994a). Thus, suppression of apoptosis by IGF-I does not require *de novo* protein synthesis, unlike mitogenesis and cell cycle progression.

From these observation emerges a novel paradigm for the control of cell proliferation that we have called the "Dual Signal" model. In this model, cell proliferation and apoptosis are obligatorily coupled, such that every cell that engages its proliferative cycle also necessarily engages a suicide "abort" pathway. This suicide programme is only forestalled if the cell then receives appropriate anti-apoptotic signals—for example, in the form of specific "survival factors." Thus, the limited availability of anti-apoptotic cytokines or survival factors limits clonal expansion in a manner analogous to that proposed for developmental control within the CNS (Raff et al., 1993). Incorporated within this "Dual Signal" hypothesis is a potent mechanism for the suppression of carcinogenesis (Evan and Littlewood., 1993; Evan et al., 1992; Harrington et al., 1994b). The coupling of the mitogenic and apoptotic pathways means that any oncogenic lesion that activates mitogenesis will be lethal as the affected cell and its progeny outgrow the paracrine environment enabling their survival. In effect, surveillance against neoplastic transformation is hardwired into the proliferative machinery of every cell.

Studies with other dominant oncogenes reinforce the notion of an obligate coupling between proliferation and cell suicide. For example, the adenovirus E1A protein is the principal early gene responsible for driving host cell cycle progression which the virus needs for its productive infection. E1A, like c-Myc, is both oncogene and also a potent inducer of apoptosis (White et al., 1991). To defeat the obligate linkage between proliferation and cell death adenovirus has evolved two polypeptides with potent anti-apoptotic activity, both encoded by the E1B gene. p55^{E1B} sequesters and inactivates p53 (Sarnow et al., 1982; Yew and Berk., 1992), a critical component of the cell suicide pathway triggered by genome damage, whereas p19^{E1B} is a functional homologue of Bcl-2 (White et al., 1991; White et al., 1992). A further example of the obligate growth/death dual function is the chimaeric homeobox oncogene *E2A-PBX1*, generated during t(1;19) chromosomal translocations in some childhood leukaemias. Transgenic mice that constitutively express *E2A-PBX1* in lymphocytes show high incidence of lymphomas, attesting to the oncogenic nature of the gene. However, they also exhibit massive lymphocyte apoptosis during the pre-malignant phase of the disease (Dedera et al., 1993). The proto-oncogene c-*fos* is also implicated in the control of apoptosis. Recent studies of the topographical expression of c-*fos* during mouse embryogenesis (Smeyne et al., 1993) suggest that sustained expression of c-*fos* maps to regions of tissues undergoing apoptosis. Finally, the G1-specific transcription factor E2F1 has also been shown to be both promoter of cell proliferation and apoptosis (Qin et al., 1994; Wu and Levine., 1994).

INTERACTIONS BETWEEN c-myc AND OTHER GENES

Activated oncogenes are associated with most cancers. However, if (as indicated above) activated oncogenes also trigger cell death, this implies that such tumours must have acquired mechanisms to suppress apoptosis. This idea has important implications for models of multistage carcinogenesis. Carcinogenesis is normally portrayed as a linear accumulation mutations that progressively lead to more "malignant" or "aggressive" phenotypes (e.g. the colon carcinoma model of Fearon and Vogelstein (Fearon and Vogelstein., 1990)). The generic induction of apoptosis by mitogenic oncogenes suggests, however, that almost all such activating mutations that trigger uncontrolled cell cycle progression will be lethal to the affected clone, through induction of apoptosis. In this scheme, most oncogenic mutations become a dead end (Figure 4). Only if the clone *immediately* acquires a complementary anti-apoptotic lesion can a proto-tumour cell survive to become a frank malignancy. Carcinogenesis must therefore involve anti-apoptotic lesions.

Indeed, several such anti-apoptotic mechanisms have recently been identified. The *bcl*-2 proto-oncogene maps to the site on chromosome translocation of the t(14,18) translocation found in many follicular B cell lymphomas in man. *bcl*-2 encodes membrane

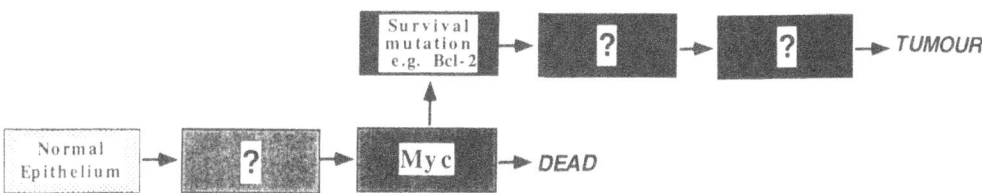

Figure 4. Alternative scheme for carcinogenesis. Activation of dominant oncogenes leads to unscheduled cell cycle progression, but also apoptosis in the absence of excess "survival factors." Thus, carcinogenic events are self-terminating unless the cell acquires, or already possesses, some anti-apoptotic lesion (e.g. *bcl*-2 dergulation).

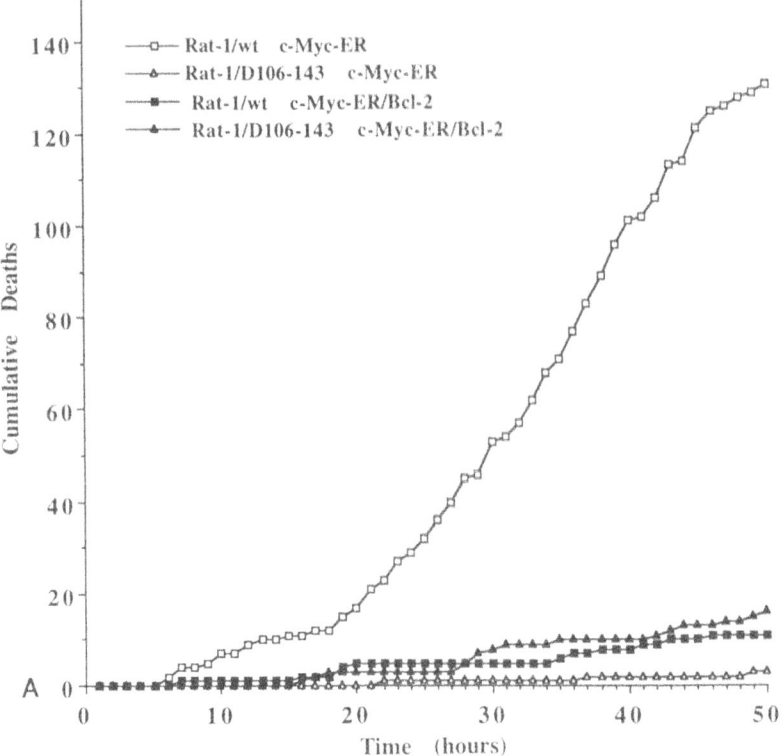

Figure 5. Suppression of c-Myc-induced apoptosis by Bcl-2. (A) Serum-deprived Rat-1 fibroblasts expressing the conditional c-MycER protein undergo apoptosis when c-Myc is activated by addition of 4-hydroxytamoxifen. In contrast, cells also expressing the Bcl-2 protein are substantially protected from apoptosis. Control cell express a defective c-Myc mutant Δ106–143 that does not induce apoptosis or proliferation. Analysis was carried out by time-lapse videomicroscopy (Fanidi et al., 1992). (B) Rat-1/Myc fibroblasts were transfected with an expression vector directing constitutive expression of human Bcl-2α. Rat-1 cells, with and without deregulated Bcl-2, were then incubated in medium containing thymidine (1 mM) or etoposide (0.1 μM) for 24 hours. c-Myc was activated by addition of 4 OHT to the growth medium and the cultures observed by time-lapse videomicroscopy.

associated polypeptides localised to most intracellular membranes (Krajewski et al., 1993; Nakai et al., 1993) bcl-2 is widely expressed during development but its expression in the adult is confined to immature and stem-cell populations and long-lived cells such as peripheral sensory neurons and resting B lymphocytes (Hockenbery et al., 1991). Targeted expression of Bcl-2 to lymphoid cells in transgenic mice leads to increase in numbers of mature resting B cells and potentiates their longevity. T cells expressing a bcl-2 transgene are markedly resistant to the cytocidal effects of glucocorticoids, radiation and anti-CD3-triggered apoptosis although general thymic censorship appears normal. As outlined above, transgenic expression of both bcl-2 and c-myc shows marked oncogenic synergy over either oncogene alone (reviewed in (Adams and Cory., 1991)). Analogous synergy between bcl-2 and c-myc is also seen in vitro (Bissonnette et al., 1992; Fanidi et al., 1992; Vaux et al., 1988; Wagner et al., 1993). The synergy occurs because bcl-2 blocks the ability of c-myc to induce apoptosis Figure 5A (Bissonnette et al., 1992; Fanidi et al., 1992; Wagner et al., 1993). Expression of Bcl-2 also blocks induction of apoptosis by other on-

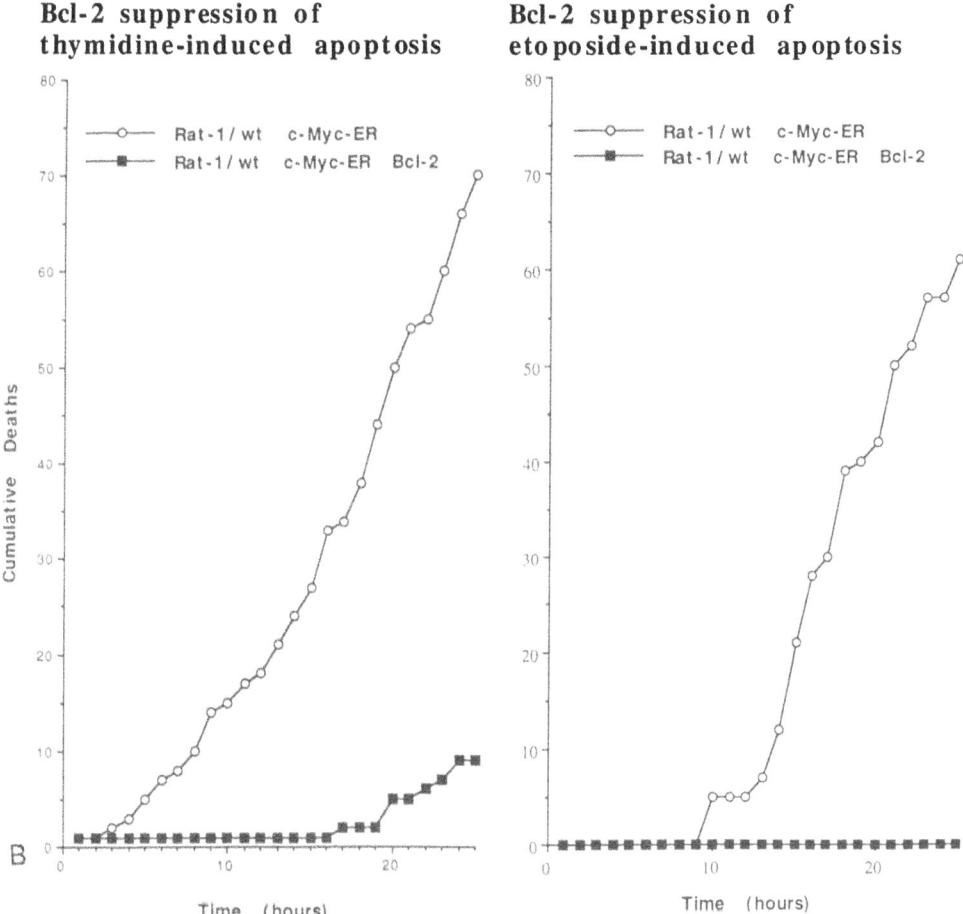

Figure 5. (*Continued.*)

cogenes; for exampl adenovirus E1A (Rao et al., 1992). *bcl*-2 also mitigates the increased sensitivity to cytotoxic and cytostatic agents elicited by expression of c-Myc (Fanidi et al., 1992) Figure 5B. However, the anti-apoptotic effect of *bcl*-2 is not mediated through enhanced capacity to exclude or metabolise drugs, nor does *bcl*-2 confer any increased physical resistance to toxic agents (Kamesaki et al., 1993) *per se*. Instead, it acts merely to suppress the inclination of damaged cells to commit suicide notwithstanding any damage they might sustain. Such direct suppression of apoptosis represents a discrete mechanism of resistance to anti-neoplastic drugs with important implications for the effective design of future cancer therapies.

bcl-2 is now known to be but one of a family of highly evolutionarily conserved genes that regulate cell death. These include *ced*-9 of C. *elegans* (Hengartner et al., 1992), the mammalian genes *bcl*-X (Boise et al., 1993), Mcl-1 (Kozopas et al., 1993), A1 (Lin et al., 1993), Bax (Oltvai et al., 1993) and *bak* (Chittenden et al., 1995; Farrow et al., 1995; Kiefer et al., 1995), and the viral proteins *BHRF1* from Epstein-Barr Virus (Pearson et al., 1987) and $p19^{E1B}$ from adenovirus (Rao et al., 1992; White et al., 1991). Functionally, these genes fall

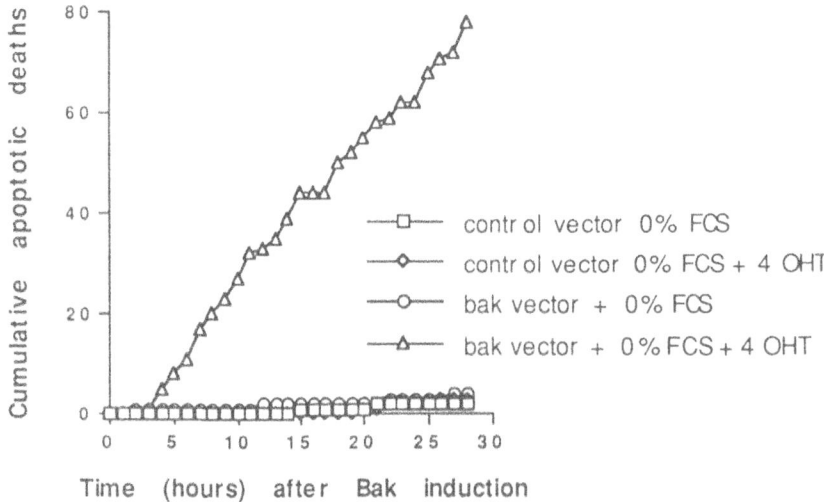

Figure 6. Induction of apoptosis in Rat-1 fibroblasts by Bak. *bak* cDNA was cloned into a pSP65 derivative containing a synthetic promoter containing Gal4 binding sites (gift of M. Busslinger) that is conditionally transactivated by the synthetic chimaeric transcription factor GalER-VP16 fusion (Braselmann et al., 1993). Rat-1/GalER-VP16 cells were co-transfected with pSP65/Bak (10 μg) so that *bak* is under the control of a GalER-VP16 responsive promoter which becomes active upon addition of 4-hydroxytamoxifen (4 OHT) to the growth medium. Control cells were transfected with an empty control vector. Sub-confluent Rat-1/puro and Rat-1/Bak cells were deprived of serum for 48 hours and Bak expression was activated by addition of 4-OHT. In parallel cultures, 4-OHT was omitted. Apoptotic cell deaths were recorded by time-lapse video microscopy (Chittenden et al., 1995).

into two groups. *bcl*-2, *bcl*-X_L, *BHRF1*, *p19*^{E1B} and *ced*-9 all suppress programmed cell death whilst *bax* and *bak* appear to promote apoptosis. The antagonistic actions of differing members of the Bcl-2 protein family appears tio be a result of their mutual interactions. Bcl-2 dimerises with Bax (Oltvai et al., 1993), whilst the favoured partner for Bcl-x is Bak (Chittenden et al., 1995; Farrow et al., 1995; Kiefer et al., 1995). However, it is not clear how such interactive dimerisations serve to regulate cell survival. Specifically, it is not known whether Bcl-2 and Bcl-x activate a "survival" pathway which Bax and Bak quench by sequestration or, alternatively, if Bax and Bak activate a "kill" programme that is mitigated by Bcl-2 and Bcl-x. Nonetheless, ectopic expression of Bak is sufficient to trigger apoptosis in various cell types (Chittenden et al., 1995) and Figure 6, perhaps favouring the latter notion. Identification of downstream targets of Bcl-2 proteins will presumably elucidate the molecular mechanisms underlying their actions. One intriguing possibility is that just as Bcl-2 can act as a dominant oncogene by suppressing apoptosis and promoting survival of cells with activated *myc*, so Bak and Bax might act as tumour suppressor genes to trigger suicide in tumour cells. Chromosomal localisation of *bak* and *bax* genes may help support or refute this idea.

SUPPRESSION OF CELL DEATH IN CARCINOGENESIS

The propensity of dominant oncogenes to drive apoptosis together with the identification of dominant oncogenes and signal transduction pathways that promote survival rather than cell proliferation all attest the importance of apoptosis as a regulator of cell number and as a major restraint against neoplastic growth. To date, only a very limited number of anti-apoptotic lesions have been identified in tumours. However, the involvement of cytokines and signalling pathways, anti-apoptotic genes like *bcl*-2, and tumour suppressor proteins such as *p53* and *Rb* (Howes et al., 1994) in apoptosis all suggest that the mechanisms regulating programmed cell death may be as diverse and complex as those regulating proliferation and differentiation. Identification of mechanisms by which tumour cells evade cell death is important because it may reveal novel targets for therapeutic intervention in cancer and degenerative diseases that are both effective and humane.

REFERENCES

Adams, J. M. and Cory, S. (1991). Transgenic models for haemopoietic malignancies. Biochim Biophys Acta., *1072*, 9–31.

Amati, B., Brooks, M., Levy, N., Littlewood, T., Evan, G. and Land, H. (1993). Oncogenic activity of the c-Myc protein requires dimerisation with Max. Cell., *72*, 233–245.

Amati, B., Dalton, S., Brooks, M., Littlewood, T., Evan, G. and Land, H. (1992). Transcriptional activation by c-Myc oncoprotein in yeast requires interaction with Max. Nature., *359*, 423–426.

Amati, B., Littlewood, T., Evan, G. and Land, H. (1994). The c-Myc protein induces cell cycle progression and apoptosis through dimerisation with Max. EMBO J., *12*, 5083–5087.

Bello, F, C., Packham, G. and Cleveland, J. L. (1993). The ornithine decarboxylase gene is a transcriptional target of c-Myc. Proc Natl Acad Sci U S A., *90*, 7804–8.

Benvenisty, N., Leder, A., Kuo, A. and Leder, P. (1992). An embryonically expressed gene is a target for c-Myc regulation via the c-Myc-binding sequence. Gene Devel., *6*, 2513–2523.

Bissonnette, R., Echeverri, F., Mahboubi, A. and Green, D. (1992). Apoptotic cell death induced by c-*myc* is inhibited by *bcl*-2. Nature., *359*, 552–554.

Boise, L., González-Garcia, M., Postema, C., Ding, L., Lindsten, T., Turka, L., Mao, X., Nuñez, G. and Thompson, C. (1993). *bcl*-x, a *bcl*-2-related gene that functions as a dominant regulator of apoptotic cell death. Cell., *74*, 597–608.

Braselmann, S., Graninger, P. and Busslinger, M. (1993). A selective transcriptional induction system for mammalian cells based on Gal4-estrogen receptor fusion proteins. Proc Natl Acad Sci U S A., *90*, 1657–61.

Chittenden, T., Harrington, E., O'Connor, R., Evan, G. and Guild, B. (1995). Induction of apoptosis by the Bcl-2 homologue Bak. Nature., *374*, 733–736.

Coppola, J. A. and Cole, M. D. (1986). Constitutive c-*myc* oncogene expression blocks mouse erythroleukaemia cell differentiation but not commitment. Nature., *320*, 760–763.

Dedera, D., Waller, E., LeBrun, D., Sen-Majumdar, A., Stevens, M., Barsh, G. and Cleary, M. (1993). Chimeric homeobox gene E2A-PBX1 induces proliferation, apoptosis and malignant lymphomas in transgenic mice. Cell., *74*, 833–843.

Denis, N., Blanc, S., Leibovitch, M. P., Nicolaiew, N., Dautry, F., Raymondjean, M., Kruh, J. and Kitzis, A. (1987). c-*myc* oncogene expression inhibits the initiation of myogenic differentiation. Exp. Cell Res., *172*, 212–7.

Dmitrovsky, E., Kuehl, W. M., Hollis, G. F., Kirsch, I. R., Bender, T. P. and Segal, S. (1986). Expression of a transfected human c-myc oncogene inhibits differentiation of a mouse erythroleukaemia cell line. Nature., *322*, 748–750.

Dyall, S. D. and Cory, S. (1988). Transformation of bone marrow cells from E mu-myc transgenic mice by Abelson murine leukemia virus and Harvey murine sarcoma virus. Oncogene Res., *2*, 403–9.

Eilers, M., Schirm, S. and Bishop, J. M. (1991). The MYC protein activates transcription of the alpha-prothymosin gene. EMBO J., *10*, 133–41.

Evan, G. and Littlewood, T. (1993). The role of c-*myc* in cell growth. Curr. Opin. Genet. & Dev., *3*, 44–49.

Evan, G., Wyllie, A., Gilbert, C., Littlewood, T., Land, H., Brooks, M., Waters, C., Penn, L. and Hancock, D. (1992). Induction of apoptosis in fibroblasts by c-*myc* protein. Cell., *63*, 119–125.

Fanidi, A., Harrington, E. and Evan, G. (1992). Cooperative interaction between c-*myc* and *bcl*-2 proto-oncogenes. Nature., *359*, 554–556.

Farrow, S., White, J., Martinou, I., Raven, T., Pun, K.-T., Grinham, C., Martinou, J.-C. and Brown, R. (1995). Cloning of a novel *bcl*-2 homologue by interaction with adnovirus E1B 19K. Nature., *374*, 731–733.

Fearon, E. R. and Vogelstein, B. (1990). A genetic model for colorectal tumorigenesis. Cell., *61*, 759–67.

Freytag, S. O. (1988). Enforced expression of the c-*myc* oncogene inhibits cell differentiation by precluding entry into a distinct predifferentiation state in G0/G1. Mol. Cell. Biol., *8*, 1614–1624.

Freytag, S. O., Dang, C. V. and Lee, W. M. F. (1990). Definition of the activities and properties of c-*myc* required to inhibit cell differentiation. Cell Growth & Diff., *1*, 339–343.

Harrington, E., Fanidi, A., Bennett, M. and Evan, G. (1994a). Modulation of Myc-induced apoptosis by specific cytokines. EMBO J., *13*, 3286–3295.

Harrington, E., Fanidi, A. and Evan, G. (1994b). Oncogenes and cell death. Curr. Opin. Genet. Dev., *4*, 120–129.

Hengartner, M. O., Ellis, R. E. and Horvitz, H. R. (1992). Caenorhabditis elegans gene ced-9 protects cells from programmed cell death. Nature., *356*, 494–9.

Hockenbery, D. M., Zutter, M., Hickey, W., Nahm, M. and Korsmeyer, S. J. (1991). BCL2 protein is topographically restricted in tissues characterized by apoptotic cell death. Proc Natl Acad Sci U S A., *88*, 6961–5.

Howes, K., Ransom, L., Papermaster, D., Lasudry, J., Albert, D. and Windle, J. (1994). Apoptosis or retinoblastoma—alternative fates of photoreceptors expressing the HPV-16 E7 gene in the presence or absence of p53. Genes & Dev., *8*, 1300–1310.

Kamesaki, S., Kamesaki, H., Jorgensen, T., Tanizawa, A., Pommier, Y. and Cossman, J. (1993). Bcl-2 protein inhibits etoposide-induced apoptosis through its effects on events subsequent to topoisomerase II-induced DNA strand breaks and their repair. Cancer Research., *53*, 4251–4256.

Kato, G. J., Barrett, J., Villa, G. M. and Dang, C. V. (1990). An amino-terminal c-myc domain required for neoplastic transformation activates transcription. Mol Cell Biol., *10*, 5914–20.

Kiefer, M., Brauer, M., VC, P., Wu, J., Umansky, S., Tomei, L. and Barr, P. (1995). Modulation of apoptosis by the widely distributed Bcl-2 homologue Bak. Nature., *374*, 736–739.

Kozopas, K. M., Yang, T., Buchan, H. L., Zhou, P. and Craig, R. W. (1993). MCL1, a gene expressed in programmed myeloid cell differentiation, has sequence similarity to BCL2. Proc Natl Acad Sci U S A., *90*, 3516–20.

Krajewski, S., Tanaka, S., Takayama, S., Schibler, M., W., F. and JC., R. (1993). Investigation of the subcellular-distribution of the Bcl-2 oncoprotein—residence in the nuclear-envelope, endoplasmic-reticulum, and outer mitochondrial-membranes. Cancer Res., *53*, 4701–14.

Kretzner, L., Blackwood, E. and Eisenman, R. (1992). Myc and Max possess distinct transcriptional activities. Nature., *359*, 426–429.

Langdon, W. Y., Harris, A. W. and Cory, S. (1988). Growth of E mu-myc transgenic B-lymphoid cells in vitro and their evolution toward autonomy. Oncogene Res., *3*, 271–9.

Lin, E., Orlofsky, A., Berger, M. and Prystowsky, M. (1993). Characterization of A1, a novel hemopoietic-specific early-response gene with sequence similarity to *bcl*-2. J. Immunol., *151*, 1979–1988.

Nakai, M., Takeda, A., Cleary, M. L. and Endo, T. (1993). The *bcl*-2 protein is inserted into the outer-membrane but not into the inner membrane of rat-liver mitochondria *in vitro*. Biochem Biophys Res Comms., *196*, 233–9.

Neiman, P. E., Thomas, S. J. and Loring, G. (1991). Induction of apoptosis during normal and neoplastic B-cell development in the bursa of Fabricius. Proc Natl Acad Sci U S A., *88*, 5857–61.

Oltvai, Z., Milliman, C. and Korsmeyer, S. (1993). Bcl-2 heterodimerizes in vivo with a conserved homolog, Bax, that accelerates programed cell death. Cell., *74*, 609–619.

Pearson, G. R., Luka, J., Petti, L., Sample, J., Birkenbach, M., Braun, D. and Kieff, E. (1987). Identification of an Epstein-Barr virus early gene encoding a second component of the restricted early antigen complex. Virology., *160*, 151–61.

Qin, X., Livingston, D., Kaelin, W. and Adams, P. (1994). Deregulated transcription factor e2f-1 expression leads to S-phase entry and p53-mediated apoptosis. Proc Natl Acad Sci U S A., *91*, 10918–10922.

Raff, M., Barres, B., Burne, J., Coles, H., Ishizaki, Y. and Jacobson, M. (1993). Programmed cell death and the control of cell survival: lessons from the nervous system. Science., *262*, 695–700.

Rao, L., Debbas, M., Sabbatini, P., Hockenberry, D., Korsmeyer, S. and White, E. (1992). The adenovirus E1A proteins induce apoptosis, which is inhibited by the E1B 19-kDa and Bcl-2 proteins. Proc Natl Acad Sci U S A., *89*, 7742–7746.

Sarnow, P., Ho, Y., Williams, J. and Levine, A. (1982). Adenovirus E1b-58kd tumor antigen and SV40 large tumor antigen are physically associated with the same 54kd cellular protein in transformed cells. Cell., *28*, 387–94.

Smeyne, R., Vendrell, M., Hayward, M., Baker, S., Miao, G., Schilling, K., Robertson, L., Curran, T. and Morgan, J. (1993). Continuous c-*fos* expression precedes programmed cell-death *in vivo*. Nature., *363*, 166–169.

Spencer, C. A. and Groudine, M. (1991). Control of c-*myc* regulation in normal and neoplastic cells. Adv Cancer Res., *56*, 1–48.

Vaux, D. L., Cory, S. and Adams, J. M. (1988). *Bcl*-2 gene promotes haemopoietic cell survival and cooperates with c-*myc* to immortalize pre-B cells. Nature., *335*, 440–2.

Wagner, A. J., Small, M. B. and Hay, N. (1993). Myc-mediated apoptosis is blocked by ectopic expression of *bcl*-2. Mol Cell Biol., *13*, 2432–2440.

White, E., Cipriani, R., Sabbatini, P. and Denton, A. (1991). Adenovirus E1B 19-kilodalton protein overcomes the cytotoxicity of E1A proteins. J Virol., *65*, 2968–78.

White, E., Sabbatini, P., Debbas, M., Wold, W., Kusher, D. and Gooding, L. (1992). The 19-kilodalton Adenovirus E1B transforming protein inhibits programmed cell death and prevents cytolysis by tumour necrosis factor α. Mol Cell Biol., *12*, 2570–2580.

Wu, X. and Levine, A. J. (1994). p53 and E2F-1 cooperate to mediate apoptosis. Proc Natl Acad Sci U S A., *91*, 3602–6.

Yew, P. R. and Berk, A. J. (1992). Inhibition of p53 transactivation required for transformation by adenovirus early 1B protein. Nature., *357*, 82–5.

DISCUSSION

M. Oren: Addressing your cycloheximide experiment, do you add cycloheximide at the same time that you take away the serum?

G. Evan: You do not need to take away the serum. So, if you add cycloheximide and/or actinomycin in situations where cells are expressing high levels of myc at the time you add the drug, you trigger massive apoptosis, but if you take the serum away, the apoptosis occurs even more rapidly. That is because IGF-1 suppresses it.

M. Oren: So that could mean that you do not need new gene activation by myc after the time you add the cycloheximide, because the program is running on.

G. Evan: Right.

M. Oren: But alternatively it could mean that in parallel with the expression of myc in those cells, you have a short lived survival gene or survival protein which has to be made all the time and when you add cycloheximide you block that, and in effect you now exacerbate myc death because you facilitate the program which before was held in check by something else. Can you distinguish between the two? And technically, what happens if you do a similar experiment except that you now add cycloheximide at the same time that you add tamoxifen? You could do that in principle now, because with tamoxifen you just activate pre-existing protein. That would really give you a better distinction if myc turns on something else, or myc does something directly as a protein in the absence of a survival function.

G. Evan: In a sense we tried to do that experiment; it is not so easy because when apoptosis occurs, even with loads of myc, it does not all happen immediately, it happens over a very protracted period, so what you are really looking at is the rate of onset of apoptosis. But it is pretty clear that if you activate myc in the presence of inhibitors of protein synthesis, then you do not sensitize the cells to apoptosis. The way that we view those things as happening is as follows: we think that when you express myc, the consequence of expressing myc and, for all we know, things downstream of myc and upstream of myc, the cell is merely made much more sensitive to triggers of apoptosis; so myc is not inducing apoptosis, it is lowering the threshold of induction by other factors that trigger apoptosis. So cells expressing myc need more survival factors to prevent apoptosis from occurring spontaneously and are acutely sensitive to things that would normally cause apoptosis at a lower level, such as DNA damage. It could work either way, it could be that myc induces the apoptosis machinery or that it suppresses a repressor of apoptosis such as BCL-2 or BCL-XL or a bit of both. We have no idea because we do not know the downstream targets of myc. Why cycloheximide triggers death is a separate question, and the most obvious simple explanation is that there is a short-lived protein which has to be made continuously to suppress a default death program. Now if one adheres to the view that death is a default program that is present all the time, one does not need to induce the death program: it is always there. In a sense that is what we have had to have in order to become multi-cellular organisms, for a variety of reasons that we have discussed and I am sure other people are aware of. We do not know what that short-lived protein is and we are a bit weary of that idea also because we know that cycloheximide does a lot of other things to cells as well as inducing distort DNA and damage DNA. I do not think that these phenomena are mutually exclusive, they can both work.

F. Rauscher: A couple of questions. Is the IGF-1 protective effect dependent on continuos presence of IGF-1 in the medium?

G. Evan: Yes, it is.

F. Rauscher: You cannot pulse it or anything like that?

G. Evan: No. It is required throughout the cell cycle. So if you remove IGF-1 in S-phase, the cell stops dying immediately after you put it back. We have also done experiments where we have asked where does IGF-1 work in the hierarchy of steps involved in apoptosis? One way that you can address this is to see how quickly does death stop when you add IGF-1 back. So, if you have got cells dying under the influence of myc, you are looking at them by videomycroscopy and they die apparently at random and then you add back IGF-1 and you ask how long is it before the cells stop dying? The answer is that from the moment you add IGF-1 back, you never see another death of a cell that has not already started to die. So that argues that there is no precommittment to death and that IGF-1 is very very far down.

F. Rauscher: So are the results concordant with the fact that you see a dose dependence for myc expression in death as well; that is, does the requirement for IGF-1 change in terms of the dose of myc?

G. Evan: Yes, it does, so the more myc you have the more serum IGF-1 you need to suppress that. Now, if you take V-myc or E1A which are like super myc's or you express enormous levels of C-myc in cells, then they die even in serum (10% serum) and you can add IGF-1 until you want, but you cannot suppress death. However, in cells transfected with more IGF-1 receptor, one can begin to see suppression of death also under those conditions. In a sense, with the fibroblast that we are using, you cannot introduce anymore survival because you run out of receptor, but if you put more receptor in, you can.

F. Rauscher: Do you have any sense of whether the IGF-1 effect at the cellular phenotypic level for protection is dominant or recessive. I mean, are you gaining anything in the cell, are you losing anything? It is a hard experiment to do, I know.

G. Evan: It is very hard. I do not think we really know. We do not even know anything about the signaling system at all that mediates survival.

M. Fried: What happens to p53 in the presence of IGF-1?

G. Evan: Nothing, although there are long term changes in p53 levels in response to mytogeneric stimulation.

T. Taniguchi: Do you have any evidence that cell death genes, for example Ice, are involved in myc-induced apoptosis? For example, did you try CrmA expression in those cells?

G. Evan: Again, I did not have time to talk about it and it is pretty preliminary data. There are at least seven different members of this family that are now known and they are all homologous to the Ice death gene. There are inhibitors of these proteases which are cell membrane permeable, some of which we have used. There is one which is called Z-VAD that can get into cells and that blocks every type of cell death that we have seen. It blocks Staurosporin, myc, DNA damage, TSp53, the works. It is probably fairly promiscuous as an inhibitor of all the Ice family members, and that means that all of these go through Ice. Now, there is an interesting corollary of this, which is that if we look at how quickly individual cells die, then nothing that we have ever been able to do to manipulate cells has affected the rate at which individual cells die, so they make lots of Bcl 2 and still die in twenty minutes. Myc, Bcl 2, IGF-1, p53, none of these make any difference in terms of the rate at which individual cells die, they just affect the tendency to which the cells engage the death mechanism. The Ice inhibitors do something different: if you add the Ice inhibitors and switch on myc or we got a new member of the Bcl 2 family called BAC that is also a killer, then the cells round up, they start to glare and they do this for hours, they just go on and on until in the end you get bored you turn myc off, then they stop, settle down and redivide. So our explanation of this is if you look carefully at what is happening inside the cell, they can undergo the cytoplasmic changes but they cannot break up the nucleus, you can come back and live another day. So that is what we know about the Ice proteases at the moment and that suggests to us that they are actually right down in the process of cell death itself.

D. Livingston: You made the point that the cycloheximide experiment rules out the possibility that the signalling runs through the nucleus. But I suppose there is still the formal possibility that the signalling actually does, in part, run to the nucleus but the end effect is not gene expression. Rather it is some effect on the structure of DNA.

G. Evan: I think you are right, I think it rules out changes in gene expression by and large. That does not mean to say that if you add IGF-1 you get partial protection, but eventually the cell will die and it will die by apoptosis, so one suspects that IGF-1 also has genetic effects as well which may further protect the cell in long term, such as down regulating p53 or up regulating Bcl 2; we do not know about that, but you do not need that for short-term protection.

D. Livingston: I am thinking of a cycloheximide effect there.

G. Evan: Yes, but all we can say about that is that Mike Jacobson has done experiments on enucleated cells and cytoplasts also undergo the process of apoptosis without a nucleus and it is blockable by Bcl 2 and also by IGF-1. So there must be, to some extent, an independent cytoplasmic read out but one would suspect that there may also be a nuclear plasmic read out as well about which we know nothing. So yes, I did not want to exclude the nucleus. The thing that is pretty clear is that the nuclear and cytoplasmic apoptosis, if you like, can be semi-independent; you do not need one to have the others.

D. Livingston: Well that is implied from your Ice inhibitor experiment.

G. Evan: Yes.

M. Green: Following up on David's experiment in which you conclude that IGF-1 protective effect is not transcriptionally related. I think I would not have said it the way that David did about changes in DNA structure, but it does not rule out any changes in phosphorylation status of any transcription factors.

G. Evan: Well, what it says is that you can change the transcription factor and activate it or repress it but it cannot turn on any genes or make any proteins, so that is all it is saying. So the simplest idea about what IGF-1 is doing is that it up-regulates Bcl 2. Well that idea is out, because you do not need to up-regulate any proteins at the transcriptional level.

M. Green: But it could certainly up-regulate it at the post transcriptional level?

G. Evan: Absolutely and activate it, yes, that is right.

M. Green: There may be another way around it, so what do you think the IGF-1 is doing, what is your best guess on the protective effect?

G. Evan: My best guess is that I have absolutely no idea. All we suspect is that the ras pathway is not involved because, ras does not suppress myc induced death, in fact, it exacerbates myc induced cell death. So ras and myc cooperation is a different type of cooperation. We can exclude, perhaps, very crudely, that pathway but the answer is that I have really no idea.

M. Green: A second question, maybe a naive one, I had an idea about what the role of myc was in cell proliferation physiologically but what do you think the role of the apoptosis induction might be?

G. Evan: The fall back position would be that myc induced apoptosis has nothing to do with normal cells at normal levels of expression. However, you cannot get away from the fact that it is important in carcinogenesis. There is loads of myc in neoplasia; it promotes anti-apoptotic lesions from being sort of optional extras that tumors might acquire that make them a bit tougher, to being absolutely mandatory components of carcinogenesis. Because essentially every dominant oncogene that people looked at also promote cell death. So you have got to block that or suppress it to some degree. The harder question is to what extent is this present in every cell all of the time. We see no difference in quality or kind between cells that make loads of myc and cells that make less myc; it is just a quantitative difference, so we would argue that this happens in every cell that expresses myc all of the time.

M. Fried: Your survival factors delay death, they do not really prevent it. Do you think there are survival factors that prevent it all the time? Are tumors that come out of real animals full of survival factors?

G. Evan: If you look at all the literature all anybody ever showed is a delay of the onset of cell death, that is the clearest indicator that you can see of death suppression. If the observations are carried out far enough—some we did, some we did not. Every cell dies. You cannot find any gene or any manipulation that people can carry out, with the exception, we think, of the Ice blocking where cells refuse to die if you hit them hard enough for long enough. But my argument would be that that is not what happens in somatic tissues where these things are sporadic and you are playing a numbers game and even when you are inducing death by chemotherapy in tumors you are not dealing with one type of cell, you are dealing with a genetically heterogeneous cell population and the question is who survives and how many survive to come back and hit you a second time?

M. Fried: Yes, but are tumors full of factors that could be survival factors, that you could test on other cells?

G. Evan: The first problem is that I do not think anybody really knows what is a survival factor and what is not. But certainly in breast cancer IGF-1 has never been very important. In mice, where the large T-antigen of SV-40 is transgenically targeted to the islet cells tumors occur. For the islet cells the major survival factor that one can find is not IGF-1 but IGF-2, which is protected by the immediate neighboring cells. So Hanan gets tumors and he can show that there is mitogenic induction by transgenic T and go through the various stages of tumorogenisis. If you now do the same experiment in the IGF-2 knockout mice, which are small but otherwise viable, then tumor formation is massively reduced. But if you look at the mitotic effects of the T-antigen within those cells it is exactly the same. So that argues that endogenous survival factors really do affect the rate at which cells can break out and acquire more mutations in cancers.

T. Graf: Two unrelated questions: the first having to do with the physiological role of myc in inducing proliferation by serum. What happens if you deplete from serum IGF-1 (and perhaps also PDGF), then trigger cells into growth, do you also see cell death?

G. Evan: Yes, we find that whenever we remove the IGF-1 or PDGF your cells are up and running and wherever they are at the cell cycle death processes are immediately initiated.

T. Graf: And that is also apoptotic death?

G. Evan: All apoptotic. Liz Harrington did some very nice experiments in which she took cells that were distributed throughout the cell cycle, then removed the IGF-1 or serum, switched on myc and the cells started to die immediately in S-phase or out of S-phase; it does not matter where they are in the cycle, they die at the same rate.

T. Graf: The other question, unrelated, refers to your grand scheme in which you propose that all oncogenes induce apoptosis. I would like to ask you: what do you think about the report that rel prevents cell death and it seems to be important in the maintenance of transformation? We recently found that the same is true for myb. Myeloid cells transformed with a ts mutant of the oncogene, when shifted to the non permissive temperature, not only differentiate into macrophages but also die by apoptosis. There is also a down regulation of Bcl-2 which can be reversed by re-activating myb. So it looks like, at least formally speaking, that Bcl-2 is regulated by myb and this might help to explain how the oncogene transforms hematopoietic cells. Would this not argue against your hypothesis?

G. Evan: No, I am sorry; what I meant to say was that it looks like dominant oncogenes that promote cell cycle progression all seem to promote also apoptosis. But clearly there is a class of oncogenes which functions at least in a major way by suppressing apoptosis and Bcl-2 is the prototype of that, which does not promote cell cycle progression; I guess your data on myb would accord as well.

T. Graf: Coming back again to your grand scheme, would you not predict that those types of tumors which are driven by the anti-apoptotic subclass of oncogenes are much more common?

G. Evan: Well, I do not know about that. The transgenic data, say with Bcl 2, show very clearly that if you transgenically target Bcl 2 to tissues it is not really oncogenic. Bcl 2 certainly does not give cells any growth advantage except under situations where you are killing them off. So it does not promote proliferation, it does not promote mutagenesis, so they may be fairly neutral except in cooperation with the growth promoting oncogenes.

F. Rauscher: If you make myc a better activator or a better, say, repressor of transcription, can you get this myc induced apoptosis at lower levels rather than not over-expressing myc? By fusing it to VP-16 or something like that?

G. Evan: The VP-16 experiment has been done, if you replace the transactivation domain of myc into VP-16 you get something which in all model systems is an absolutely brilliant transactivator. It is dead as an oncogene and, in fact, as a tumor suppressor gene and it is dead as an inducer of apoptosis. The only thing I can say is that if you take V-myc, which is like a super myc or you take the myc's from BL which also have the same sort of mutation which act as super myc's, then what you see is that they are much more effective at both promotion of growth and promotion of apoptosis. So you get this phenotype which is much more like E1A where even 10% serum can not prevent massive apoptosis from occurring.

P. Comoglio: Your idea that there might be a signal transducer that directly links the IL-2 or IL-.1 receptor to the prevention of apoptosis is, I say, very challenging. Did you, or anyone else, ever try if tyrosine kinase inhibitors would interfere with IGF-1 protection?

G. Evan: A number of studies have been done with agents like cyclosporin and they are all incredibly effective inducers of apoptosis so that the cells die before you can get around to doing the experiment. What needs to be done is a systematic dissection of the internal domain of say, the IGF-1 receptor, and try to find the bits that are responsible for survival. There is no reason to belive that there is an overlap between the mitogenic signalling and the survival signalling and there is no reason to believe that there is not. Clues may come from experiements by which we and others are trying to ask whether the insulin receptor, which differs in important domains from the IGF-1 receptor, can also propogate a survival signal. I think the hints are that it may not.

B. Brandt: Your talk offers many very exciting data if I think about their possible clinical implications. First, what is the interaction between differentiation of cells and the mechanism of myc? Recently, new drugs causing cancer cell differentiation like phenol acetic acid and phenol butyric acid for new cancer therapy regimen have been reported.

G. Evan: Differentiated cells are different from each other by definition and therefore you cannot make broad categorical statements. The difficulty we have with the myc experiments and myc expression is that you can get these cells to differentiate. When they do so, they turn off myc. But they become something else, and the survival of this other cell, therefore, clearly is not affected by myc because myc is no longer expressed, but is now in the realms of the factors that would normally regulate the viability of that differentiated cell type. So, for example, I am not saying that myc is required for all apoptosis. Neurons die very easily when you deprive them of NGF, and there is no myc, and I presume it is not the same mechanism at all. What I am saying however, is that the expression of myc and presumably things up and downstream of it is tightly coupled to apoptosis.

B. Brandt: My second question is: you said that it makes sense to interfere downstream in the myc intracellular cascade. ErbB receptors are in the beginning of a signal transduction cascade which leads beside other ways to a myc interaction. In your opinion, does it make sense to interfere at erbB signal transduction on that background?

G. Evan: I do not know what Erb B-2 does because I do not know that anybody systematically evaluated oncogenes for survival potentiation versus mitogenic potentiation. I think it is a part of what Thomas was saying. There are assays that look at focus formation or tumor formation in animals and there are an awful lot of oncogenes known that really are not particularly mitogenic and people just say well, who knows? Maybe some of them are potent survival factors, I do not know. The point with myc, however, I think is more important. Where does this splitting of these two functions of myc occur? Does it occur at myc? So myc regulates a set of death genes and a set of proliferation genes or does myc regulate one set of genes from which assorted function can be derived by other factors? So I would say that myc has nothing to do with the decision the biforcation is not myc. And that is why I put it downstream of myc, downstream of the transcriptional programs. There are data from David Livingston's lab that the E2F also induces apoptosis: maybe that is downstream of myc. It is certainly in cell cycle. So the answer is that we do not know, because we do not know the downstream targets of myc. We have to find that out. But just blocking myc may be counterproductive.

D. Livingston: Following up on your suggestion that activated ras does not perturb the ability of myc to kill or to induce a state that leads to killing, can one do a Land—Weinberg experiment and determine whether such cells are inured to death despite the fact that they are immortal as a result of myc overexpression?

G. Evan: Land-Weinberg experiments require very high levels of serum to work.

D. Livingston: Now take the immortal cells and subject them, for example, to low serum assault. They die.

G. Evan: The ones we have looked at certainly die. The problem is that if you grow them for very long, presumably you are getting other mutations and you select out the ones that do not die anymore. There is very strong selectioning culture against the death process.

D. Livingston: That is what I am asking. Have those cells made it because they cannot die and are they inured to death because of some mutation or collection of mutations in the pathway downstream of myc for example?

G. Evan: That is certainly what we believe from the data looking at the immediate responsiveness or dependence of serum on the ras myc co-transfection.

E. Mihich: A very interesting cytokine is TNF because it can replace EGF in some cell systems for growth sustainment and also can induce apoptosis in other cells. Do you know whether there are any relationships between some actions of TNF and myc?

G. Evan: I can just say this: the more myc is expressed, the more sensitive to TNF a cell becomes. There is a report in the literature using antisense technology, that TNF killing is, at least in part, dependent upon myc expression. We have not done these experiments. There are problems with antisense technology particularly referring to myc. It turns out that the antisense that people use for myc, at the start of translation, have clusters of four G's in them. It turns out that all of the polynucleotides with four G's are pretty toxic. Antisense is always a minefield. The problem you are really bearing on, I think, is a very fundamental problem: it is pretty clear that EGF is not a survival factor in some cells, but it is so for other cells. IGF-1, on the other hand, seems to be a survival factor in every cell type that we have ever looked at. We are back to the basic problem of signal transduction which is that the same bits of information are used by different cells for different purposes.

G. Dranoff: Regarding your notion that targeting myc may not be a very good cancer therapeutic strategy, have you looked at the sensitivity to DNA-damage of fibroblasts transfected with dominant negative myc constructs?

G. Evan: The problem there is, of course, that they stop.

G. Dranoff: Yes, but that does not mean that you cannot read out cell death.

G. Evan: We have not done that, what we have done is to express high levels of MAD in these cells and they stop and they become quite resistant to induction of cell death, not completely but they lose the increased sensitivity that myc affords them.

G. Dranoff: So then if cells are arrested in cycle, the link between myc expression and susceptibility to death is less clear?

G. Evan: I cannot tell you anything at the moment about the molecular coupling between program cell death and proliferation. We do not know whether cells have to actually physically move through the cycle in order to become sensitive or whether just induction of myc is enough. But we suspect it is the latter, because as soon as myc is expressed, cells become sensitized to death within about ten to fifteen minutes. Enough for some sort of transcriptional program to come on long before the cells ever go into S, or any of the G-1 processes occur.

M. Oren: In lymphoid tumors you have a very nice natural paradigm for Bcl-2 overexpression and myc overexpression. Now, what happens in tumors where you have myc amplification,e.g., lung cancer with C or N or L-myc. Is it known what happens there? Is Bcl-2 activated? Is there an autocrine loop of any survival factor?

G. Evan: The prediction is, and it is only a prediction at the moment, that cells that have lots of myc, tumors that have lots of myc by definition have some potent, anti-apoptotic mechanism: the question is what that might be. The answer is nobody knows. One of the big projects in the lab at the moment is to take cDNA's in expression vectors from those high myc expressing tumor lines and dump them into our myc cells and look for protection from cell death. That is, we would suspect that there is a repertoire, we have no idea how big, of anti-apoptotic lesions out there and we have got to find out what they may be.

D. Livingston: So tumors do experience some apoptosis?

G. Evan: Right. A very important point. Nothing we have ever found blocks apoptosis, all it does is suppress it. There is not a tumor that has ever been found by anyone in which you cannot induce apoptosis with the same kinetics. All that happens is that all these genes that we find suppress the tendency of the tumors to engage the apoptosic machinery. I think that is a very hopeful sign because it means that suicide mechanism is there but the tumor is somehow undergoing some active indulgence—suppression of that.

D. Livingston: So you want to bring the balance the other way?

G. Evan: That is right and then the tumor should involute.

2

CONTROL OF INVASIVE CELL GROWTH BY THE MET FAMILY ONCOGENES

Francesco Galimi and Paolo M. Comoglio

Institute for Cancer Research and Treatment (I.R.C.C.)
University of Torino School of Medicine

The Hepatocyte Growth Factor receptor, encoded by the *MET* proto-oncogene (Naldini et al., 1991b, 1991c; Bottaro et al., 1991), is the prototype of a growing family of tyrosine kinases whose members share structural features of crucial functional relevance. Recently, two molecules have joined the family: the *RON* and the *SEA* gene products (Ronsin et al., 1993; Huff et al., 1993; Gaudino et al., 1994). Interestingly, the *Ron* protein was shown to be the specific receptor for Macrophage Stimulating Protein (MSP), a growth factor highly homologous to Hepatocyte Growth Factor (Gaudino et al., 1994; Wang et al., 1994). Therefore, the ligands for receptors of the *MET* family form a family themselves (the "HGF family"). So far, the ligand for the putative receptor encoded by the *SEA* proto-oncogene is elusive.

The Hepatocyte Growth Factor (HGF) is a paracrine factor secreted by tissues of mesodermal origin. It elicits a variety of biological responses in several organs, ranging from liver regeneration to control of hematopoiesis (for a review, see Zarnegar and Michalopoulos, 1995). However, the hallmark of the HGF biological activities, both *in vitro* and *in vivo,* is the induction of coordinated cell proliferation and movement, and the resulting control of invasive growth and morphogenesis. In fact, HGF is a powerful angiogenic factor (Bussolino et al., 1992), it is able to dissociate epithelial sheets and can promote progression of epithelial neoplasms toward malignant phenotypes (Weidner et al., 1990). Significantly, the *MET* gene is overexpressed in a relevant fraction of primary and metastatic tumors (Di Renzo et al., 1991 and 1992); in the latter case, overexpression is often associated to amplification (Di Renzo 1995b). Deregulation of the HGF receptor function appears to be a crucial step in the progression of epithelial neoplasms (Zhen et al., 1994).

HEPATOCYTE GROWTH FACTOR CONTROLS CELL GROWTH AND MOTILITY

Hepatocyte Growth Factor (HGF), also known as Scatter Factor, is a soluble molecule with the unusual property of inducing an invasive growth pattern in target cells.

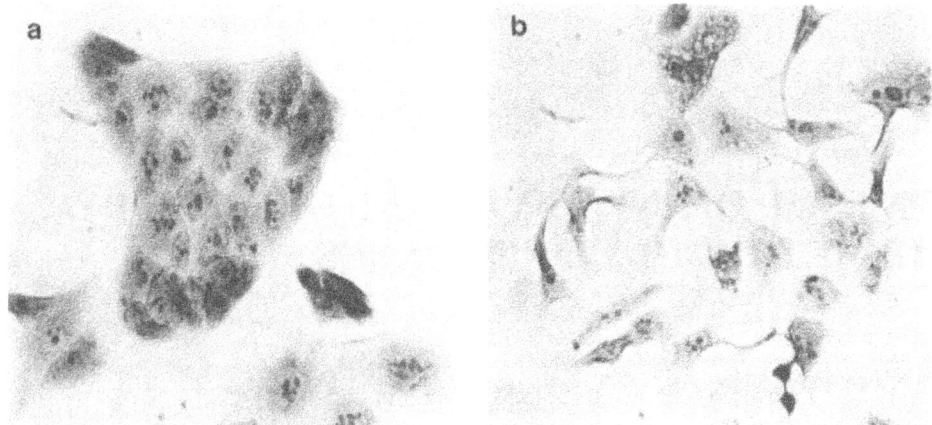

Figure 1. Dissociation of epithelial sheets or "cell scattering" is the hallmark of HGF-induced motogenesis. MDCK (Madin Darby Canine Kidney) cells cultured in standard medium (a) grow in islands; after 18 h incubation with pro-HGF 10 ng/ml (b) cells dissociate, moving apart from each other and acquiring a spindle-shaped appearance.

Among its recognized effects are: (i) dissociation of epithelial sheets, or "cell scattering" (figure 1; Stoker et al.,1987; Gherardi et al., 1989; Weidner et al.,1990 and 1991; Naldini et al.,1991b); (ii) increased motility and chemotaxis of dissociated cells (Morimoto et al.,1991; Bussolino et al.,1992; Giordano et al.,1993); (iii) mitogenesis (Michalopoulos et al.,1984; Nakamura et al.,1984); (iv) invasion of extracellular matrices (Weidner et al., 1990, Naldini et al.,1991b); (v) organization of invading cells into complex structures such as branching tubules (figure 1, Medico et al., submitted; Montesano et al., 1991; Bussolino et al., 1992). Both physiological processes (such as morphogenesis of epithelial organs, angiogenesis and tissue repair) and invasive neoplasm growth require coordinated execution of these events. In fact, HGF is a powerful angiogenetic factor *in vivo* (Bussolino et al., 1992, Grant et al., 1993) and it is involved in kidney and liver regeneration (Nagaike et al., 1991; Higuchi et al., 1991). HGF is thought to act in a paracrine fashion, being produced by mesenchymal/stromal cells (Stoker et al., 1987), and acting on neighbouring *MET*-expressing epithelial cells (Sonnemberg et al., 1993a).

BIOSYNTHESIS AND BIOLOGICAL ACTIVATION OF PRO-HGF

HGF is secreted as a single-chain inactive precursor of 92 kDa (pro-HGF: Naldini et al.,1992; Naka et al.,1992; Mizuno et al.,1992). Pro-HGF is bound to the cell surface or to the extracellular matrix, presumably via low-affinity high-capacity sites on heparin-like glycosaminoglycans (Naldini et al.,1991b; Kobayashi et al., 1994). Pro-HGF weakly binds the *Met* receptor, without triggering its kinase activity (Naldini et al.,1992; Hartmann et al.,1992; Lokker et al.,1992).

The mature factor derives from pro-HGF after proteolytic cleavage at the Arg[494]-Val[495] bond, yielding a disulfide-linked heterodimer of a 60 kDa (α) and a 32–36 kDa (β) chain ($\alpha\beta$HGF; Nakamura et al.,1987; Zarnegar and Michalopoulos,1989; Weidner et al.,1990). The molecular structure of HGF is very similar to that of proteolytic enzymes of the blood clotting cascade; the α chain consists of a putative hairpin loop and four triple-disulfide structures called kringles (Patthy, 1984); the β chain is homologous to the catalytic domain of serine proteases but lacks enzymatic activity (Nakamura et al., 1989; Myazawa et al., 1989). The dimeric mature HGF binds the *Met* receptor with high affinity, triggers its kinase activity and elicits the biological responses in target cells (Naldini et al., 1991a and 1991b; Bottaro et al.,1991).

The maturation of pro-HGF to functional HGF is a crucial point in the physiology of the factor. The proteolytic cleavage takes place in the extracellular environment, and is mediated by either urokinase-type plasminogen activator (uPA: Naldini et al., 1992) or a factor-XII-like serum protease (Miyazawa et al.,1993).

The cleavage of pro-HGF to the active dimeric form by uPA is a stoichiometric reaction, reproducible *in vitro* and occurring *in vivo* (Naldini et al., 1995). In a standard catalytic reaction, given enough time, virtually all the substrate is processed and the total yield of product is independent from the concentration of enzyme. The reaction is only limited by the initial substrate concentration. On the contrary, for uPA and HGF the limiting factor is the amount of enzyme and not the amount of substrate. The stoichiometric reaction of uPA with pro-HGF could be due either to the formation of a stable complex between the reaction products or to an irreversible modification of uPA in the course of its reaction with pro-HGF. The level of bioactive HGF in a tissue microenvironment is titrated by the extent of activity of uPA. This, in turn, is subject to strict spatial and temporal regulation by the level of expression of the protein and its interplay with activators, inhibitors and cellular receptors (reviewed in Blasi et al., 1987). Extracellular activation by a protease is envisaged as a critical regulatory step in signalling mediated by morphogenic factors since it provides a mechanism for the local production of intercellular signals.

Coordination of cell growth, movement and matrix invasion occurs not only in physiological events but also in the progression of cancer cells towards malignancy. Several growth factors, including HGF (Pepper et al., 1992, Boccaccio et al., 1994), induce expression of uPA and its receptor as an early event in the course of the mitogenic response (reviewed in Saksela and Rifkin, 1988). A correlation between surface uPA activity and tumor cell invasion and metastasis has been well documented (Ossowski L, and Reich E., 1983; Kirchheimer et al., 1987 and 1989; Ossowski L., 1988a and 1988b; Hearing et al.,1988; Axelrod et al., 1989; Pyke et al., 1991; Meissauer et al., 1991). The induction of uPA is therefore an indirect mechanism through which HGF promotes cell invasiveness.

STRUCTURE, BIOSYNTHESIS AND SUBCELLULAR DISTRIBUTION OF THE HGF RECEPTOR

The HGF receptor is the tyrosine kinase encoded by the *MET* proto-oncogene. It is a two-chain oligomer, composed of a 50 kDa (α) chain disulfide linked to a 145 kDa (β) chain in an $\alpha\beta$ complex of 190 kDa (Giordano et al., 1989a). The α chain is extracellular and the β chain spans the plasma membrane; the latter contains a tyrosine kinase domain (Gonzatti et. al., 1988) as well as sites for tyrosine auto-phosphorylation (Ferracini et al., 1991, Ponzetto et al., 1993).

The HGF receptor is synthesized as a large single-chain precursor (pr170). The mature dimeric molecule is derived from the precursor by cotranslational glycosylation and proteolytic cleavage (Giordano et al., 1989a). Under normal conditions the single chain precursor is not exposed at the cell surface: core glycosylation is crucial for further processing since the aglycoproreceptor, produced in the presence of tunicamycin, is neither cleaved into the mature chains nor inserted into the plasma membrane. Disulfide bond formation between α and β chains takes place before the cleavage (Giordano et al.,1989b). The cleavage site[*] (K^{303} RKKR-S^{308}) is a canonical consensus for the endoplasmic reticulum protease furin (Barr, 1991), and is crucial for the correct cleavage of the receptor, as shown by site directed mutagenesis experiments involving the two arginines in position 304 and 307 (Mark et al., 1993).

After synthesis, the HGF receptor is targeted from the Trans Golgi Network to the basolateral plasma membrane domain of polarized epithelial cells. The receptor is concentrated around cell-cell contacts, showing a distribution pattern overlapping that of the cell-adhesion molecule E-cadherin and, in polarized cells, interacts with detergent-insoluble cytoskeleton components (Crepaldi et al., 1994b).

THE HGF RECEPTOR KINASE ACTIVITY IS REGULATED BY TYROSINE OR SERINE PHOSPHORYLATION

The earliest detectable consequence of HGF stimulation of target cells is the tyrosine autophosphorylation of its receptor (Naldini et al., 1991b). As with other growth factor receptors, this indicates activation of the receptor kinase. Autophosphorylation of the receptor β subunit was observed both in cells showing growth as response to HGF and in cells showing increased motility.

The HGF receptor tyrosine kinase is up-regulated by an autocatalytic mechanism. Unlike other growth factor receptors (e.g.EGF or PDGF receptors), tyrosine autophosphorylation increases by several fold the catalytic activity of the kinase domain (Naldini et al., 1991a). The major tyrosine autophosphorylation site of the $p190^{MET}$ receptor was identified with the tyrosine residue 1235 (Ferracini et al., 1991). Tyr ^{1235} is located within the tyrosine kinase domain and is part of a "three tyrosine" motif, including Y^{1230}, Y^{1234} and Y^{1235}, conserved in the Insulin and Insulin-like receptors (Tornqvist et al., 1987, 1988; Hanks et al., 1988). The role of these tyrosines in positively regulating the HGF receptor enzymatic activity has been studied with site-directed mutagenesis by replacement with phenylalanine (Longati et al., 1994). We observed that both Y^{1234} and Y^{1235} are essential for full activation of the enzyme. Phosphorylation of both residues may be required for maximal activation of the HGF receptor kinase. Alternatively, given that Y^{1235} has been identified as the major phosphorylation site, Y^{1234} may facilitate phosphorylation of the nearby residue, or may stabilize the activated form of the enzyme via its phenolic side group. This tyrosine doublet is present at homologous locations in the proteins encoded by *RON* and *SEA*, the other two members of the *MET* family (Ronsin et al., 1993; Huff et al., 1993).

Phosphorylation on serine and/or treonine residues by protein kinase-C is a well known modulation mechanism for several membrane receptors (for a review see Nishizuka et al., 1988). Also in the case of HGF, stimulation of protein kinase-C by phorbol esters is followed by serine phosphorylation of the receptor and consequent decrease in tyrosine kinase activity (Gandino et al., 1990). An independent negative regulatory pathway is triggered by increasing the intracellular Ca^{2+} concentration, either experimen-

---

* Aminoacid numbers are derived from the sequence of the major *MET* transcript: Ponzetto et al., 1991. (EMBL/GenBank Accession number: X54559).

tally or by physiological agonists. The enzyme involved is a serine kinase with the biochemical properties of Ca^{2+}-Calmodulin kinase III (Gandino et al., 1991). Interestingly, the target residue phosphorylated in both instances is Ser^{985}, located within the juxtamembrane domain of the HGF receptor, in a canonical consensus sequence for phosphorylation by protein kinase-C and Ca^{2+}-Calmodulin kinase III (Kennelly and Krebs, 1991). The substitution of Ser^{985} with an alanine residue by site-directed mutagenesis abolishes the inhibitory effects of either TPA or calcium ionophores on the HGF receptor activity (Gandino et al., 1994).

THE HGF RECEPTOR ACTIVATES INTRACELLULAR SIGNAL TRANDUCERS VIA AN UNCONVENTIONAL DOCKING SITE

The HGF receptor activates multiple intracellular signal transduction pathways, in line with HGF capability of evoking complex biological responses such as mitogenesis, motogenesis and morphogenesis (figure 2). Stimulation of responsive cells induces activation of PI 3-kinase (Graziani et al., 1991; Ponzetto et al., 1993), of a *Ras* nucleotide exchanger (Graziani et al., 1993) and of a tyrosine phosphatase (Villa-Moruzzi et al., 1993). Moreover in epithelial cells, upon phosphorylation of the receptor, PLCγ and MAP kinase become phosphorylated on tyrosine (Ponzetto et al., 1994). For PLCγ this modification is essential for activation of the enzyme and hydrolysis of inositol phospholipids generating second intracellular messengers (Kim et al., 1991), whereas MAP kinase phosphorylation has been correlated to activation of the *Ras* pathway (Pelech and Sanghera, 1992). HGF also induces tyrosine phosphorylation and stimulation of the cytoplasmic tyrosine kinase $pp60^{Src}$ (Ponzetto et al., 1994). Finally, after ligand-induced tyrosine phosphorylation, the HGF receptor associates with the *Shc* adaptor protein and phosphorylates it on $Y^{317}VNV$, generating a high affinity binding site for *Grb2* (K_d=15 nM). This duplicates the high affinity binding site for *Grb2* present on the HGF receptor itself ($Y^{1356}VNV$: see below). Thus, HGF stimulation triggers the *Ras* pathway by recruiting *Grb2* either directly, through the receptor, or indirectly, through *Shc*. Overexpression of wild-type *Shc*, but not

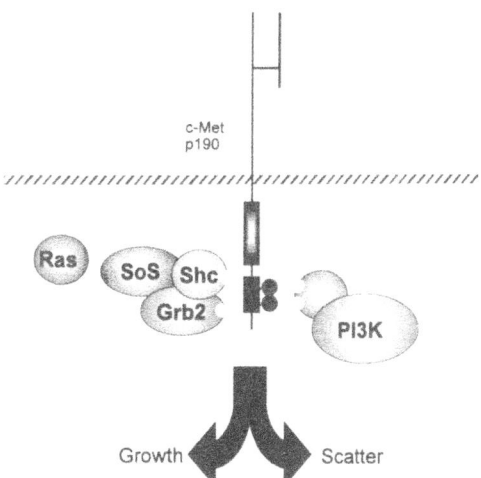

Figure 2. The HGF receptor transductosome. The activated receptor triggers cell growth and movement ("scattering") by activating different intracellular transducers *via* the bidentate docking site in its C-terminal tail.

of the $Y^{317} \rightarrow F$ mutant, enhances cell migration and growth in response to HGF, showing that *Shc* is a relevant substrate of the HGF receptor, and works as an "amplifier" of the motogenic as well as the mitogenic response (figure 2).

The currently accepted mechanism for coupling tyrosine kinase receptors with cytoplasmic signalling molecules involves ligand binding, receptor dimerization, and reciprocal transphosphorylation of each monomer at multiple sites. Some of the phosphorylated residues are "docking" sites for cytoplasmic transducers, which bind specific phosphotyrosines *via* conserved structural modules known as Src homology 2 (SH2) domain (Cantley et al., 1991; Koch et al., 1991). SH2 domains are found in one or two copies in molecules involved in signal transduction such as PI 3-kinase, *Ras* GAP, PLCγ, *Src*-related tyrosine kinases, the tyrosine phosphatase SHPTP2 and the *Shc* and *Grb*-2 adaptors (for a review see Pawson and Schlessinger, 1993). In a number of tyrosine kinase receptors, distinct phosphotyrosine residues have been identified, responsible for binding either PI 3-kinase, PLCγ, *Ras* GAP, or pp60^{c-Src} (for a review, see Pawson, 1995).

We have shown that two phosphotyrosines located in the HGF receptor C-terminal tail are responsible for mediating its interactions with SH2-containing cytoplasmic effectors (Ponzetto et al., 1994). Unlike other tyrosine kinases, members of the HGF receptor family contain a sequence

$$Y\ V\ (N,H,Q)\ (V,L) - X_3 - Y\ (V,M)\ N\ (V,L),$$

known as the "bidentate super-site," capable interacting with high affinity and activating PI 3-kinase, PLCγ, pp60^{c-Src}, the *Shc* adaptor and the *Grb-2*/SOS complex. All these molecules, with the only exception of *Grb*-2, interact directly with either phosphotyrosine in the "bidentate" site. Comparison of the sequence YV(H,N,Q)V with the optimal binding motifs listed by Songyang et al. (1993), indicates that it represents a degenerate consensus potentially permissive for a number of SH2 domains. By BIAcore biosensor measurings, we showed that the SH2 domains of p85, PLCγ, and pp60^{c-Src}, interact directly with either version (YVHV or YVNV) of the HGF receptor "super-site." *Grb-2*, which has a strong requirement for asparagine in the +2 position (Songyang et al., 1993), specifically interacts with the sequence YV<u>N</u>V. The affinities of the bidentate site for all the different SH2's were similar to the corresponding canonical sequences, with the exception of p85 which showed a K_d one order of magnitude apart from that for the optimal sequence YXXM (Ponzetto et al., 1993).

The multifunctional "super-site" represents a variation from the common theme of sequence specificity in the recognition process between SH2 domains and phosphotyrosine residues in tyrosine kinase receptors. We propose as an explanation to how such a site may work, that a number of factors will concur in determining which transducer binds at any moment. Listed among these factors are differences in affinity, variations in local concentration of effectors, and in levels of receptor phosphorylation. At very low levels of receptor phosphorylation (early times after stimulus), only the highest affinity interactions will occur and thus only a few transductional pathways will be activated. As the number of phosphorylated receptors increases, the formation of additional complexes involving molecules capable of binding with lower affinities may become possible. Through this mechanism, additional pathways can be superimposed onto those already operating. Different cell types contain significantly different amounts of receptor and transducers. This may explain why HGF activates some pathways (e.g. mitogenesis or motogenesis) in some cells and not in others.

THE HGF RECEPTOR GENE (*MET*) IS ONCOGENIC *IN VITRO*

MET was originally described as a human oncogene activated *in vitro* after treatment of a cell line with a chemical carcinogen (Cooper et al., 1984). The cloned oncogene is a hybrid between 5' sequences of a gene named *TPR*, derived from chromosome 1, and 3' sequences of *MET*, located on chromosome 7 (Park et al., 1986; Tempest et al., 1986; Dean et al., 1987; Mitchell et al., 1992b). Moreover, it has been reported that transfection of a full size *MET* cDNA can induce transformation upon establishment of an autocrine circuit (Rong et al., 1994).

To study the molecular mechanisms underlying *MET*-induced transformation, a number of deletion or point mutants of the HGF receptor were created (Zhen et al., 1994). Similarly to other tyrosine kinase receptors, such as the EGF receptor (Downword et al., 1984; Khazaie et al., 1988), the SCF receptor (Qiu et al., 1988) and the Insulin receptor (Shoelson et al., 1988), truncation of the extracellular and transmembrane domains of the HGF receptor deregulates its tyrosine kinase activity; such mutated HGF receptors are both transforming and tumorigenic. Under physiological conditions, the HGF receptor catalytic activity is latent unless the extra-cellular domain binds the cognate ligand (Naldini et al., 1991a and b). While deletion of the α chain is not sufficient to induce deregulation of the tyrosine kinase activity (Zhen et al., 1994), lack of cleavage between the α and the β chain can cause constitutive activation (Mondino et al., 1991).

Deletions involving the juxtamembrane domain of the HGF receptor do not constitutively activate its kinase activity and are devoid of transforming ability (Zhen et al., 1994). The oncogenic potential is restored by replacing the juxtamembrane domain with 5' sequences derived from the *TPR* gene (Mitchell et al., 1992a; Mitchell et al., 1992b). Comparing the first 39 amino acids of the HGF receptor juxtamembrane domain to the *TPR* moiety does not reveal obvious structural similarities. It is generally agreed that receptor tyrosine kinases are activated by conformational changes induced by ligand binding, resulting in receptor oligomerization which stabilizes the interactions between contiguous cytoplasmic domains (Heldin et al., 1989; Seifert et al., 1989). According to this activation mechanism, it is conceivable that a critical segment of the juxtamembrane domain may be necessary to stabilize the formation of kinase dimers leading to transactivation. A role of *TPR* sequences in the dimerization of the *Tpr-Met* hybrid kinase has been shown (Rodrigues et al., 1993).

Like all receptor, as well as non-receptor, tyrosine kinases, the transforming potential of the intracellular domain of the HGF receptor relies on its tyrosine kinase activity. The catalytic domain entails a number of critical residues whose mutation can abolish transformation. (i) Substitution of the lysine residue responsible for ATP binding invariably results in a loss of catalytic function and transforming activity (Snyder et al., 1985). (ii) The two tyrosines Y^{1234} and Y^{1235}, known to positively regulate the receptor enzymatic activity upon autophosphorylation (Ferracini et al., 1991; Longati et al., 1994), are indispensable. The HGF receptor is, in fact, "autocatalytic" since autophosphorylation dramatically increases the V_{MAX} of the phosphate transfer reaction (see above, Naldini et al., 1991c). This mechanism of up-regulation is critical for unleashing the oncogenic potential of the MET oncogene.

THE HGF RECEPTOR GENE (*MET*) IS A HARMFUL ONCOGENE *IN VIVO*

The first evidence for amplification of the *MET* proto-oncogene came from a cell line derived from a metastasis of a human gastric carcinoma, where the gene was amplified and overexpressed, and the tyrosine kinase constitutively activated (Giordano et al., 1989a). No alteration in the sequence was found in the cloned cDNA (Ponzetto et al., 1991), showing that constitutive activation of the *MET* kinase may be caused by simple overexpression. Since then, *MET* has been found to be amplified and/or overexpressed in a significant number of human tumors of epithelial origin (Di Renzo et al., 1991; Prat et al., 1991a; Di Renzo et al., 1992; Liu et al., 1992). In thyroid tumors overexpression of *MET* is observed in a significant proportion (~ 70%) of carcinomas derived from the follicular epithelium and correlates with the aggressive phenotype (Di Renzo et al., 1992). While the *MET*-encoded receptor is detectable only in the acinar cells of the normal human exocrine pancreas, it is up-regulated in the majority of pancreatic ductal adenocarcinomas (Di Renzo et al., 1995a). In most cases the HGF receptor found in the malignant cells has features of the normal receptor. In overexpressing cell lines, the *Met*/HGF receptor is phosphorylated in the absence of ligand, suggesting that activation of the *MET* gene may be involved in the growth of pancreatic cancer and may contribute to the ductal phenotype of these tumors.

Of particular interest are the changes of *MET* gene expression occurring during the progression of colorectal tumors from adenomas to primitive carcinomas and liver metastases. In several examples it was possible to compare same patient samples of normal colon mucosa to primary tumor and primary carcinoma to synchronous metastasis (Di Renzo et al., 1995b). The expression of the *MET* gene was increased from five to fifty-fold in about 50% of tumors, at any stage of progression, and in 70% of liver metastases. Overexpression was associated to amplification of the *MET* gene in only few primary carcinomas, but in a significant proportion of the metastases examined. These data suggest that overexpression of *MET* contributes a selective growth advantage to neoplastic colorectal cells at any stage of tumor progression. Moreover, amplification appears to give a further selective advantage for the acquisition of metastatic potential.

Normal and neoplastic ovary tissue provide further evidence for the implication of the *MET* oncogene in tumor progression. DNA level and expression of the *Met*/HGF receptor gene were studied in human ovary, benign ovarian tumors and epithelial ovarian carcinomas (Di Renzo et al. 1994). The *Met*/HGF receptor is detectable in the surface epithelium in normal ovary. The level of expression is unchanged in benign ovarian tumors of various origin, but about 30% of malignant carcinomas show a three to ten-fold increase in expression. The *Met*/HGF receptor protein can sometimes be found over-expressed over fifty-fold without *MET* gene amplification. Most interestingly, a correlation can be found between the clinical aggressive behaviour of ovarian tumors and the overexpression of the *MET* gene.

MET has long been considered to affect only tumors derived from epithelial tissues. A growing amount of evidence, however, suggests that the *MET*/HGF receptor might also have a role in the growth of sarcomas. In fact, *MET* was originally identified as an oncogene activated upon artificial rearrangement in a human osteosarcoma cell line (Cooper et al., 1984, Park et al., 1986). Moreover, the murine *met* homologue was found to be amplified and overexpressed in spontaneously transformed fibroblasts grown *in vitro* (Cooper et al., 1986). It was reported that NIH/3T3 fibroblasts that co-express the *Met* receptor and its ligand HGF are tumorigenic (Rong et al., 1992, 1994). It has been recently shown that the creation of an HGF autocrine loop either in fibroblasts or in epithelial cells induces invasive properties *in vitro* and metastatic ability *in vivo* (Bellusci et al., 1994; Rong et al., 1994). This prompted us to study the expression of the *Met*/HGF receptor and its ligand in human bone tumors. A significant percentage of human osteosarcomas and all the osteosarcoma cell lines examined expressed the *Met*/HGF receptor, in some cases together with HGF itself. HGF stimulated cell motility and penetration in extracellular matrices ("scattering"), suggesting that inappropriate *Met*/HGF receptor activation might provide osteosarcoma cells with the capacity to invade neighboring tissues (Ferracini et al., 1995).

THE HGF RECEPTOR FAMILY

The HGF receptor is a prototype for a class of receptor-type tyrosine kinases. The HGF receptor family includes the two receptors encoded by the oncogenes *RON* and *SEA* (Ronsin et al., 1993; Huff et al., 1993; Gaudino et al., 1994). Structural features common to the members of the family can be found both in the extracellular and in the intracellular domains (figure 3). (i) They are heterodimers (Giordano et al., 1989a; Gaudino et al., 1994); (ii) they have two neighbouring tyrosine residues in the kinase domain, responsible for regulation of the receptor kinase activity upon autophosphorylation (Ferracini et al., 1991; Longati et al., 1994); (iii) they share the eleven-aminoacid motif in the C-terminal tail (the "bidentate super-site," see above) acting as a multifunctional dock for SH2-containing signal transducers (Ponzetto et al., 1994). In the extracellular domain, (iv) the three receptors share the cleavage site between the α and β chains and (v) the location of

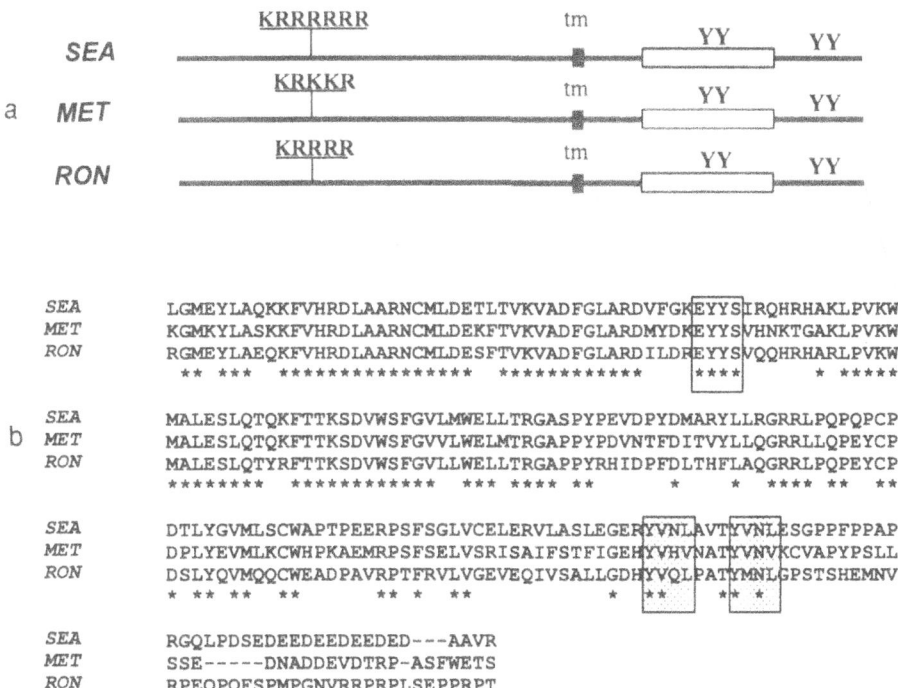

Figure 3. (a) Schematic representation of the sequence similarities among the *Met*, *Sea* and *Ron* receptors. tm: transmembrane domain; the white rectangle indicates the kinase domain, containing the major phosphorylation site (YY); YY in the C-terminal tail indicate the bidentate docking site. The arginine-rich cleavage site in the extracellular domain is also shown. (b) Sequence alignment of the three receptors' intracellular domain aminoacid sequences. The asterisks (*) indicate the conserved residues. The empty box shows the major phosphorylation site in the kinase domain; the dotted boxes entail the two tyrosine residues forming the bidentate docking site in the C-terminal tail.

the cysteine residues (Park et al., 1987; Ronsinet al., 1993). The homology between *Met*, *Ron* and *Sea* is concentrated in the kinase domain and in the bidentate SH2-docking site; these domains are directly involved in eliciting the biological responses distinctive to the *Met*-family of RTK's. The extracellular portion, the juxtamembrane domain and the C-terminal tail are quite divergent between *Met*, *Ron* and *Sea*.

While the ligand for the putative receptor encoded by the *SEA* protooncogene still remains elusive, the ligand for the *RON* receptor has been recently identified with MSP (Macrophage Stimulatory Protein; Gaudino et al., 1994; Wang et al., 1994).

THE *RON* GENE PRODUCT IS THE RECEPTOR FOR MACROPHAGE STIMULATORY PROTEIN (MSP)

The *RON* receptor is a 185-kDa heterodimer, consisting of two subunits linked by disulphide bonds: β, of 150 kDa and α, of 35 kDa. The receptor is synthesised in a single-chain precursor form of 170 kDa (p170); proteolytic cleavage occurs at a site for furin-like proteases, highly conserved among the members of the HGF receptor family. In cells expressing physiological amounts of endogenous *RON*, only the mature dimeric p185^{RON} is exposed at the cell surface. In COS-1 cells over-expressing the transfected *RON* cDNA, a fraction of uncleaved precursor can be found at the cell surface. The intracellular portion of the *Ron* β chain contains a fully functional kinase domain, as shown by *in vitro* tyrosine autophosphorylation under appropriate conditions (Gaudino et al., 1994).

The ligand for the *Ron* receptor is Macrophage Stimulatory Protein (MSP), closely related to HGF and originally isolated as a chemotactic factor for peritoneal macrophages ((Friezner-Degen et al., 1991; Skeel et al., 1991). Stimulation of responsive cells with MSP results in *Ron* receptor phosphorylation and DNA synthesis (Gaudino et al., 1994). It should be noted that also in the case of MSP, the factor is secreted as a single-chain inactive precursor which is cleaved to the bioactive dimer by serum-derived proteases (Wang et al., 1994).

The expression of the *Ron* receptor was studied in adult and developing mouse tissues (Gaudino et al., submitted). Specific *RON* transcripts were detectable in the mouse liver from early embryonal life (day 12.5 p.c.) through adult life. Adrenal gland, spinal ganglia, skin, lung and - unexpectedly - ossification centers of developing mandible, clavicle and ribs were also positive at later stages (day 13.5–16.5 p.c.). From day 17.5 *RON* was expressed in the gut epithelium and in a specific area of the central nervous system, corresponding to the nucleus of the hypoglossus. In adult mouse tissues *RON* transcripts were observed in brain, adrenal glands, gastro-intestinal tract, testis and kidney. Epithelial, osteoclast-like and neuroendocrine cells express the *Ron* receptor and respond to MSP *in vitro*. In PC12 cells, while NGF induced growth arrest and morphological differentiation, MSP behaved as a strong mitogen.

Altough the receptors for MSP and HGF share a common ancestry and strong structural homologies, the pattern of expression of the *RON* gene during development shows only few overlapping features with that reported for *MET* (Sonnenberg et al., 1993), suggesting that the two genes play separate roles in morphogenesis. The two receptors are concurrently expressed in the developing and adult liver: however "knock-out" mice defective for *MET* expression develop lethal liver abnormalities at day 15 p.c. (Schmidt et al., 1995); at this stage *RON* is expressed but can not replace *MET* functions. Moreover, *MET* has been found expressed at early stages in endodermal epithelia, forming tubules or branching cavities (e.g., lung, pancreas, salivary gland and kidney) while *RON* is expressed at a late stage in these organs. Conversely, *RON* appears critical in the development of epithelial organs derived from the ectoderm (e.g. the skin and the neuro-endocrine systems). Finally, the localization of the two receptors in the nervous system are different, MET being expressed in the spinal cord and in the rostral brain (telencephalon) (Sonnenberg et al., 1993).

ACKNOWLEDGMENTS

The experimental work reviewed in this paper is the result of the collaborative effort of our co-workers M.F. Di Renzo, G. Gaudino, C. Ponzetto, M. Prat, T. Crepaldi, S. Giordano, A. Graziani, L. Naldini, C. Boccaccio, G. Gambarotta, E. Medico, P. Longati and E. Vigna, who are gratefully acknowledged. The manuscript has been written with the excellent assistance of A. Cignetto and E. Wright. Supported by grants from the Associazione Italiana Ricerche Cancro (AIRC) and from the Italian National Research Council (CNR), progetto finalizzato ACRO.

REFERENCES

Axelrod, J.H., Reich, R. and Miskin, R. (1989). Expression of human recombinant plasminogen activators enhances invasion and experimental metastasis of H-ras-transformed NIH 3T3 cells. Mol. Cell. Biol. 9, 2133–2141.

Barr. J. (1991). Mammalian Subtilisins: the long-sought dibasic processing endoproteases. Cell, 66, 1–3.

Bellusci, S., Moens, G., Gaudino. G., Comoglio, P.M., Nakamura, T., Thiery J.P and Jouanneau. J. (1994). Creation of an hepatocyte growth factor/scatter factor autocrine loop in carcinoma cells induces invasive properties associated with increased tumorigenicity. Oncogene, 9, 1091–1099.

Blasi, F., Vassalli, J-D. and Dano, K. (1987). Urokinase-type plasminogen activator: proenzyme, receptor, and inhibitors. J. Cell. Biol. 104, 801–804.

Boccaccio, C., Gaudino, G., Gambarotta, G., Galimi, F., and Comoglio P.M. (1994) Hepatocyte Growth Factor (HGF) receptor expression is inducible and is part of the delayed-early response to HGF. J. Biol. Chem. 269, 12846–12851.

Bottaro, D.P., Rubin, J.S., Faletto, D.L., Chan, A.M.L., Kmiecick, T.E., Vande Woude, G.F. and Aaronson, S.A. (1991) Identification of the hepatocyte growth factor receptor as the c-met proto-oncogene. Science 251, 802–804.

Bussolino, F., Di Renzo, M.F., Ziche, M., Bocchietto, E., Olivero, M., Naldini, L., Gaudino, G., Tamagnone, L., Coffer, A., Marchisio, P.C., and Comoglio, P.M. (1992). Hepatocyte growth factor is a potent angiogenic factor which stimulates endothelial cell motility and growth. J. Cell Biol., 119:629–641.

Cantley, L.C., Auger, K., Carpenter, C., Duckworth, B., Graziani, A., Kapeller, R. and Soltoff, S. (1991) Oncogenes and signal transduction. Cell 64, 281–302.

Science 254, 1382–1385.

Cooper C.S.,Tempest P.R.,Beckman M.P.,Heldin C-H. and Brooks P.(1986). Amplification and overexpression of the *met* gene in spontaneously transformed NIH3T3 mouse fibroblasts. EMBO J., 5, 2623–2628.

Cooper, C.S., Park, M., Blair, D.G., Tainsky, M.A., Huebner, K., Croce, C.M. and Vande Woude, G. (1984). Molecular cloning of a new transforming gene from a chemically transformed human cell line. Nature 311, 29–33.

Crepaldi, T., Pollack, A.L., Prat, M., Zborek, A., Mostov, K. and Comoglio, P.M. (1994b) Targeting of the SF/HGF receptor to the basolateral domain of polarized epithelial cells. J. Cell Biol. 125, 313–320.

Dean, M., Park, M., Vande Woude, G.F. (1987). Characterization of the rearranged *tpr-met* Oncogene Breakpoint. Mol. Cell. Biol. 7, 921–924.

Di Renzo, M.F., Narsimhan, R.P., Olivero, M., Bretti, S., Giordano S., Medico, E., Gaglia, P., Zara, P., and Comoglio, P.M. (1991). Expression of the *met*/HGF receptor in normal and neoplastic human tissues. Oncogene 6, 1997–2003.

Di Renzo, M.F., Olivero, M., Ferro, S., Prat, M., Bongarzone, I., Pilotti, S., Pierotti, M.A., and Comoglio, P.M. (1992). Overexpression of the c-met/hgf receptor gene in human thyroid carcinomas. Oncogene 7, 2549–2553.

Di Renzo, M.F., Poulsom, R., Olivero, M., Comoglio, P.M. and N.R. Lemoine (1995a). Expression of the Met/Hepatocyte Growth Factor Receptor in human pancreatic cancer. Cancer Res., 55, 1129–1138.

Di Renzo, M.F., Olivero, M., Giacomini, A., Porte, H., Chastre, E., Mirossay, L., Nordlinger, B.,Bretti, S., Bottardi, S., Giordano, S., Plebani, M., Gespach C. and P.M. Comoglio. (1995b) Overexpression and amplification of the met/hgf receptor gene during the progression of colorectal cancer. Clin. Cancer Res., 1, 147–154.

Di Renzo, M.F., Olivero, M., Katsaros, D., Crepaldi, T., Gaglia, P., Zola, P., Sismondi P. and P.M. Comoglio (1994). Overexpression of the met/HGF receptor in ovarian cancer. Int. J. Cancer, 58, 658–662.

Downword, J., Yarden, Y., Mayes, E., Scrace, G., Totty, N., Stockwell, P., Ullrich, A., Schlessinger, J. and Waterfield, M.D. (1984). Close similarity of epidermal growth factor receptor and v-erb-B oncogene protein sequences. Nature 307, 521–527.

Ferracini, R., Longati, P., Naldini, L., Vigna, E. and Comoglio, P.M. (1991) Identification of the major phosphorylation site of the Met/Hepatocyte Growth Factor receptor tyrosine kinase. J. Biol. Chem. 266, 19558–19564.

Ferracini, R., Di Renzo M.F., Scotlandi, K., Baldini, N., Olivero, M., Lollini, P., Cremona, O., Campanacci, M. and Comoglio P.M. (1995). The met/hgf receptor is overexpressed in human osteosarcomas and is activated by either a paracrine or an autocrine circuit. Oncogene, 10, 739–749.

Friezner-Degen, S.J., Stuart, L.A., Han, S. and Jamison, C.S. (1991). Characterization of the mouse cDNA and gene coding for a hepatocyte growth factor-like protein: expression during development. Biochemistry 30, 978–9791.

Gandino, L., Di Renzo, M.F., Giordano, S., Bussolino, F. and Comoglio, P.M. (1990) Protein kinase-C activation inhibits tyrosine phosphorylation of the c-Met protein. Oncogene 5, 721–725.

Gandino, L., Longati, P., Medico, E., Prat, M. and Comoglio, P.M. (1994) Phosphorylation of ser^{985} negatively regulates the hepatocyte growth factor receptor kinase. J. Biol. Chem. 269, 1815–1820.

Gandino, L., Munaron, L., Naldini, L., Ferracini, R., Magni, M. and Comoglio, P.M. (1991) Intracellular calcium regulates the tyrosine kinase receptor encoded by the MET oncogene. J. Biol. Chem. 266, 16098–16104.

Gaudino, G., Follenzi, A., Naldini, L., Collesi,C.Santoro, M., Gallo, K.A., Godowski P.J. and Comoglio P.M. (1994). Ron is a heterodimeric tyrosine kinase receptor activated by the HGF-homolog MSP. EMBO J., 13, 3524–3532.

Gherardi, G., Gray, J., Stoker, M., Perryman, M., and Furlong, R. (1989). Purification of scatter factor, a fibroblast-derived basic protein that modulates epithelial interaction and movement. Proc. Natl. Acad. Sci. USA 86, 5844–5848.

Giordano, S., Di Renzo, M.F., Narsimhan, R.P., Cooper, C.S., Rosa, C. and Comoglio, P.M. (1989b) Biosynthesis of the protein encoded by the c-MET proto-oncogene. Oncogene 4, 1383–1388.

Giordano, S., Ponzetto, C., Di Renzo, M.F., Cooper, C.S. and Comoglio, P.M. (1989a) Tyrosine kinase receptor indistinguishable from the c-Met protein. Nature 339, 155–156.

Giordano, S., Zhen, Z., Medico, E., Gaudino, G., Galimi, F. and Comoglio, P.M. (1993) Transfer of motogenic and invasive response to scatter factor/hepatocyte growth factor by transfection of human MET protooncogene. Proc. Natl. Acad. Sci. USA 90, 649–653.

Gonzatti-Haces, M., Seth, A., Park, M., Copeland, T., Oroszlan, S. and Vande Woude, G.F. (1988). Characterization of the TPR-MET oncogene p65 and the MET protooncogene p140 protein-tyrosine kinases. Proc. Natl. Acad. Sci. USA, 85, 21–25.

Grant, D.S., Kleinmann, H.K., Goldberg, I. D., Bhargava, M., Nickoloff. B.J., Kinsella, J.K., Polverini, P.J. and Rosen, E.M. (1993). Scatter Factor induce blood vessel formation in vivo. Proc. Natl. Acad. Sci. U.S.A. 90, 1937–1941.

Graziani, A., Gramaglia, D., dalla Zonca, P. and Comoglio, P.M. (1993) Hepatocyte growth factor/scatter factor stimulates the Ras-guanine nucleotide exchanger. J. Biol. Chem. 268, 9165–9168.

Graziani, A., Gramaglia, D., Cantley, L.C. and Comoglio, P.M. (1991) The tyrosine phosphorylated hepatocyte growth factor/scatter factor receptor associates with phosphatidylinositol 3-kinase. J. Biol. Chem. 266, 22087–22090.

Hanks, S.K., Quinn, A.M. and Hunter, T. (1988) The protein kinase family: conserved features and deduced phylogeny of the catalytic domains. Science 241, 42–52.

Hartmann, G., Naldini, L., Weidner, M., Sachs, M., Vigna, E., Comoglio, P. and Birchmeier, W. (1992). A functional domain in the heavy chain Of Scatter Factor/Hepatocyte Growth Factor binds the c-Met receptor and induces cell dissociation but not mitogenesis. Proc. Natl. Acad. Sci.USA, 89, 11574–11578.

Hearing, V.J., Law, L.W., Corti, A., Appella, E. and Blasi, F. (1988). Modulation of metastatic potential by cell surface urokinase of murine melanoma cells. Cancer Res. 48, 1270–1278.

Heldin, C.H., Ernlund, A., Rorsman, C. and Ronnstrand,L. (1989). Dimerazation of B-typr platelet-derived Growth Factor Receptors is closely associated with receptor kinase activation. J.Biol.Chem., 264, 8905–8912.

Higuchi O. and Nakamura T. (1991). Identification and change in the receptor for hepatocyte growth factor in rat liver after partial hepatectomy or induced hepatitis. Biochem. Biophys. Res. Commun. 176, 599–607.

Huff, J.I., Jelinek, A.M., Borgman, C.A., Lansing, T.J. and Parsons, J.T. (1993) The protooncogene c-sea encodes a transmembrane protein-tyrosine kinase related to the Met/hepatocyte growth factor/scatter factor receptor. Proc. Natl. Acad. Sci. USA 90, 6140–6144.

Kennelly, P.J. and Krebs, E.G. (1991) Consensus sequences as substrate specificity determinants for protein kinases and protein phosphatases. J. Biol. Chem. 266, 15555–15558.

Khazaie, K., Dull, T.J., Graf, T., Schlessinger, J., Ullrich, A., Beug, H. and Vennstrom, B. (1988).Truncation of the human EGF receptor leads to differential transforming potentials in primary avian fibroblasts and erythroblasts. EMBO J., 7, 3061–3071.

Kim, H.K., Kim, J.W., Zilberstein, A., Margolis, B., Kim, J.G., Schlessinger, J. and Rhee, S.G. (1991) PDGF stimulation of inositol phospholipid hydrolysis requires PLC 1 phosphorylation on tyrosine residues 783 and 1254. Cell, 65, 435–441.

Kirchheimer, J.C., Wojta, J., Christ, G., and Binder, B.R. (1989). Functional inhibition of endogenously prodeced urokinase decreases cell proliferation in a human melanoma cell line. Proc. Natl. Acad. Sci. USA 86, 5424–5428.

Kirchheimer, J.C., Wojta, J., Christ, G., and Binder, B.R. (1987). Proliferation of a human epidermal tumor cell line stimulated by urokinase. FASEB J. 1, 125–128.

Kirchhmeier J.C. and Remold H.G. (1989). Functional characteristic of receptor-bound urokinase on human monocytes: catalytic efficiency and susceptibility to inactivation by plasminogen activator inhibitors. Blood 74, 1396–1402.

Kobayashi, T., Honke, K., Miyazaki, T., Matsumoto, K., Nakamura, T., Ishizuka, I. and Makita, A. (1994). Hepatocyte growth factor specifically binds to sulfoglycolipids. J. Biol. Chem. 269, 9817–21.

Koch, C.A., Anderson, D., Moran, M.F., Ellis, C. and Pawson, T., (1991) SH2 and SH3 domains: elements that control interactions of cytoplasmic signaling proteins. Science, 252, 668–674.

Liu, C., Park, M., and Tsao, M.-S. (1992). Overexpression of c-*met* proto-oncogene but not epidermal growth factor receptor or c-*erb*B-2 in primary colorectal carcinomas. Oncogene, 7, 181–185.

Lokker, N.A., Mark, M.R., Luis, E.A., Bannet, G.L., Robbins, K.A., Baker, J.B. and Godowski, P.J. (1992). Structure function analysis of hepatocyte growth factor: identification of variants that lack mitogenic activity yet retain high affinity receptor binding. EMBO J. 11, 2503–2510.

Longati, P., Bardelli, A., Ponzetto, C., Naldini, L. and Comoglio, P.M. (1994). Tyrosines 1234–1235 are critical for activation of the tyrosine kinase encoded by the MET protooncogene (HGF receptor). Oncogene 9, 49–57.

Mark, M.R., Lokker N.A., Zioncheck T.F., Luis, E.A. and Godowski P.J. (1993). Expression and Characterization of Hepatocyte Growth Factor Receptor-IgG Fusion Proteins. J Biol Chem, 267, 26166–26171.

Meissauer, A., Kramer, M.D., Hofmann, M., Erkell, L.J., Jacob, E., Schirrmacher, V. and Brunner, G. (1992). Generation of cell surface-bound plasmin by cell-associated urokinase-type or secreted tissue-type plasminogen activator: a key event in melanoma cell invasiveness in vitro. Exp. Cell. Res. 199, 179–90.

Michalopoulos, G., Houck, K.A., Dolan, M.L., and Luetteke, N.C. (1984). Control of hepatopoietic replication by two serum factors. Cancer Res. 44, 4414–4419.

Mitchell, P.J. and Cooper, C. (1992b). The human *tpr* gene encodes a protein of 2094 amino acids that has extensive coiled-coil regions and an acisic C-terminal domain. Oncogene, 7, 2329–2333.

Mitchell, P.J. and Cooper, C. (1992a). Nucleotide sequence analysis of human *tpr* cDNA clones. Oncogene, 7, 383–388.

Miyazawa, K., Tsubouchi, H., Naka, D., Takahashi, K., Okigaki, M., Arakaki, N., Nakayama, H., Hirono, S., Sakiyama, O., Takahashi, K., Gohda, E., Daikuhara, Y., and Kitamura, N. (1989). Molecular cloning and sequence analysis of cDNA for human Hepatocyte Growth Factor. Biochem. Biophys. Res. Commun. 163, 967–973.

Miyazawa, K., Shimomura, T., Kitamura, A., Kondo, J., Morimoto, Y., Kitamura, N. (1993). Molecular cloning and sequence analysis of the cDNA for a human serine protease responsabile for activation of hepatocyte growth factor. J. Biol. Chem. 268, 10024–10028.

Mizuno K., Takehara T., Nakamura T. (1992). Proteolytic activation of a single-chain precursor of hepatocyte growth factor by extracellular serine-protease. Biochem. Biophys. Res. Comm. 189, 1631–1638.

Mondino, A., Giordano, S. and Comoglio, P.M. (1991). Defective post-translational processing activates the tyrosine kinase encoded by the *met* proto-oncogene (Hepatocyte Growth Factor Receptor). Mol. Cell. Biol., 11, 6084–6092.

Montesano, R., Matsumoto, K., Nakamura, T. and Orci, L. (1991) Identification of a fibroblast-derived epithelial morphogen as hepatocyte growth factor. Cell 67, 901–908.

Morimoto, A., Okamura, K., Hamanaka, R., Yasufumi, S., Shima, N., Higashio, K. and Kuwano, M. (1991). Hepatocyte growth factor modulates migration and proliferation of human microvascular endothelial cells in culture. Bioch. Bioph. Res. Comm. 179, 1042–1049.

Nagaike M., Hirao S., Tajima H., Noji S., Taniguchi S. Matsumoto K., Nakamura T. (1991). Renotropic functions of hepatocyte growth factor in renal regeneration after unilateral nephrectomy. J. Biol. Chem. 266, 22781–22784.

Naka D., Ishii T., Yoshiyama Y., Miyazawa K., Hara H., Hishida T., Kitamura N. (1992). Activation of hepatocyte growth factor by proteolytic conversion of a single chain form to a heterodimer. J. Biol. Chem. 267, 20114–20119-

Nakamura, T., Nishizawa, T., Hagiya, M., Seki, T., Shimonishi, M., Sugimura, A., Tashiro, K. and Shimizu, S. (1989) Molecular cloning and expression of human Hepatocyte Growth Factor. Nature 342, 440–443.

Nakamura, T., Nawa, K., Ichihara, A. (1984). Partial purification and characterization of hepatocyte growth factor from serum of hepatectomized rats. Biochem. Biophys. Res. Commun. 122, 1450–1459.

Nakamura, T., Nawa, K., Ichihara, A, Kaise A., Nishino, T. (1987). Purification and subunit structure of hepatocyte growth factor from rat platelets. FEBS Lett. 224, 311–318.

Naldini, L., Tamagnone, L., Vigna, E., Sachs, M., Hartmann, G., Birchmeier, W., Daikuhara, Y., Tsubouchi, H., Blasi, F. and Comoglio, P.M. (1992) Extracellular proteolytic cleavage by urokinase is required for activation of hepatocyte growth factor/scatter factor. EMBO J. 11, 4825–4833.

Naldini, L., Vigna, E., Bardelli, A., Follenzi, A., Galimi, F. and Comoglio, P.M. (1995). Biological activation of pro-HGF (Hepatocyte Growth Factor) by urokinase is controlled in vivo by a stoichiometric reaction. J. Biol. Chem. 70, 603–611.

Naldini, L., Weidner, K.M., Vigna, E., Gaudino, G., Bardelli, A., Ponzetto, C., Narsimhan, R.P., Hartmann, G., Zarnegar, R., Michalopoulos, G.K., Birchmeier, W. and Comoglio, P.M. (1991c) Scatter factor and hepatocyte growth factor are indistinguishable ligands for the *Met* receptor. EMBO J. 10, 2867–2878.

Naldini, L., Vigna, E., Ferracini, R., Longati, P., Gandino, L., Prat, M. and Comoglio, P.M. (1991a) The tyrosine kinase encoded by the MET proto-oncogene is activated by autophosphorylation. Mol. Cell. Biol. 11, 1793–1803.

Naldini, L., Vigna, E., Narshiman, R.P., Gaudino, G., Zarnegar, R., Michalopoulos, G. and Comoglio, P.M. (1991b) Hepatocyte Growth Factor (HGF) stimulates the tyrosine kinase activity of the receptor encoded by the proto-oncogene c-MET. Oncogene 6, 501–504.

Nishizuka, Y. (1988). The molecular heterogeneity of protein kinase C and its implications for cellular regulation. Nature, 334, 661–665.

Ossowski, L. (1988a). In vivo invasion of modified chorioallantoic membrane by tumor cells: the role of cell surface-bound urokinase. J. Cell. Biol. 107, 2437–2445.

Ossowski, L. and Reich, E. (1983). Antibodies to plasminogen activator inhibit human tumor metastasis. Cell 35, 611–619.

Ossowski, L. (1988b). Plasminogen activator dependent pathways in the dissemination of human tumor cells in the chick embryo. Cell 52, 321–328.

Park. M., Dean, M., Kaul, K., Braun, M.J., Gonda, M.A., and Vande Woude G.(1987). Sequence of *MET* protooncogene cDNA has features characteristic of the tyrosine kinase family of growth-factor receptor. Proc. Natl. Acad. Sci. USA, 84, 6379–6383.

Park.M., Dean.M., Cooper C.S., Scmidt M., O'Brien S.J., Blair D.G., and Vande Woude G.F. (1986). Mechanism of *met* oncogene activation. Cell 45, 895–904.

Patthy, L., Trexler, M., Vali, Z., Banyai, L. and Varadi, A. (1984). Kringles: modules specialized for protein binding. Homology of the gelatin-binding region of fibronectin with the kringle structures of proteases. FEBS letters 171, 131–136.

Pawson, T. and Schlessinger, J. (1993) SH2 and SH3 domains. Current Biology 3, 434–442.

Pawson, T. (1995). Protein modules and Signalling networks. Nature, 373, 573–576.

Pelech, S.L. and Sanghera, J.S. (1992). MAP kinases: charting the regulatory pathways. Science 257, 1355–1356.

Pepper M.S. Matsumoto K., Nakamura T., Orci L., Montesano R. (1992). Hepatocyte growth factor increases urokinase-type plasminogen activator (uPA) and uPA receptor expression in Madin-Darby canine kidney epithelial cells. J. Biol. Chem. 267, 20493–20496.

Ponzetto, C., Giordano, S., Peverali, F., Della Valle, G., Abate, M., Vaula, G., and Comoglio, P.M. (1991). c-*MET* is amplified but not mutated in a cell line with an activated *met* tyrosine kinase Oncogene 6, 553–559.

Ponzetto, C., Bardelli, A., Maina, F., Longati, P., Panayotou, G., Dhand, R., Waterfield, M.D. and Comoglio, P.M. (1993) A novel recognition motif for phosphatidylinositol 3-kinase binding mediates its association with the hepatocyte growth factor/scatter factor receptor. Mol. Cell. Biol. 13, 4600–4608.

Ponzetto, C., Bardelli, A., Zhen, Z., Maina, F., dalla Zonca, P., Giordano, S., Graziani, A., Panayotou, G. and Comoglio, P.M. (1994) A multifunctional docking site mediates signalling and transformation by the hepatocyte growth factor/scatter factor receptor family. Cell 77, 261–271.

Prat, M.P., Narsimhan, R.P., Crepaldi, T., Nicotra, M.R., Natali, P.G., and Comoglio, P.M. (1991a.) The receptor encoded by the human *c-MET* Oncogene is expressed in hepatocytes, in epithelial cells and in solid tumors. Int. J. Cancer 49, 323–328.

Pyke, C., Kristensen, P., Kalfiaer, E., Grondahl-Hansen, J., Eriksen, J., Blasi, F. and Dano, K. (1991). Urokinase-type plasminogen activator is expressed in stromal cells and its receptor in cancer cells at invasive foci in human colon adenocarcinomas. Am. J. Pathol. 138, 1059–1067.

Qiu, F., Ray, P., Brown, K., Barker, E., Jhanwar, S., Ruddle, F.H., Besmer, P. (1988).Primary structure of *c-kit*: relationship with the CSF-1/PDGF receptor kinases family-oncogenic activation of *v-kit* involves deletion of extracellular domain and C terminus. EMBO. J., 7, 1003–1011.

Rodrigues, G.A. and Park, M. (1993). Dimerization mediated through a leucine zipper activates the oncogenic potential of the met receptor tyrosine kinase. Mol. Cell. Biol., 13, 6711–6722.

Rong S., Segal S., Anver M., Resau J.H., Vande Woude G.F. (1994). Invasiveness and Metastasis of NIH 3T3 cells induced by Met-Hepatocyte Growth Factor/Scatter Factor Autocrine Stimulation. Proc Natl. Acad. Sci. 91, 4731–4745.

Rong, S., Bodescot, M., Blair, D., Dunn, J., Nakamura, T., Mizuno, K., Park, M., Chan, A., Aaronson, S., Vande Woude, G.F. (1992). Tumorigenicity of the met proto-oncogene and the gene for hepatocyte growth factor. Mol. Cell. Biol., 12 (11), 5152–5158.

Ronsin, C., Muscatelli, F., Mattei, M.G. and Breathnach, R. (1993) A novel putative receptor protein tyrosine kinase of the met family. Oncogene 8, 1195–1202.

Saksela, O. and Rifkin, D.B. (1988). Cell-associated plasminogen activation: regulation and physiological functions. Ann. Rev. Cell. Biol. 4, 93–126.

Schmidt, C., Bladt, F., Goedecke, S., Brinkmann, S., Zschiesche, W., Sharpe, M., Gherardi, E., and Birchmeier, C. (1995). Scatter factor/Hepatocyte Growth Factor is essential for liver development. Nature, 373, 699–701.

Seifert, R.A., Hart, C. E., Philips, P.E. (1989). Two different subunits associate to create isoform-specific platelet-derived Growth Factor. J. Biol. Chem., 264, 8771–8778.

Shoelson, S.E., White, M.F., Kahn, C.R. (1988). Tryptic activation of the insulin receptor. J. Biol. Chem., 10, 4852–4860.

Skeel, A., Yoshimura, T., Showalter, S.D., Tanaka, A., Appella, E. and Leonard,E.J. (1991). Macrophage stimulating protein: purification, partial amino acid sequence, and cellular activity. J. Exp. Med. 173, 1227–1234.

Snyder, M.A., Bishop, J.M., McGrath, J.P., Levinson. (1985).A mutation at the ATP-binding site of pp60^{v-src} abolishes kinase activity, transformation and tumorigenicity. Mol. Cell. Biol., 5, 1772–1779.

Songyang, Z., Shoelson, S.E., Chaudhuri, M., Gish, G., Pawson, T., Haser, W.G., King, F., Roberts, T., Ratnofsky, S., Lechleider, R.J., Neel, B.G., Birge, R.B., Fajardo, J.E., Chou, M.M., Hanafusa, H., Schaffhausen, B. and Cantley, L.C. (1993) SH2 domains recognize specific phosphopeptide sequences. Cell 72, 1–20.

Sonnenberg, E., Meyer, D., Weidner, K.M. and Birchmeier, C. (1993a) Scatter factor/hepatocyte growth factor and its receptor, the c-*met* tyrosine kinase, can mediate a signal exchange between mesenchyme and epithelia during mouse development. J. Cell Biol. 123, 223–235.

Stoker, M., Gherardi, E., Perryman, M., and Gray, J. (1987). Scatter Factor is a fibroblast-derived modulator of epithelial cell mobility. Nature 327, 239–242.

Tempest P.R., Reeves, B.R., Spurr, N.K., Rance, A.J., Chan, M-L. and Brooks, P. (1986). Activation of the *met* oncogene in the human mnng-hos cell line involves a chromosomal rearrangement. Carcinogenesis, 7, 2051–2057.

Tornqvist, H.E. and Avruch, J. (1988) Relationship of site-specific β subunit tyrosine autophosphorylation to insulin activation of the insulin receptor (tyrosine) protein kinase activity. J. Biol. Chem. 263, 4593–4601.

Tornqvist, H.E., Pierce, M.W., Frackleton, A.R., Nemenoff, R.A. and Avruch, J. (1987). Identification of insulin receptor tyrosine residues autophosphorylated *in vitro*. J. Biol. Chem. 262: 10212–10219.

Villa-Moruzzi, E., Lapi, S., Prat, M., Gaudino, G. and Comoglio, P.M. (1993) A protein tyrosine phosphatase activity associated with the hepatocyte growth factor/scatter factor receptor. J. Biol. Chem. 268, 18176–18180.

Wang, M.H., Ronsin, C., Gesnel, M.C., Coupey, L., Skeel, A., Leonard, E.J., Breathnach, R. (1994). Identification of the ron gene product as the receptor for the human macrophage stimulating protein. Science 266, 117–119.

Weidner, K.M., Behrens, J., Vandekerckove, J. and Birchmeier, W. (1990). Scatter Factor: molecular charac-
teristics and effect on the invasiveness of epithelial cells. J. Cell Biol. 111, 2097–2108.
Weidner, K.M., Arakaki, N., Vandekerchove, J., Weingart, S., Hartmann, G., Rieder, H., Fonatsch, C., Tsubouchi,
H., Hishida, T., Daikuhara, Y. and Birchmeier, W. (1991) Evidence for the identity of human Scatter Factor
and Hepatocyte Growth Factor. Proc. Natl. Acad. Sci. USA 88, 7001–7005.
Zarnegar, R. and Michalopoulos, G. (1989). Purification and biological characterization of human hepatopoietin
A, a polypeptide growth factor for hepatocytes. Cancer Res. 49, 3314–3320.
Zarnegar, R. and Michalopoulos, G.K. (1995). The many faces of Hepatocyte Growth Factor:from hepatopoiesis
to hematopoiesis. J. Cell Biol. 129, 1177–1180.
Zhen, Z., Giordano, S., Longati, P., Medico, E., Campiglio, M., Comoglio, P.M.(1994) Structural and functional
domains critical for constitutive activation of the HGF receptor (*Met*). Oncogene 9, 1691–1697.

DISCUSSION

M. Oren: I have two questions: One; your data would suggest that any tyrosine kinase receptor which provides a good anchor for PI3 kinase would, in fact, be a scatter factor. Is
that the case and it has just been overlooked by people working with other receptors, or do
you need something else in the met receptor, in addition, to make a good scatter response?

P. Comoglio: Good question. Scattering, for some reason that we do not understand, is a
sort of unique for the receptor of the HGF family. So for MET and for RON there is a little bit of scattering made by either the PDGF receptor AA or BB, one of the two, alpha or
beta, but it is more a chemotactical response than a scattering response. Let me point out
that scattering is not only movement, scattering is activation of a genetic program that includes production of proteolytic enzymes that destroy the extra cellular matter. The PDGF
receptor alpha or beta (I forgot) is more chemotactic than scattering.

M. Oren: The other question is concerning angiogenesis. Did you test the types of MET
receptor, whether angiogenesis also requires both pathways or only one; and related to
that, how tight is the correlation between angiogenesis induced by this oncogene and its
metastatic capacity?

P. Comoglio: First of all let me make this clear; MET is not HGF. HGF is the ligand and
is angiogenic and MET is the receptor. So MET has nothing to do, HGF does. I can answer using an indirect experiment. We have done and published an experiment where we
chopped HGF which is an enormous molecule and made it smaller, smaller and smaller.
So, as I told you, if we remove the beta chain, the protease-like chain, cells scatter but do
not grow. And the same if we remove the two kringles and the same is that if we save the
hairpin loop and the first kringle. So we have a minimal segment which contains the first
loop, the first kringle domain of the N-terminal portion of the alpha chain which induces
scattering but not mitogenesis. Bussolino in the lab has tried to see if this is angiogenic
and the answer is no. Actually, it is an inhibitor of angiogenesis.

D. Livingston: Is the p13 kinase the real ligand which contributes to scattering?

P. Comoglio: This is a good point. For the sake of simplicity, I would say PI3 kinase is
Rho upstream. So what we know is the Rho pathway. And evidence from Alan Hall,
Courtneidge and others, tends to put PI3 kinase upstream Rho. The only clear piece of evidence I can provide to you besides the trick that we really induce the scattering pathway
making an artificial super-PI3 kinase binding site, so receptor only will bind and activate

PI3 kinase, are the experiments with the inhibitors wortmannin and in the presence of wortmannin we fully abolish the scattering.

D. Livingston: Again, that is not absolutely specific.

P. Comoglio: Absolutely not.

T. Graf: I have a somewhat related question: You are saying that the two mutated MET receptors, which display selective binding specificity for cytoplasmic ligands, by themselves do not cause tumors. Have you tried to put the two mutated receptors separately into the same cell to see whether they synergize for oncogenesis in trans?

P. Comoglio: No, not yet. But I bet it would not work because this is what happened with another receptor. One receptor can activate RAS and the other neighbor receptor can activate the PI3 kinase. So there is something magic that we do not understand in this supersite. But this is definitely an experiment that we are doing right now.

S. Courtneidge: Have you got any evidence for hetero-dimerization between say MET and RON or SEA to explain those differences that you see between scattering and mitogenesis with the different forms of the growth factor?

P. Comoglio: This is something that Gianni Gaudino is doing. So far, we have not seen anything really shocking. But we cannot exclude - on the other side - the only piece of evidence that I can report is that RON and MET synergize. If you add sub-optimal concentration of MSP which is a ligand for RON and suboptimal concentration of HGF which is a ligand for met you get a terrific response. Whether or not this has any meaning in terms of hetero-dimerization I do not know.

S. Courtneidge: The other question relates to your observation about over-expression of MET in tumors. Do you have any idea whether that is always going to be an autocrine loop or a receptor activation or is this going to be an interaction between the epithelial cells that express the receptor to a high level and mesenchymal cells that make the growth factor?

P. Comoglio: MET can be activated in a number of ways. Let us start with the most complicated - the most complicated one is lack of cleavage between alpha and beta chain. We have found very few tumors where there is a mutation in KRK site which is specific consensus for furin. And furin is required to separate the alpha chain from the beta chain. And we have shown and published - this is old stuff - that the uncleaved alpha-beta receptor goes to the membrane and this is constitutively activated. This is a fancy one or two possibilities: three patients out of several hundred we have examined. Second there are autocrine-loops; there are reports that it can make an artificial autocrine-loop in fibroblast and obtain transformation. I do not really understand the mechanism of this because HGF is in the serum and Riccardo Ferracini has published very recently that this indeed may happen in cells that express normally HGF but normally do not express the MET receptor. And this happens to be in human osterosarcomas. And although the statistics were very limited (only twenty or thirty cases) in more than half of the osteosarcomas that normally express HGF, because HGF is very important in bone formation, by mistake, they expressed MET, so there is an autocrine-loop whether or not it is functional, I do not know, but it is there. But the point I wanted to stress, that MET is activated by over-expression because if you immunoprecipitate MET you activate it. It is enough is to put in close contact two MET receptors and due to the autocatalytic mechanism they activate like -zap. In fact, we and others have found that you got over-expression of met in roughly half of the tumors of the GI tract.

S. Courtneidge: Have you tried the dominant negative approach to ask whether those tumors are growing because of that dimerization, can you interrupt that with a dominant negative?

P. Comoglio: Yes, I think that Enzo Medico has done this sort of classical experiment and in experimental system with a dominant negative lysine minus mutant dimerization was abolished.

E. Nigg: Following up on this over-expression business: It used to be a very important question whether mere over-expression of an oncogene was oncogenic, or whether you needed mutation. You certainly emphasized that, in the case of MET, over-expression is sufficient; yet on your slide which you showed to illustrate this point, you have, what looked to me, a truncation of the MET receptor in at least one of the tumors. How confident are you that over-expressing alone is the predominant way for activating MET in tumors?

P. Comoglio: It is because we are working like crazy since five years to find out that mutation and we never got one. So I have a strong feeling that over-expression alone is enough. We did all kinds of experiments. My slide might be misleading because since this is a rare event out of three to four hundred patients we got one patient with a recombination. So on top of that we cloned the MET promoter and we have found out that it is inducible. So, Gambarotta, in my lab, is looking whether he could put a finger on a sequence which may be genetically altered in these tumors, which is a sequence upstream of the promoter.

E. Nigg: Second question about RON: Is its chromosonal localization known? is it implicated in tumor formation and, if so, in what kind of tumors?

P. Comoglio: RON behaves quite differently from met. It may turn out that it is sort of a counterpart. The super-site which is slightly different not in terms of the two tyrosines but in terms of the neighbor amino acid and in our hands is not terrifically transforming *in-vitro,* and although we have started this work only a few months ago, we have not been able to get amplification. So, I have a strange feeling about RON. It may not be an oncogene.

G. Dranoff: First, I want to return to the angiogenesis issue; have you looked for MET expression in endothelial cells specifically?

P. Comoglio: Yes, of course.

G. Dranoff: What was the result?

P. Comoglio: It is absolutely expressed there. Endothelial cells do express MET.

G. Dranoff: So then, in your study of expression of MET in human tumors, have you looked to see whether the MET is on the endothelial cells or on the tumor cells?

P. Comoglio: Again, remember that MET is the receptor, it is not the factor. So endothelial cells do express the MET receptor constitutively. And tumor cells do. And do not forget that HGF is a growth factor that is sort of a circulating hormone and we are loaded. So it is not the rate limiting step either for angiogenesis or for transformation. We have studied and published that pro-HGF, a single chain inactive precursor, circulates and accumulates in extra-cellular matrix. So, in transformation, development, angiogenesis my prejudism is that the HGF gene is by-standing--it is always there. The factor is secreted in an inactive form. So, like TGF-beta or whatever, stromal cells produce a lot of inactive pro-HGF which is secreted and it binds to a low affinity receptor on the surface of cells. It is then activated by a specific enzyme which is urokinase. So what turn on probably angiogenesis or differentiation or other phenomena are many things.

G. Dranoff: My second issue related to the effects on macrophages of MSP. Could you tell us what those are and whether HGF also has those effects?

P. Comoglio: Yes, very similar. We have found that macrophages do express very, very little RON and very, very little MET in resting conditions. As I showed you, Carla Boccaccio has shown that MET is an inducible gene. So when the macrophages are activated by a number of things they do express a lot of MET, and although I have not done it, but I bet that they also express RON. Actually, a paper, not by our group, will soon show that also the MET promoter is inducible. So, when you take monocytes or resting macrophages, if they exist, they almost have no receptor and do not respond either to MSP or HGF. If you stimulated them with what you want, in the case of MET it is very easy to switch on the receptor and then the macrophages will move or scatter - of course, not grow - but move. In the case of RON, I can tell you only as a joke -- but it is a real thing -- that my complement does not activate the macrophages, not the complement of the people in the lab, except for the complement of Luigi Nardini - who is a guy in the lab. So we were able to repeat other people's experiments but using the complement of Luigi Nardini.

G. Dranoff: Do the macrophage activators you study also stimulate urokinase production?

P. Comoglio: Yes, we will publish this in JBC early this year.

T. Graf: Is it possible to transplant the super site into another tyrosine-kinase receptor and induce scattering properties in the receptor?

P. Comoglio: I do not know about scattering properties. This is what we are doing, we are swapping the super-site between MET and RON and with EGF and PDGF, see what happens and I can anticipate that something can be transplanted but something not. For example, prevention of apoptosis.

G. Gilliland: I would like to come back to the over-expression question again to make sure I understand the experiments. If you over-express a wild type MET receptor in the absence of ligand - that is a transforming event?

P. Comoglio: Yes.

G. Gilliland: It is a very interesting finding if that is the case because that certainly is different from any of the other receptors tyrosine kinases, where over-expression at very high levels does not lead to signal transduction or to transforming events. And I was curious whether you had any sense of what the number of receptors is that need to be expressed for that phenomenon and, secondly, whether you think there might be a transmembrane interaction motif between this receptor that is different from other receptors tyrosine kinases?

P. Comoglio: I went a little bit too quickly in my presentation. MET has something that other tyrosine kinase receptors have not. And this is a doublet of tyrosines that are right in the middle of the catalytic site. And a few years ago we have shown that these tyrosines up-regulate the activity of one hundred fold upon phosphorylation. The only other receptor that has the two tyrosines is the insulin receptor which is non-transforming so probably it will be activated by over-expression as well, but that is a problem in transformation because of the downstream signal transduction cascade. Now what happens, when we over-express artificially or when we observe that a natural tumor is over-expressed naturally MET is that the number of receptors into the membrane is enough to make spontaneous cluster that induces transphosphorylation. And this is unique to this family of receptors. And, for example, C is another tyrosine kinase receptor that has the two activated. So we think that his is the mechanism because MET has two very dangerous features: one is the autocatalytic site and two, because it has the super site.

E. Mihich: You said that in the scattering there are two components - at least two components - the proteolytic one and the motion one. Are really these two components? Is it active motion per se or is it a motion by default following the proteolytic function? And if they are two components, is it possible to dissociate them mechanistically?

P. Comoglio: That is definitely dissociated. And mitogenic - we have observed mitogenic without proteolytic and we have not observed, of course, proteolytic without mitogenesis because this would not work into the test. But they are definitely two different mechanisms: and there are cells that only respond with the mitogenesis and others that only respond with proteolytic function. We set up a diving test in a Transwell chamber with a Millipore filter and then there is a basal membrane; and if you put the basal membrane you measure both mitogenic and the proteolytic functions. And if you do not put the basal membrane you only measure the mitogenic function and can be disassociation in different cell lines.

E. Mihich: But in the same cell line, are they dissociable molecularly in terms of the signal pathways?

P. Comoglio: Yes, I think that we published a paper together with Alan Hall, where every one of these steps has been studied and we have shown that the so-called scattering process is first, that the cells flatten, then that the cells move, then the cell disassociates, then the cells move. And Alan used, actually it was Ann Ridley, micro-injected cells with different inhibitors like antibodies against ras, antibodies against Rho and against rac and then cycloheximide. And, for example, if you add some cycloheximide you have the mitogen pathway without matrix invasion. So the proteolytic enzyme need to be synthesized.

M. Oren: If you compared the downstream signaling that you get by activation of the VEGF receptor by VEGF and then downstream signaling of the activated MET receptor by HGF, can you draw any parallels that would identify what is angiogenic?

P. Comoglio: I am simply ignorant about VEGF; I apologize. I have no answer to that question.

D. Livingston: What is known about the potential role of MET and/or the ligand in the development of ductal structures, for example, in the mouse?

P. Comoglio: A lot. I can tell you the results of the trangenesis experiments. We have been scooped by our collaborators and friends - Carmen Birchmeyer - and she succeeded in knocking out the HGF before we succeeded in knocking out the receptor. But the two phenotypes are identical, and either by knocking out completely the ligand or the receptor there is a very interesting phenotypes. Mice have problems with the placenta, but if they can overcome the problems with the placenta they develop at day 15.5 and they have a liver. In the absence of either HGF or the receptor at day 16 they have no more liver. So the liver is gone by apoptosis. So this is something interesting to what we had discussed this morning. Since we do not like to be scooped we decided to do something more sophisticated and Carola Ponzetto succeeded in making a knockout mouse. So what she has done in the lab is to change the famous N in third position with an H. So we make knockout mice that now have perfectly normal HGF receptor which is phosphorylated that activates all the downstream pathways but one: the Grb-2 pathway. And the mouse is living, it burns up and that is what is the phenotype. As muscular dystrophy, no muscle in the shoulder, no muscle in the neck, no muscle in the tongue. So what in the hell is happening? But apparently there is a window of differentiation where not only HGF is required in muscles, but the Grb-2 pathway is required in muscles because you do not observe it unless you really knock-out this third residue substitution.

D. Livingston: But in the complete knock-out animals, are there some normally developed ductal structures?

P. Comoglio: Everything develops normally. At day 16, everything disappears. Do not forget that as I showed you here the apoptotic progenitors also express RON. And RON is able to induce differentiation of the liver. So it probably differentiates normally through RON, but then at a certain point RON is not able to prevent apoptosis.

3

SRC FAMILY KINASES AND THE CELL CYCLE

Sara A. Courtneidge

SUGEN, Inc.,
515 Galveston Drive, Redwood City,California 94063
Telephone: 415 306 7700; Telefax: 415 306 7613.

INTRODUCTION

The Src family of protein tyrosine kinases consists of at least nine enzymes in birds and mammals. Src family kinases share a high degree of structural similarity, including domain architecture and regulation. Topographically (from amino to carboxy terminus) they have: amino terminal acylation sites (responsible for membrane anchoring); a unique domain (40–80 amino acids that distinguish each member of the family); a Src Homology (SH) 3 domain; an SH2 domain; the catalytic domain; and carboxy terminal regulatory sequences ("the tail") All members of the family are negatively regulated by the phosphorylation of a tyrosine residue in the tail. This phosphorylation is carried out by an enzyme called Csk. The importance of the tail is demonstrated by two observations: firstly, in the many cases tested, mutation of the tail such that it can no longer be phosphorylated is sufficient to convert proto-oncogene to oncogene; secondly, mice lacking Csk have constitutively active Src family kinases and die during embryogenesis (reviewed in [1,2,3]).

A number of studies have contributed to our understanding of how phosphorylation of the tail regulates Src family kinases (reviewed in [4]). Our current view is that the phosphorylated tyrosine in the tail interacts intramolecularly with the SH2 domain. This interaction is stabilized by a second intramolecular interaction between the SH3 domain and an unidentified region in the protein. Both of these intramolecular contacts must form for stable repression of kinase activity. Since it is the ligand binding surfaces of the SH2[4] and SH3[5] domains that are involved in the intramolecular interactions, this model predicts that in the repressed state, neither SH2 nor SH3 are available to bind to other proteins. The model further predicts that there are a number of ways in which Src family kinases may become activated. The most obvious is by dephosphorylation of the tail, which would release both the SH2 and the SH3 domain to interact with other proteins, as well as increase catalytic activity. But were high affinity ligands for either the SH2 or the SH3 domain to become available in the cell, these would have the potential to compete for the intramolecular interactions, and activate the enzyme without dephosphorylation of the tail. Subsequent dephosphorylation, however, could stabilize the activated form of the enzyme.

Cancer Genes, edited by Mihich and Housman
Plenum Press, New York, 1996

Activation by competition for the SH2 domain is probably how some members of the Src family are activated by the PDGF and CSF-1 receptors (see below).

In recent years, much attention has been focused on the activity of Src family kinases in normal cells. Many members of the Src family are highly restricted in their tissue expression, often to haematopoietic cells. By physical association, they confer kinase activity to a number of receptors that themselves lack kinase activity, for example cytokine receptors, the co-stimulatory molecules CD4 and CD8, the T cell receptor etc. Many experiments, including those using cell lines deficient in members of the Src family, as well as gene knockout techniques, have demonstrated the functional importance of some of these interactions (reviewed in [6, 7]).

For the last several years work in my own laboratory has concentrated on those three members of the Src family (Src, Fyn and Yes) that are more ubiquitously expressed. These three kinases are activated by a number of stimuli in fibroblasts grown in tissue culture [8]. For example, growth factors whose receptors are themselves tyrosine kinases also activate members of the Src family. The best studied example of this is the response of quiescent fibroblasts to PDGF, which will be discussed in much more detail later. In addition to the receptor tyrosine kinases, receptors that are coupled to G proteins, for example those for thrombin and lysophosphatidic acid (LPA) also activate members of the Src family, although in this case the mechanism of activation is not known. It is not only the stimulation of quiescent fibroblasts with growth factors that elicits changes in Src family kinases; both UV irradiation and the passage of cell from G2 into mitosis also increase their activity[8]. The mechanism of activation in each case is unclear.

As mentioned above, all members of the Src family can be classified as proto-oncogenes. This, together with the observation that many members of the Src family were first identified in mutated form as the transforming agents of retroviruses, demonstrates that they are capable of malignantly transforming cells [1]. But to date evidence for their involvement in human malignancy is limited. Overexpression of Lck as a result of chromosome rearrangement has been noted in leukaemia[9], and overexpression/hyperactivity of Src has been reported in both breast and colon cancer[10, 11, 12]. Whether the Src family kinases are critical for the disease state has not yet been addressed. But the fact that Src family kinases are hyperexpressed, along with the demonstration that Src family kinases are often required for growth of cells in culture (see below) suggests that they may be relevant therapeutic targets in some cancers.

RESULTS AND DISCUSSION

Src Family Kinases and the Response to Growth Factors

In recent years we have been using mouse fibroblasts as a model system to study the involvement of the Src family kinases, Src, Yes and Fyn, in signal transduction processes in normal cells. We first studied the activation of Src, Fyn and Yes by stimulation of quiescent cells with PDGF[13, 14, 15]. We could show that activation is accompanied by association with the activated receptor[15]; association requires the SH2 domains of the Src family kinases[16], and tyrosines 579 and 581 in the juxtamembrane domain of the receptor[17] (which represents a high affinity binding site for the SH2 domains of Src family kinases). As mentioned previously, association with the receptor is probably sufficient to cause activation of the Src family kinases.

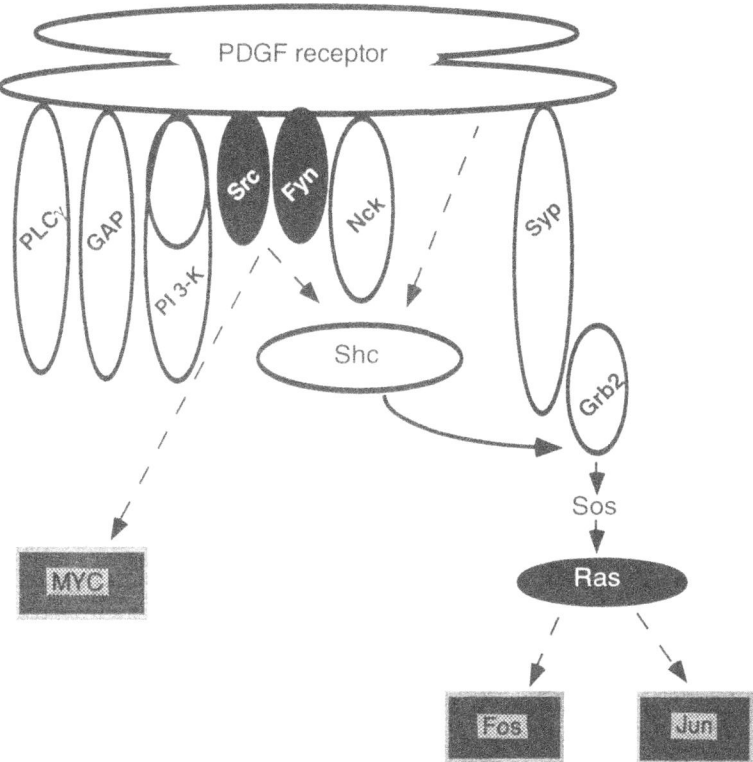

Figure 1. A schematic representation of signaling through the PDGF receptor. An activated PDGF receptor, and some of the signalling molecules shown to associate with it, are depicted. Also shown are the immediate gene products Myc, Fos and Jun. The arrows represent pathways believed to result in the production of these transcription factors.

It is known that the activated PDGF receptor interacts with a large number of SH2 domain-containing proteins, including phospholipase Cγ, rasGAP, the phosphatidylinositol 3-K, the tyrosine phosphatase Syp, members of the Src family, as well as "adaptors" (proteins that have SH2 and/or SH3 domains but lack catalytic activity) such as GRB2 and Nck (reviewed in [18, 19, 20]). With this complicated array of proteins, it was important to ask which of these associations were required for the receptor to function (defining function in this case as the ability of PDGF to promote S phase entry in quiescent fibroblasts). We used a microinjection approach, in which quiescent cells were microinjected with antibodies that inhibit all three members of the Src family expressed in either these cells (anti-cst.1), or with "dominant negative" constructs of Src or Fyn (that lack catalytic activity but retain the ability to bind to the receptors, and therefore when highly expressed prevent the endogenous Src family kinases from interacting with and being activated by the PDGF receptor). After microinjection, the cells were stimulated with PDGF, and 18–24 hours later an assessment was made as to whether the cells had entered S phase. We found that both the inhibitory antibodies and the dominant negative constructs significantly inhibited the response of the cells to PDGF, suggesting that they were indeed required for full functioning of the receptor[21]. Furthermore, the use of chimeric proteins containing individual domains of Src linked to a portion of ß-galactosidase demonstrated that inhibition could

Table 1. Signaling requirements for various growth factors

Signaling molecule required?[a]	Growth factor				
	PDGF	EGF	CSF-1	Bombesin	LPA
Ras	yes	yes	yes	yes	yes
Src family	yes	yes	yes	no	no
PI 3-Kα	yes	yes	no	no	no

[a]In each case, following microinjection of neutralizing antibodies and/or dominant negative constructs, cells were stimulated with the appropriate growth factor. 18–24 hours later bromodeoxyuridine incorporation was used to monitor entry into S phase. "yes" means that >75% of cells were inhibited by neutralizing antibody and/or dominant negative "no" means <10% inhibition.

be achieved by overexpressing just the SH2 domain, whereas overexpression of just the SH3 domain had no effect.

More recently, we used the same microinjection approach to study other growth factors able to elicit DNA synthesis in fibroblasts. These included epidermal growth factor (EGF) and colony stimulating factor-1 (CSF-1 - in cells engineered to express the receptor), whose receptors are both tyrosine kinases, as well as bombesin and lysophosphatidic acid (LPA) whose receptors are G protein-coupled but nevertheless elicit a large increase in tyrosine phosphorylated proteins. We found that both EGF and CSF-1 required Src family kinases for function, but neither LPA nor bombesin did[22] [Table 1]. We concluded that functional Src family kinases are important for several, but not all, growth factors to be able to elicit the induction of S phase.

It has been shown in several cases that the response to growth factors is complex. This is well illustrated by the case of the PDGF receptor. As mentioned above, the activated PDGF receptor associates with an array of signaling molecules. A variety of experiments from several laboratories has shown that many of these molecules are required for full functioning at the receptor (reviewed in [18, 19, 20]). One important feature of receptor activation is that it leads to activation of Ras, and subsequent activation of the MAP kinase pathway, which is required for DNA synthesis[23]. Ras, which is a membrane protein, becomes activated by an exchange protein called Sos. In quiescent cells, Sos is found in association with the adaptor protein GRB2, in the cytoplasm. The GRB2:Sos complex is recruited to the membrane to activate Ras in a number of ways after growth factor stimulation. For example, some activated receptors bind GRB2 directly, via its SH2 domain. In other cases, GRB2 is recruited to receptors via association with other proteins, for example the PDGF receptor-associated phosphatase Syp, and the adaptor protein Shc, which becomes heavily tyrosine phosphorylated and able to bind GRB2 after some growth factor stimuli (reviewed in [19]). In the case of the PDGF receptor, the activation of Ras could be initiated via indirect association of GRB2 with the receptor, and by tyrosine phosphorylated Shc (for review on Ras activation, see[24]).

Why are the Src family kinases also required for full functioning of the PDGF receptor? It is known that in Src transformed cells, Ras activation is initiated by the tyrosine phosphorylation of Shc by Src[25]. Nevertheless, the redundancy of Ras activation pathways after PDGF stimulation mentioned above seemed to preclude an absolute requirement for Src family kinases in Ras activation by growth factors. This was borne out by our observations that a dominant negative form of Src (SrcK-) did not interfere with the ability of PDGF to elicit the transcriptional activation of Fos (M. Vittoria Barone and Sara A. Courtneidge, submitted), which is a readout of the Ras pathway[26]. As expected, a dominant negative form of Ras (N17Ras) did block the production of Fos (M. Vittoria Barone

Table 2. Complementation of block to PDGF signaling by immediate early gene products

Block caused by	Rescued by?	
	Fos	Myc
Dominant negative Ras[a]	yes	no
Dominant negative Src[b]	no	yes

[a]N17Ras was microinjected together with plasmids encoding either Fos or Myc. After PDGF stimulation, bromodeoxyuridine incorporation was assessed. Rescued means that >80% of the cells entered S phase when compared to control non-injected cells.
[b]SrcK- was microinjected together with plasmids encoding either Fos or Myc. The data were assessed as above.

and Sara A. Courtneidge, submitted) [Table 2]. We therefore suspected that the Src family kinases initiated a signal transduction cascade separate from the Ras pathway.

Growth factor stimulation results in the transcriptional activation of many immediate early genes, several of which are transcription factors. Apart from Fos, mentioned above, the Myc protein is also produced early in G1 in response to growth factors, and may be required for commitment to S phase[27, 28, 29]. It had previously been shown that a mutant form of the CSF-1 receptor defective in signaling could be complemented by constitutive expression of Myc[30], and we had shown that one of the defects of this mutant receptor was a failure to fully activate Src family kinases[31]. We therefore tested whether the S phase block caused by SrcK- could be rescued by forced expression of Myc. We found that it could [Table 2]. In contrast, Myc could not rescue the block caused by N17Ras (M. Vittoria Barone and Sara A. Courtneidge, submitted). These data together support a model in which activation of Src family kinases by PDGF stimulation activates a signal transduction cascade that results in the transcriptional activation of *myc* in a Ras-independent fashion.

Src Family Kinases and the G2/M Transition

It was Shalloway's laboratory that first showed that Src becomes activated at the G2/M transition in mammalian fibroblasts[32]. Subsequent studies in our own laboratory showed that Fyn and Yes were also activated[33]. During mitosis, Src becomes phosphorylated on serine and threonine residues in the unique domain, probably by cdc2 kinase. The activation of Src does not occur as a direct consequence of these phosphorylations, but rather appears to occur via transient dephosphorylation of the regulatory tyrosine in the tail. The serine and threonine phosphorylations may serve to make Src more susceptible to a tyrosine phosphatase, or a less efficient substrate for Csk (reviewed in [34, 35]). The mechanism of activation of Fyn and Yes during mitosis is unknown.

The fact that Src family kinases are activated during mitosis, and that at least one mitosis-specific substrate of Src exists[36, 37], suggests that these enzymes may play important roles during mitosis. To address this, we again used the microinjection approach. We introduced the anti-cst.1 antibody, that binds to and inhibits Src, Fyn and Yes, into cells in G2, and then measured the ability of the microinjected cells to divide[33]. We determined that cell division was inhibited by approximately 75% in the presence of the cst.1 antibody, with most of the cells being arrested in G2. Control antibodies, as well as antibodies specific for the PI 3-K, had no such inhibitory effect. Interestingly, in NIH-3T3 cells, that contain Src, Fyn and Yes, an antibody that recognized only Src did not inhibit the entry

Table 3. The requirement for Src family kinases in G2 for entry into mitosis

	Cells arrested in G2?	
Protein microinjected	NIH 3T3	"Src fibroblasts"
Pre-immune-IgG	no	no
Anti-cst.1	yes	yes
Anti-cst.1 + peptide	no	no
Anti-PI 3-K	no	no
Anti-Src.1	no	yes
GST-Fyn SH3	no	no
GST-Fyn SH2	yes	yes
GST-p85 SH2	no	no

A defined number of cells in the G2 phase of the cell cycle were injected with the proteins shown.
10-12 hours later the microinjected cells were counted, and a determination made of whether they
were arrested in G2, or had divided.

into mitosis. This result could mean that it was in fact Fyn or Yes that was required, or that these three members of the Src family are redundant in this function. To address this, we made use of a cell line, derived from "knockout" mice, in which the only catalytically active member of the Src family present is Src itself[33]. In these cells, both the anti-cst.1 and the anti-Src antibody blocked cells in G2. We concluded therefore that Src, Fyn and Yes have redundant functions that are required in G2 for fibroblasts to enter mitosis.

To begin to address why Src family kinases might be required in G2, we also asked which domains were necessary for function[33]. We found that whereas high expression of the SH3 domain of Fyn had no effect, high expression of the SH2 domain of Fyn arrested cells in G2. SH2 domains from other proteins (phospholipase Cγ, PI 3-K and rasGAP) were without effect. We surmise that during G2, a protein (or proteins) that associates with the SH2 domains of Src family kinases is phosphorylated and then has an obligate function for entry into mitosis. Overexpression of an isolated SH2 domain acted to bind all this protein, so preventing its phosphorylation by endogenous, activated Src family kinases.

CONCLUSIONS

In the future, we will continue our work in the two areas I have described here today. Firstly, we will address how the activation of Src family kinases by PDGF results in the transcriptional activation of Myc. We have but a few clues at present. We have recently observed that high expression of a Src molecule that has catalytic activity, but lacks an SH3 domain, blocks the ability of PDGF to induce DNA synthesis (Thorsten Erpel, Gema Alonso and Sara A. Courtneidge, submitted). This suggests that, once bound to the PDGF receptor via their SH2 domains, Src family kinases recruit and phosphorylate critical signaling molecules via their SH3 domains. We are therefore in the process of examining tyrosine phosphorylated proteins that have the ability to associate with the SH3 domains of Src, Fyn and Yes shortly after PDGF stimulation.

Secondly, we do not yet understand why the Src family kinases are required during G2 for entry into mitosis. We have demonstrated that their SH2 domains are required for this function. Since the association of Src with the cytoskeleton has been shown to be mediated by its SH2 domain, one possibility is that Src family kinases are responsible for initiating the cytoskeletal rearrangements that must occur for a cell to be able to round up prior to dividing. We are beginning these studies by searching for G2 proteins that are both tyrosine phosphorylated and able to associate with the SH2 domains of the Src family kinases.

Finally, our laboratory has investigated in detail the function of the Src family of tyrosine kinases in normal cells. In the future, we will also explore whether they play pivotal roles in tumor cells. For example, it is known that some tumors have amplified and hyperactive receptor tyrosine kinases. We will determine whether this leads to an activation of Src family kinases, and whether this in turn is required to maintain the transformed phenotype. If this is the case, then the Src family of protein tyrosine kinases might represent good therapeutic targets in some tumor types.

REFERENCES

1. J.A. Cooper, The *src* family of protein-tyrosine kinases. *Peptides and Protein Phosphorylation*. 104–113. 1990.
2. J.A. Cooper and B. Howell, The when and how of Src regulation. *Cell*. 73: 1051–1054 (1993)
3. S.A. Courtneidge, Protein tyrosine kinases, with emphasis on the Src family. *Sem. in Cancer Biol.* 5: 239–246 (1994)
4. G. Superti-Furga and S.A. Courtneidge, Structure-function relationships in Src family and related protein tyrosine kinases. *Bioessays*. 17: 321–30 (1995)
5. T. Erpel, G. Superti-Furga and S.A. Courtneidge, Mutational analysis of the Src SH3 domain: the same residues of the ligand binding surface are important for intra- and intermolecular interactions. *EMBO J.* 14: 963–975 (1995)
6. C.E. Rudd, O. Janssen, K.V. Prasad, M. Raab, A. da Silva, J.C. Telfer and M. Yamamoto, *src*-related protein tyrosine kinases and their surface receptors. *Biochem. Biophys. Acta*. 1155: 239–266 (1993)
7. J.B. Bolen, R.B. Rowley, C. Spana and A.Y. Tsygankov, The src family of tyrosine protein kinases in hemopoietic signal transduction. *FASEB J.* 6: 3403–3409 (1992)
8. T. Erpel and S.A. Courtneidge, Src family protein tyrosine kinases and cellular signal transduction pathways.q. *Current Op. Cell Biol.* 7: 176–182 (1995)
9. D.D. Wright, B.M. Sefton and M.P. Kamps, Oncogenic activation of the Lck protein accompanies translocation of the LCK gene in the human HSB2 T-cell leukemia. *Mol. Cell. Biol.* 14: 2429–2437 (1994)
10. A.E. Ottenhoff-Kalff, G. Rijksen, E.A. van Beurden, A. Hennipman, A.A. Michels and G.E. Staal, Characterization of protein tyrosine kinases from human breast cancer: involvement of the c-*src* oncogene product. *Cancer Res.* 52: 4773–4778 (1992)
11. C.A. Cartwright, A.I. Meisler and W. Eckhart, Activation of the pp60^{c-src} protein kinase is an early event in colonic carcinogenesis. *Proc. Natl. Acad. Sci. USA*. 87: 558–562 (1990)
12. J. Park, A.L. Meisler and C.A. Cartwright, c-Yes tyrosine kinase activity in human colon carcinoma. *Oncogene*. 8: 2627–2635 (1993)
13. R. Ralston and J.M. Bishop, The product of the proto-oncogene c-*src* is modified during the cellular response to platelet-derived growth factor. *Proc. Natl. Acad. Sci. U.S.A.* 82: 7845–7849 (1985)
14. K. Gould and T. Hunter, Platelet-derived growth factor induces multisite phosphorylation of pp60^{c-src} and increases its protein-tyrosine kinase activity. *Mol. and Cell. Biol.* 8: 3345–3356 (1988)
15. R.M. Kypta, Y. Goldberg, E.T. Ulug and S.A. Courtneidge, Association between the PDGF receptor and members of the *src* family of tyrosine kinases. *Cell*. 62: 481–492 (1990)
16. G. Twamley, B. Hall, R. Kypta and S.A. Courtneidge, Association of Fyn with the activated PDGF receptor: requirements for binding and phosphorylation. *Oncogene*. 7: 1893–1901 (1992)
17. S. Mori, L. Rönnstrand, K. Yokote, A. Engström, S.A. Courtneidge, L. Claesson-Welsh and C.-H. Heldin, Identification of two juxtamembrane autophosphorylation sites in the PDGF ß-receptor. Involvement in the interaction with Src family tyrosine kinases. *EMBO J.* 12: 2257–2264 (1993)
18. W.J. Fantl, D.E. Johnson and L.T. Williams, Signalling by receptor tyrosine kinases. *Annu. Rev. Biochem.* 62: 453–481 (1993)
19. T. Pawson and J. Schlessinger, SH2 and SH3 domains. *Curr. Biol.* 3: 434–442 (1993)
20. J. Schlessinger and A. Ullrich, Growth factor signalling by receptor tyrosine kinases. *Neuron*. 9: 383–391 (1992)

21. G.M. Twamley-Stein, R. Pepperkok, W. Ansorge and S.A. Courtneidge, The Src family tyrosine kinases are required for platelet-derived growth factor-mediated signal transduction in NIH-3T3 cells. *Proc. Nat. Acad. Sci. USA.* 90: 7696–7700 (1993)

22. S. Roche, M. Koegl, V.M. Barone, M. Roussel and S.A. Courtneidge, DNA synthesis induced by some, but not all, growth factors requires Src family protein tyrosine kinases. *Mol. Cell. Biol.* 15: 1102–1109 (1995)

23. M.R. Smith, Y.-L. Liu, H. Kim, S.G. Rhee and H.-F. Kung, Inhibition of serum- and ras-stimulated DNA synthesis by antibodies to phospholipase C. *Science.* 247: 1074–1077 (1990)

24. S.E. Egan and R.A. Weinberg, The pathway to signal achievement. *Nature.* 365: 781–783 (1993)

25. J. McGlade, A. Cheng, G. Pelicci, P.G. Pelicci and T. Pawson, Shc proteins are phosphorylated and regulated by the v-Src and v-Fps protein-tyrosine kinases. *PNAS.* 89: 8869–8873 (1992)

26. D.W. Stacey, T. Watson, H. Kung and T. Curran, Microinjection of transforming *ras* protein induces c-*fos* expression. *Mol. Cell. Biol.* 7: 523–527 (1987)

27. S. Biro, Y.-M. Fu, Z.-X. Yu and S.E. Epstein, Inhibitory effects of antisense oligodeoxynucleotides targeting c-*myc* mRNA on smooth muscle cell proliferation and migration. *PNAS.* 90: 654–658 (1993)

28. E.L. Wickstrom, T.A. Bacon, A. Gonzalez, D.L. Freeman, G.H. Lyman and E. Wickstrom, Human promyelocytic leukemia HL-60 cell proliferation and c-*myc* protein expression are inhibited by an antisense pentadecadeoxynucleotide targeted against c-*myc* mRNA. *PNAS.* 85: 1028–1032 (1988)

29. G.P. Studzinski, Z.S. Brelvi, S.C. Feldman and R.A. Watt, Participation of c-*myc* protein in DNA synthesis of human cells. *Science.* 234: 467–470 (1986)

30. M.F. Roussel, J.L. Cleveland, S.A. Shurtleff and C.J. Sherr, *Myc* rescue of a mutant CSF-1 receptor impaired in mitogenic signalling. *Nature.* 353: 361–363 (1991)

31. S.A. Courtneidge, R. Dhand, D. Pilat, G.M. Twamley, M.D. Waterfield and M. Roussel, Activation of Src family kinases by colony stimulating factor-1, and their association with its receptor. *EMBO J.* 12: 943–950 (1993)

32. I. Chackalaparampil and D. Shalloway, Altered phosphorylation and activation of pp60$^{c\text{-}src}$ during fibroblast mitosis. *Cell.* 52: 801–810 (1988)

33. S. Roche, S. Fumagalli and S.A. Courtneidge, Requirement for Src family protein tyrosine kinases in G2 for fibroblast cell division. *Science.* in press: (1995)

34. S.T. Taylor and D. Shalloway, The cell cycle and c-Src. *Current Opinion in Genetics and Development.* 3: 26–34 (1993)

35. S.A. Courtneidge and S. Fumagalli, A mitotic function for Src? *Trends in Cell Biol.* 4: 345–347 (1994)

36. S. Fumagalli, N. Totty, J.J. Hsuan and S.A. Courtneidge, A target for Src in mitosis. *Nature.* 368: 871–874 (1994)

37. S.T. Taylor and D. Shalloway, An RNA-binding protein associated with Src through its SH2 and SH3 domains in mitosis. *Nature.* 368: 867–871 (1994)

DISCUSSION

M. Oren: You have told us that PDGF and IGF-1 operate through Src and upregulate myc. Gerard told us that IGF-1 and PDGF are survival factors against myc-induced apoptosis. That would kind of fit a nice scenario with PDGF having a dual action in terms of making the cell proliferate and survive. Now, questions along that line to you or to Gerard: Question number one: Will activated Src substitute for IGF-1 as a survival factor in cells over-expressing myc? The other question: Will a negative dominant Src block the survival effect of IGF-1 in myc over-expressors?

S. Courtneidge: We have not done those experiments yet; they are very good experiments. I was trying to be very careful about the IGF-1 receptor experiments, we did those under conditions where the cells expressed half a million IGF-1 receptors so the way the cells respond in that case is with DNA synthesis and as Gerard mentioned, that is an inappropriate response, in a way, and I do not want us to think that the Src involvement means that Src is induced in the survival functions of IGF-1 receptor, but obviously it is something we are testing at the moment. The PDGF experiments we do are with the natural levels of PDGF receptors in the cell we do not manipulate these cells to over-express in that case. So I am a lot more comfortable that Src family kinases are needed in that response. In terms of the other experiments, I can tell you that Src transformed cells have very high levels of myc on the whole time, and in fact, Src transformed cells do not need any serum or other growth factors.

M. Oren: That would support Src being a survival factor for myc overproducers.

S. Courtneidge: Yes.

Xiong: Do you know whether cell cycle kinases are activated in cells arrested in G2 by cst-1 antibodies?

S. Courtneidge: I cannot tell you the answer, but one way that was suggested to me is that one could look at the translocation, of cyclin-B into the nucleus, because that is an event that will correlate with cdc2 activation, and we are in the process of doing that right now. To ask whether we have stopped whatever the pathway is at that early stage that is about the only experiment that I think we can do, until we can get inducible expression of a dominant negative in a way that we can do some biochemistry, which of course we would love to do. But we are very limited with the microinjection. We also cannot, in this case, do the plasmid microinjection because an indeterminate number, but between 10–30% of cells that you microinject with plasmids express the protein, and you do not know what that number will be so, for the mitosis experiments we rely upon microinjecting a definitive number of cells and then ask how many we have later. So if we do not know how many are going to express our plasmids that becomes an impossible experiment. So we are limited to doing experiments with antibodies and with proteins that we can purify to microinject for rescues which is pretty limited.

Y. Xiong: Can you microinject purified cdc2 kinase?

S. Courtneidge: Yes, that would be one of those things we could do, in fact, providing we could get it in a concentrated enough form, soluble, which I am not sure about. It is not the easiest thing in the world to get proteins that actually live inside the cell somewhere between 5–10mg/ml for microinjection but it is certainly something we could try, absolutely.

T. Graf: I was not entirely clear what your thoughts are about the function of the mitotic substrate of Src family kinase. Your experiment with the anti-unique Src domain antibodies which inhibit Src function but not that of other Src family members would suggest, although not prove, that Src contains a specific-substrate binding site.

S. Courtneidge: When we identified SAM-68 that was the first and the most abundant substrate that you see during mitosis. It is a very abundant protein and you see it in Src and Fyn and Yes transform cells during mitosis. So it is certainly a substrate for all three of them. But as I say I think it is a nuclear protein that I do not think really gets a chance to see these enzymes until after the nuclear envelope has broken down, so for that reason alone it is unlikely to be the critical substrate that we are looking for the G2/M transition. It could be required later on and indeed if we ablate it we may find out that there are other functions during mitosis. Src's activity stays high for quite a while during mitosis, it is not like is goes down again immediately. I would suspect, and we have seen hints in our laboratory, that there are going to be other substrates for Src kinases during G2 and M, it is just that they are not going to be as abundant and are not going to be as easy to find as this one was. I just should mention something I did not which is that Serge Roche has also microinjected GST fusion proteins during G2. He knows that if he microinjects the GSTSH3 domain of Fyn or Src or any other SH3 domain he does not block this G2 to M transition. And we know that SAM-68 is an SH3 domain binding protein. On the other hand if he microinjects the GST construct containing the SH2 domain of Fyn, he does block G2 to M. He does not block it with the SH2 domains of GAP or PLC gamma or PI-3 kinase or any other that we have looked at. So our suspicion is that this pathway is initiated by something binding to the SH2 domain of Src family kinases. Obviously, what we are looking for are tyrosine phosphorylated proteins late in G2 that we can pull out with the GSTSH2, as the candidates. I think there will be multiple substrates.

D. Livingston: Is there any evidence that cells in the presence of anti-Src family antibodies, or in the Fyn, yes minus cells injected with the anti-Src antibodies itself, progress anywhere into M by, for example, looking for evidence of chromatin condensation or something like that?

S. Courtneidge: That, we have not seen. It is a very difficult experiment. You can, of course, wait a long time then you will start to see things, but is that because your antibody is now being degraded to below a critical level that is needed to do the inhibition. Maybe I will answer for Tony Hunter -- Martin Broone in his laboratory has generated a cell line that does express a kinase inactive form of Src and he knows in that cell line that PDGF signaling is very low. Those cells sort of are pretty strange looking and do grow. Now they looked more carefully since they heard about our data and they find that their cells, many of those cells, are multi-nucleate, they grow very slowly and poorly. So I think there will be some creep through, but there will be other blocks later on during mitosis.

D. Livingston: But there are some antibodies that will allow you to detect antigens, for example, which occur prior to meta-phase or at meta-phase like MDM-1. For which there are good monoclonal antibodies that would allow you do the injection experiment.

S. Courtneidge: Right. If they are monoclonal we can do it. We have not done them yet, I mean this is early days, I think we need to look at all of those and get that block set better. The cyclin-B experiment, I think, is also a good one because in the past, a lot of these things are based on the morphology of cells. Exactly where is the start of mitosis and the end of G2. What we need are more accurate markers, I would say, so that we can place the block caused by lack of Sr in the context of known things that regulate the G2 to M transition.

D. Livingston: Do you have to inject the antibody into the nucleus for this?

S. Courtneidge: No. This is antibody injected into the cytoplasm.

D. Livingston: And if you try injecting the antibody into the nucleus do you get the same effect?

S. Courtneidge: We have not done it. Although it is easy to do.

G. Lenaz: You mentioned that oxidative stress activates Src: Is there anything known about the mechanism?

S. Courtneidge: Not that I am aware of, no. It is a very rapid activation--within a minute. It is not something that we have studied. What Michael Karin has published, however, is that both tyrosine kinase inhibitors and a dominant negative form of Src will block the cell's ability to recover from that insult, suggesting that it is an important part of the recovery pathway from UV radiation. But how Src gets activated I do not know.

E. Nigg: You proposed cytoskeletal changes as possible common consequences of Src activation at the Go to S and G2 to M transitions. But you also emphasized myc induction at the Go to S transition. So, is there any evidence that myc functions is required at G2/M?

S. Courtneidge: Gerard could comment on that maybe as well as I can. Myc is required, as he said, all the time once cells are growing. You just have it there the whole time. So I think it would be hard to time it and say there is a requirement here rather than there.

E. Nigg: What would happen if you inject anti-myc antibodies into G2 cells, will they go into mitosis?

G. Evan: I can sort of answer that. In experiments we have done, which actually agree with a lot of early experiments done by people like Zeta Burg. If you do not regulate myc or remove mitogens in the post commitment stage of the cell cycle, you divide on schedule, she has now effect on the efficiency with which the cells divide or the timing that they do so. However, even if you do not regulate myc temporarily, even if you switch it back on again and add mitogens back on again so that by the time the cells divide - this is fibroblast - by the time the cells divide, myc is back on and they are back in 10% serum, then what you seen is a delay in the next cell cycle. You can block that by keeping myc on, and the bits of myc required to block the function of the bits and make it look like a transcription factor. So the inference from that when myc levels fall, is that there is a transcriptional program that comes into play that triggers growth arrest and I would argue that where the cells arrest depends upon types, though some cells will arrest in G2.

S. Courtneidge: Let me just expand a little bit because I was being a bit cryptic about the cytoskeletal changes in G1 as well. What I concentrated on today was the ability to induce DNA synthesis only and it is clear that you need Src kinases for that in some cases but not others. And I should say, that we have done the myc experiments with CSF-1 and EGF and it is the same story as with PDGF. But we also know from Vittoria Barone in the lab that if you take those growth factors where you do not need Src kinases for DNA synthesis and that is LPA and bombesin for example, you get very rapid cytoskeletal changes in response to those growth factors. The cst-1 antibody will block those cytoskeletal changes so of course, by the way that we are defining requirement, I am saying the ability to drive past a restriction point, but of course those cytoskeletal changes in terms of the growth of the cell are going to turn out to be equally important. So we do have evidence for pleiotropic effects of Src family kinases in G1. I think these are going to be different pathways. The ability to induce myc and the ability to change the cytoskeleton are likely to be different. And that is something that we are looking at now. And so that is why, at this point, we are thinking a little bit about cytoskeletal changes in G2 as well.

P. Comoglio: Most of us started this business looking at Src because it is a terrific bird oncogene what about in man - something happens?

S. Courtneidge: In tumors you mean? One of my new interests. There is limited information in the literature on the involvement of Src family kinases in human tumors but I think what is there is getting more compelling. The best examples at this point are in breast cancer (in cell lines and in primary tumors). It is not really clear yet whether it is hyperactivity of Src or hyperactivity and overexpression. And also, of course, the original work from Jo Bolen and Chris Cartwright and a number of others suggesting that in colon cancer cell lines and more recently from Chris Cartwright with tumor samples, show that some good percentage have an activation of Src. Now what is interesting with Chris' work on colon cells and tumors is that in almost all cases where she sees as activation of Src she also sees as activation of Yes. So I think most people in the field think that there is not going to be any mutation of Src involved in colon tumors, but rather that the Src family kinase are getting activated. Perhaps in those tumors that have amplified growth factors receptors where they are known to be involved in the responses. Perhaps because the phosphatases and the kinases that regulate Src are misbalanced, because one of those activities changed or is mutated. But there is no direct involvement of a mutation of Src itself. The only other member of Src family, where there is some evidence, is now in some T-cell tumors that there has been some rearrangements that have resulted in activation of Lck. What has not been done, to my knowledge as yet, is a test of whether hyperactivity of Scr is important for tumor growth, what we have been looking at now with these signaling pathways, for example with the PDGF receptors in normal cells. I think the next question really is whether in a tumor that is driven by PDGF receptor amplification (for example, glioma) whether all those pathways are critically required in that case as well, or whether one pathway dominates in the case where the receptors are amplified. And I think that is unknown at this point--whether at high levels of receptors you require all of these different signaling pathways or whether they now lose the need to have all of those check points in place. That is obviously experiments that we want to do in the future.

T. Taniguchi: In our hematopoietic system we have been working on these signals induced by IL2 and activated Src kinases. So far we have no supporting indications that Src kinases are involved in myc induction. So a possible explanation would be cell type dependence?

S. Courtneidge: As I understand it, your data says the opposite, in a sense, as to what induces myc and what induces for in hematopoietic cells compared to fibroblasts. At this point, yes, all we can say is that these are different cell types and we probably do not know enough about the pathways that pertain to those cell types yet. So in that context with tumors it is of course, going to be very important to look at epithelial cells rather than always using a fibroblast cell model for the signaling that we are doing. But I think it is very curious that the involvement of these pathways is quite distinct in these different cell types.

p16 FAMILY INHIBITORS OF CYCLIN-DEPENDENT KINASES

Yan Li,[1] Christopher W. Jenkins,[2] Michael A. Nichols,[2] Xiaoyu Wu,[5] Kun-Liang Guan[5] and Yue Xiong[1–4]

[1] Department of Biochemistry and Biophysics
[2] Curriculum in Genetics and Molecular Biology
[3] Lineberger Comprehensive Cancer Center
[4] The Program in Molecular Biology and Biotechnology
The University of North Carolina at Chapel Hill
Chapel Hill, North Carolina 27599–3280
[5] Department of Biological Chemistry and Institute of Gerontology
The University of Michigan
Ann Arbor, Michigan 48109–0606

INTRODUCTION

The origin and development of human tumors begins at the molecular level and involves a complex multi-step process. A feature common to many tumor cells is their ability to enter and progress through the cell division cycle under conditions where normal cells would either be quiescent or proliferating at a reduced rate. Therefore, the molecular pathways controlling the cell division cycle must inevitably interact with pathways which regulate cell growth, and are a very likely target of oncogenic events. It was not until very recently, however, that experimental evidence became available to bring such a connection to light.

It is now well established that the primary control of the eukaryotic cell cycle is provided by a family of serine/threonine protein kinase complexes consisting of a catalytic subunit, a CDK (cyclin-dependent kinase); and a regulatory subunit, a cyclin. In unicellular yeast cells, the prototype CDK gene, *cdc2* of the fission yeast *Schizosaccharomyces pombe* or *CDC28* in the budding yeast *Saccharomyces cerevisiae*, in conjunction with the various types of cyclins controls both the G1/S(START) and G2/M transitions. In humans and other higher eukaryotes, CDKs constitute a multigene family. Seven CDK genes have been identified in human cells, CDC2 (or CDK1), CDK2, 3, 4, 5, 6, and 7. In general, each of these CDKs can form binary complexes with several different cyclins, and *vice versa*, although often with a predominant association between a particular CDK and cyclin[31,57]. Cyclins were originally discovered in invertebrate eggs as proteins whose abundance after fertilization oscillated during early cleavage divisions owing to their active synthesis and abrupt proteolytic degradation at mitosis [17]. Subsequently, cyclin genes have been isolated from virtually all eukaryotic species that have been studied and found to constitute a multigene family as well [reviewed in [68]]. Thus, the cyclin-CDKs comprise a very large family of related protein kinase complexes whose whole range is probably still not yet fully appreciated.

CDK subunits by themselves are inactive and binding to a cyclin protein is required for their activity as well as their regulation. CDKs are also regulated intrinsically by activating and inhibitory phosphorylations [reviewed in [60]]. In addition to cyclin activation and subunit phosphorylation, it has become clear recently that CDK activity is also negatively regulated by a number of small proteins that physically associate with cyclins, CDKs or their complexes. In mammalian cells, the number of small cell cycle inhibitory proteins identified by virtue of their ability to physically interact with cyclin or CDK proteins is rapidly increasing. Currently, two distinct families of CDK inhibitors, represented by two prototype CDK inhibitors, p21 and p16, have been identified [reviewed in [31,57]]. Although these small CDK inhibitors were only identified very recently, their biochemical and biological properties are being characterized very quickly. Most importantly, a striking connection between some of these newly discovered CDK inhibitors and tumor growth suppression has been discovered.

The first evidence that a CDK inhibitor may play an important role in tumor growth suppression came from studies of the *p21* CDK inhibitor. p21, first identified in normal human fibroblast cells as a component of cyclin D-CDK quaternary complexes that also contain proliferating cell nuclear antigen [PCNA, [70]], was subsequently identified as a universal component of all cyclin-CDK complexes in normal human fibroblasts [71,72]. p21 protein was not detected in cyclin-CDK complexes in cells transformed by a variety of tumor viruses or in p53 deficient Li-Fraumeni cells [71]. *p21* was later isolated by a large scale immunopurification and protein microsequencing [69], as a gene whose transcription was induced by wild type, but not mutant p53 gene expression [*WAF1*, [15]], through a yeast two-hybrid screen for proteins that interact with CDK2 [*Cip1*, [26]], and in a search for cDNAs corresponding to mRNAs preferentially expressed in senescent human cells that can block growing young cells from entering S phase when overexpressed by transient transfection [*Sdi1*, [49], reviewed in [58]]. The discovery that the *p21* gene is transcriptionally activated by the tumor suppressor p53 provides a critical link between the tumor suppression function of *p53* and cell cycle control [[15,39,69], reviewed in [31,57]]. *p53* is the most frequently mutated gene in human cancers with a 50% overall mutation frequency [4,29,47]. Mutations in *p53* appear to eliminate a G1-S cell cycle checkpoint that is activated in normal cells when their DNA is damaged, presumably allowing the cells time for DNA repair prior to S phase replicative DNA synthesis [reviewed in [27,38]]. Tumor cells with p53 deficiency, or having dominant mutant forms of p53, lack the G1-S delay when exposed to DNA damaging agents, perhaps resulting from failure to induce the expression of *p21* and thus to inhibit cyclin-CDK activity and/or PCNA-dependent DNA replication. Inactivation of this pathway involving p53 and p21 in tumor cells would therefore permit the accumulation of genetic alterations and deregulate growth. Expression of the *p21* gene can be induced by a wide range of cell growth regulatory signals, including the DNA damage and tumor suppressor p53 [13,15,69], cellular senescence [49], the antiproliferative growth factor TGF-β [12], and the myogenic factor MyoD [24]. Studies from both in vitro cell culture and in vivo mice have further provided intriguing data correlating accumulation of p21 with the withdrawal of cells from the division cycle during differentiation of a number of cell types [24,34,44,50,62], supporting a broad role for p21 in normal cell differentiation. *p21* regulates cell cycle through at least four different pathways: inhibiting the kinase activity of cyclin-CDK enzymes [21,26,69], interacting with PCNA to inhibit DNA replication [19,65], blocking activating phosphorylation of CDK by CDK-activating kinase [CAK, [3,37]], and interacting with and potentially regulating the activity of E2F transcription factor complexes via its interaction with cyclin-CDK proteins [1].

The involvement of CDK inhibitors in cancer development is further illustrated by the studies of *p16*. p16 was first identified as a CDK4-specific associated protein in virally transformed cells that lack p53 and pRB function [71]. The gene encoding p16, *p16^INK4* (also known as *MTS1*, *CDK4I* and *CDKN2*) was subsequently isolated by yeast two-hybrid screening and shown to form specific binary complexes with CDK4 and CDK6 and inhibit the kinase activity of D-type cyclin-dependent CDK4 [55]. *p16* was recently found not only to be homozygously deleted or mutated at a high frequency in a wide variety of human tumor-derived cell lines [35,48], but also in several specific types of primary tumors [10,32,36,45,61], demonstrating that *p16* is a *bona fide* tumor suppressor. The extent to which *p16* is involved in tumorigenesis is currently under intensive investigation.

The major, if not the only, targets of p16's inhibitory activity are CDK4 and CDK6. Both CDK4 and CDK6 have been strongly implicated as physiological kinases of the retinoblastoma gene product pRb whose growth suppressing activity is known to be down-regulated by cell cycle dependent phosphorylation [see two most recent reviews in [18,58]]. Elucidation of the mechanism by which the activities of CDK4 and CDK6 are regulated is important to our understanding of cell cycle control, cell growth regulation and tumor suppression. Toward this goal, we have investigated the regulation and function of the p16 family CDK inhibitors.

RESULTS AND DISCUSSION

Transcriptional Repression of *p16* Gene by pRb

p16 was initially identified as a CDK4-associated protein in cells transformed by a variety of DNA tumor viruses including SV40, papilloma- and adenoviruses [71]. It is present in CDK4 complexes at a high level in transformed cells as determined by immunoprecipitation, but in normal untransformed cells the level of CDK4-associated p16 is extremely low or undetectable. A common property shared by these DNA tumor viruses is their ability to bind to and consequently inactivate the function of two tumor suppressors, pRb and p53, suggesting the possibility that pRb and/or p53 may regulate the expression of *p16*. To test this hypothesis, we first analyzed the steady state level of *p16* mRNA [40].

Total RNA was prepared from a number of tumor-derived cell lines whose pRb and/or p53 status has been previously characterized. Two such examples are shown in Figure 1. Saos-2 and U-2OS cell lines were both derived from human osteosarcomas. Northern analysis revealed a high level of *p16* mRNA in Saos-2 cells, but *p16* mRNA was undetectable in U-2OS cells (Figure 1B). Failure to detect the *p16* mRNA in U-2OS cells is not due to homozygous deletion of the *p16* locus as is observed in many cultured tumor cell lines [35,48], since we have verified the presence of the *p16* gene in both cell lines by PCR (data not shown). Whether the *p16* gene in U-2OS (and Saos-2) cells contains point mutation(s) in the coding region or promoter sequences has not been determined. The high level of *p16* mRNA in Saos-2 cells is correlated with a high level of *p16* protein and its association with CDK4 and CDK6, as shown in Figure 1C. One of the obvious genetic differences between these two osteosarcoma cell lines is their pRb status. While an apparently normal p105^pRb protein was readily detectable in U-2OS cells, it was not detected in Saos-2 cells—apparently due to a deletion in exons 21–27 of the *RB1* gene [59] (Figure 1A).

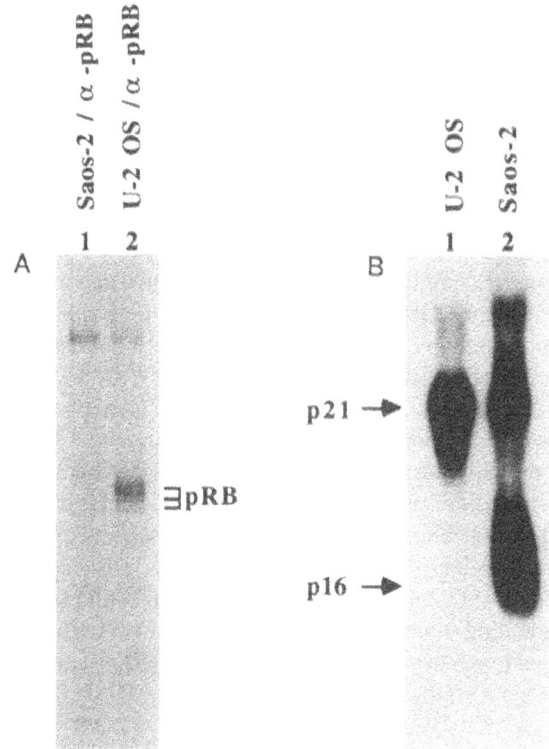

Figure 1. Analysis of p16 mRNA and protein in human osteosarcoma cells. **(A)** Analysis of pRb protein. [^{35}S]-methionine-labeled cell lysates were prepared from Saos-2 and U-2 OS cells and were immunoprecipitated with antisera specific to pRb protein [XZ77, [30]]. pRb protein was not detected in Saos-2 cells using this antibody due to a deletion in exons 21–27 of the *RBI* genes [59]. **(B)** Expression of p16 mRNA in Saos-2 and U-2 OS cells. 20 micrograms of total RNA samples prepared from each cell line were resolved on a 1% agarose gel. Equal amounts of RNA were loaded as determined by hybridization with a rat GAPDH probe (data not shown). Resolved RNA samples were transferred to an nitrocellulose filter and the blot was hybridized with a probe derived from full length human *p16* [55] and *p21* cDNA [69]. **(C)** Analysis of CDK4, CDK6 and p16 immunocomplexes. [^{35}S]-methionine-labeled cell lysates were prepared from both Saos-2 and U-2 OS cells and immunoprecipitated with antisera specific to CDK4, CDK6 and p16 with or without prior incubation with a competing antigen peptide as indicated at the top of each lane and resolved by SDS-PAGE. The relative position of proteins whose identities have been established and potential CDK4 and CDK6 interacting proteins are marked.

Similarly, when total RNA was prepared from normal human fibroblasts (HSF43) and their SV40 large T antigen transformed derivative (CT10) and hybridized with the *p16* probe, a 10-fold increase in the steady-state level of *p16* mRNA was observed in transformed CT10 cells (Figure 2A). The same result was also obtained with several additional pairs of normal human fibroblasts and their virally transformed derivatives (e.g. WI-38 vs. VA13, data not shown). These findings are consistent with the previously observed higher level of p16 protein associated with CDK4 and CDK6 in virally transformed cells[55,71] (and our unpublished observation). Taken together the data suggest that inactivation of the function of pRb and/or p53 activates the transcription and/or induces the stabilization of *p16* mRNA.

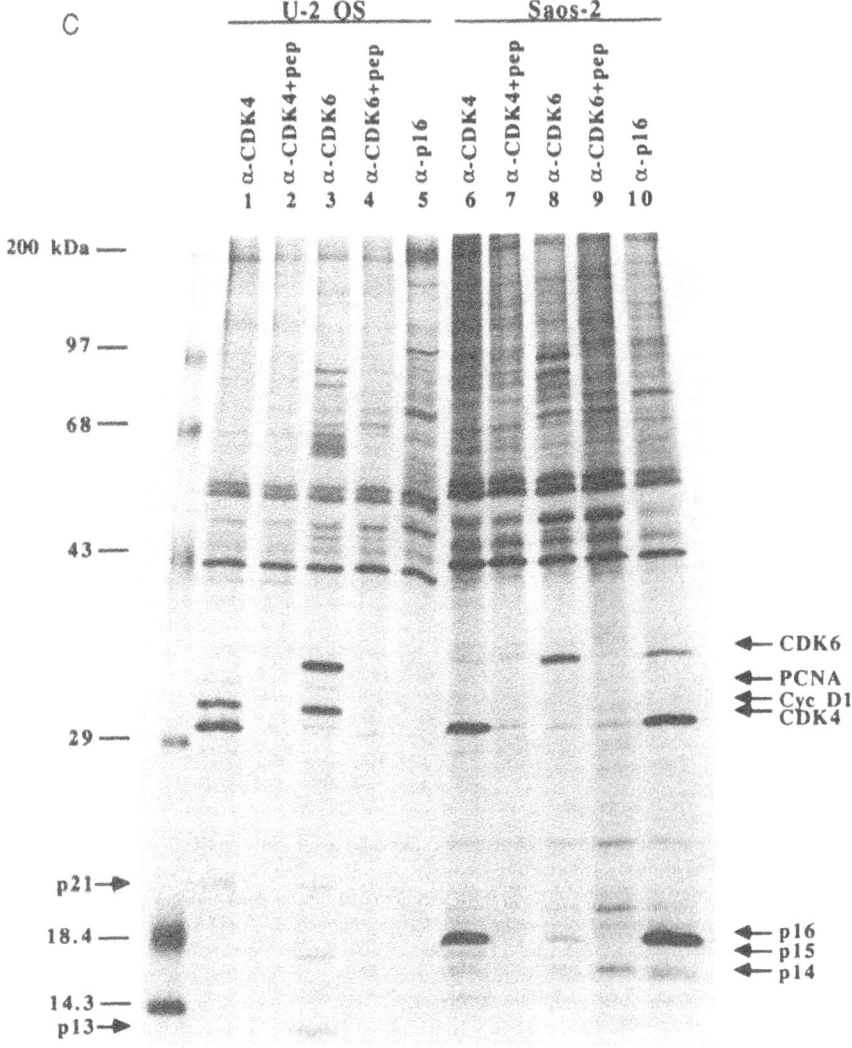

Figure 1. (*Continued.*)

To distinguish which tumor suppressor, pRb or p53, regulates the level of *p16* mRNA, we analyzed the level of *p16* mRNA in normal human fibroblast IMR-90 cells and IMR-90 cells expressing type 16 papilloma viral oncoprotein E6 (16E6), E7 (16E7), or E6 together with E7 [56]. 16E6 and 16E7 bind to and inactivate the functions of p53 and pRb, respectively [14,54]. Compared to the parental IMR-90 cells, the level of *p16* mRNA was increased by 2.7-fold in IMR-90 cells expressing 16E6, 4.2-fold in IMR-90 cells expressing 16E7, and 4.7-fold in IMR-90 cells expressing both 16E6 and 16E7 (Figure 2A). The increased level of *p16* mRNA in cells expressing viral oncoproteins also correlates closely with an increased level of p16 protein and its increased association with CDK4 and CDK6 as determined by immunoprecipitation in metabolically-labeled cells with antibodies specific to CDK4, CDK6 or p16 (Figure 2B). They further demonstrate that the expression of either E6 or E7 oncoprotein leads to an increased level of *p16* mRNA, with E7

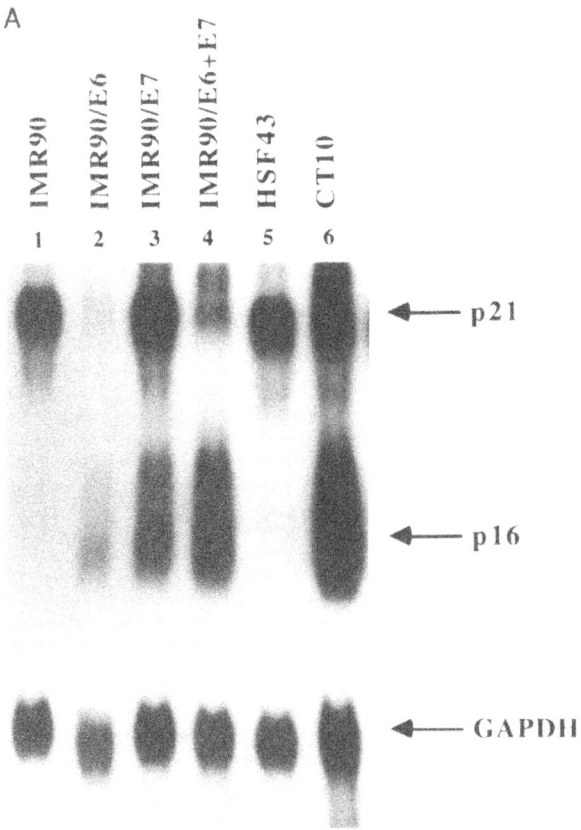

Figure 2. Increased expression of p16 mRNA and association of p16 protein with CDK4 and CDK6 in cells lacking pRb function. (**A**) Northern analysis of p16. The procedures on cell culture, RNA preparation and Northern blotting were the same as described previously [39]. Total RNA was prepared from normal human diploid fibroblasts IMR-90 cells and IMR-90 cells expressing type 16 papilloma viral oncoprotein E6, E7, and E6 together with E7 [56], and from a different strain of normal human fibroblasts (HSF43) and its SV40 large T antigen transformed derivative [CT10, [71]]. 20 micrograms of each of the RNA samples were resolved on a 1% agarose gel. Similar amounts of RNA were loaded for each sample as determined by hybridization with a rat GAPDH probe (lower panel). Resolved RNA samples were transferred to a nitrocellulose filter and the blot was hybridized with a probe derived from full length human *p16* cDNA [upper panel, [55]]. As a comparison, the same blot was also hybridized with a probe derived from full length human *p21* cDNA whose expression is drastically reduced as the result of inactivation of p53 function by the E6 oncoprotein of type 16 papillomavirus [15,54,69]. The positions of p16 , *p21* and GAPDH mRNA were indicated at left. The steady state level of p16 mRNA accumulation was determined on a PhosphoImager (Molecular Dynamics, ImageQuant software version 3.3). (**B**) Analysis of CDK4, CDK6 and p16 immunocomplexes. [^{35}S]-methionine-labeled cell lysates were prepared from parental IMR-90 cells and IMR-90 cells infected with retroviral vectors containing the type 16 HPV E6 (IMR-90 / E6), E7 (IMR-90 / E7) or E6 plus E7 (IMR-90 / E6+E7) oncogene. Labeled cell lysates were immunoprecipitated with antisera specific to CDK4 [71], CDK6 [43] and p16 [55] with or without prior incubation with a competing antigen peptide as indicated at the top of each lane and resolved by SDS-PAGE. The relative position of proteins whose identities have been established are marked at left.

being a more potent stimulus, indicating that both p53 and pRb can down regulate the expression of *p16* mRNA. Subsequent experiments were focused on the regulation of the level of *p16* mRNA by pRb. As a comparison, the same blot was also hybridized with a probe derived from the human CDK inhibitor *p21*'s cDNA. While expression of 16E7 protein had little effect, expression of 16E6 (and 16E6 together with 16E7) dramatically reduced the level of *p21* mRNA (Figure 2A) that is also correlated closely with a reduced

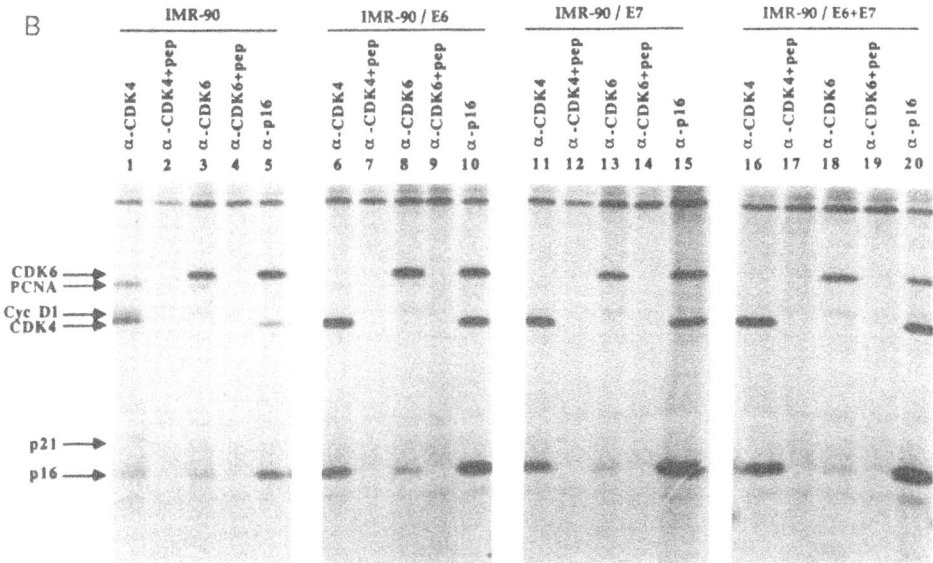

Figure 2. (*Continued.*)

level of p21 protein in these cells (data not shown). These results are entirely consistent with the previous finding that the expression of *p21* mRNA is transcriptionally activated by p53, and with the absence of p21 protein from cyclin and CDK complexes in virally transformed cells [15,69,71].

We next investigated whether transcriptional activation of *p16* contributed to the higher level of *p16* mRNA seen in virally transformed or Rb-deficient cells. Genomic fragments containing *p16* sequences were isolated from a human placenta genomic library and a 1.1 kb genomic fragment corresponding to the 5′ upstream region of *p16* cDNA was subcloned into a promoter-less luciferase expression plasmid (pGL2-Basic). The resultant plasmid, p16-Luc, gave rise to considerable luciferase activity as compared to the parental promoterless luciferase construct pGL2-Basic when it was transiently expressed in several cell lines including Saos-2 and U-2OS (Figure 3A). To allow comparison of luciferase activity in cells transfected with p16-Luc, a SV40-Luc plasmid was transiently expressed in parallel as a control for normalizing the transfection efficiency between the different cells. In five independent experiments, we have reproducibly observed an average of 10-fold higher luciferase activity in Saos-2 cells than in U-2OS cells (Figure 3A), indicating that the higher level of *p16* mRNA seen in Saos-2 cells was most likely the result of transcriptional activation of the *p16* promoter.

To determine whether pRb can directly repress transcription through the *p16* promoter, the p16-Luc reporter plasmid was co-transfected into Saos-2 cells with wild-type pRb cDNA under the control of the strong immediate-early promoter of CMV [pCMV-Rb, [28]]. Ectopic expression of pRb in these Rb-deficient cells reproducibly resulted in an average 40% reduction in luciferase activity from the *p16* promoter (Figure 3B), but had no detectable effect on the SV40 promoter (data not shown). Similar results were also obtained in separate experiments using mouse NIH 3T3 cells. Co-transfection of the p16-Luc plasmid with an increasing amount of pCMV-pRb repeatedly led to a progressive reduc-

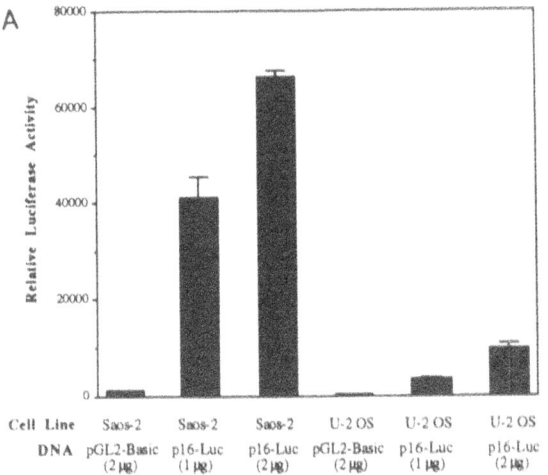

A

Relative Luciferase Activity

Cell Line	Saos-2	Saos-2	Saos-2	U-2 OS	U-2 OS	U-2 OS
DNA	pGL2-Basic (2 µg)	p16-Luc (1 µg)	p16-Luc (2 µg)	pGL2-Basic (2 µg)	p16-Luc (1 µg)	p16-Luc (2 µg)

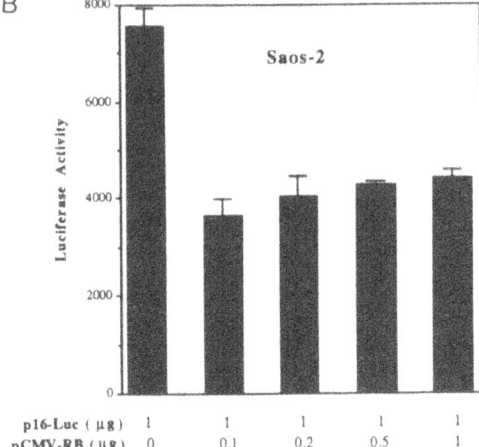

B

Saos-2

Luciferase Activity

p16-Luc (µg)	1	1	1	1	1
pCMV-RB (µg)	0	0.1	0.2	0.5	1

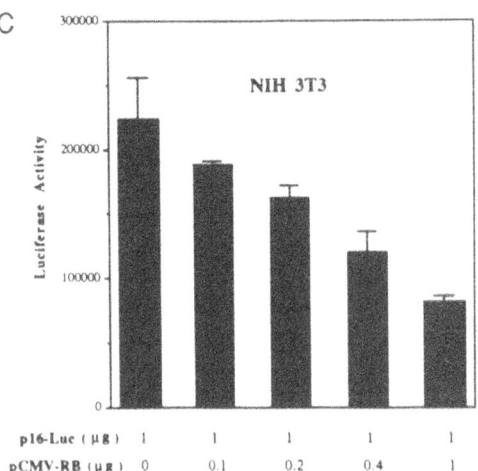

C

NIH 3T3

Luciferase Activity

p16-Luc (µg)	1	1	1	1	1
pCMV-RB (µg)	0	0.1	0.2	0.4	1

Figure 3. Transcriptional repression of the p16 promoter by pRb. Transcriptional repression of the p16 promoter by pRb. (**A**) Genomic fragments containing p16 were isolated from a human placenta genomic library using p16 cDNA as a probe and a 1.1 kb genomic fragment corresponding to the 5′ upstream region of p16 cDNA was subcloned into a promoter-less luciferase expression plasmid [pGL2-Basic (note)]. The resultant plasmid, p16-Luc, and parental pGL2-Basic DNA were transiently expressed in both human osteosarcoma Saos-2 and U-2 OS cells. Luciferase activities were measured as relative light units 28 hours after transfection. The relative luciferase activity of each transfection was calculated by dividing individual light emission values with the values obtained from a parallel transfection with pSV40-Luc DNA to normalize the transfection efficiency between two cell populations. Error bars show the standard deviation of three separate readings of triplicate transfections in a single experiment. (**B**) Ectopic expression of pRb suppresses the p16 promoter activity. The p16-Luc reporter plasmid was co-transfected with the wild type pRb cDNA under the control of strong immediate early promoter of CMV [pCMV-Rb, [28]] into the Rb-deficient Saos-2 cells as described in (note). (**C**) Repression of p16 promoter activity by the ectopic expression of pCMV-RB in mouse NIH3T3 cells.

Figure 4. A feedback regulatory loop showing transcriptional repression of p16 by pRb. A transcription factor such as E2F1 bound to the hypophosphorylated pRb is released after the phosphorylation of pRb by the cyclin D-associated CDK4 or CDK6 and activates the transcription of p16. The increasing amount of p16 protein binds to the catalytic subunit CDK4 and CDK6 and dissociates the complexes, thus inhibiting the activity of cyclin D-CDK4 and CDK6 enzymes.

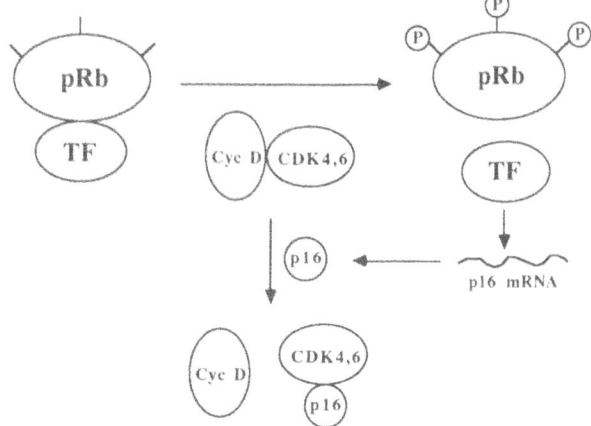

tion of luciferase activity up to 40% of the full activity from the *p16* promoter (Figure 3C). These results provide direct evidence for the repression of the *p16* promoter by pRb. We have not determined why a maximum of only 40% reduction of luciferase activity is obtained upon co-expression of pRb. A number of cellular transcription factors such as E2F-1 have been identified as the functional targets of pRb [reviewed in [18,46]]. We have determined more than 3 kb of nucleotide sequence upstream of the *p16* gene, including the 1.6 kb region used in the transfection assay, and found no apparent E2F binding site [46], nor conventional TATA sequences (M.N. and Y.X., unpublished). Whether the *p16* gene contains a weak E2F binding site or pRb represses *p16* transcription by a mechanism independent of E2F factors is currently under investigation.

The function of pRb is known to be down-regulated by cell cycle-dependent phosphorylation and both D-type cyclins and their associated kinases (primarily CDK4 and CDK6) have been strongly implicated as physiological pRb kinases [see two most recent reviews in [18,58]]. Biochemical analyses have indicated that p16 acts as an inhibitor of CDK4 [and likely CDK6 as well, [55]]. Our results demonstrate that transcription of *p16* is repressed by pRb, providing evidence for a regulatory feedback loop involving pRb, CDKs, *p16* and an as yet unidentified transcription factor (Figure 4). In this model, phosphorylation of pRb by cyclin D-CDK4 or cyclin D-CDK6 results in the release of a transcription factor (e.g. E2F-1) which is inactive when bound to hypophosphorylated Rb. Dissociation of the pRB-transcription factor complex would then activate *p16* transcription. As levels of *p16* mRNA increase, increased binding of p16 to CDK4 and CDK6 would result in inhibition of the cyclin D-CDK4 and cyclin D-CDK6 kinase activities. Ultimately, phosphorylation of pRb would decrease, as would the level of *p16* expression. This model is consistent with, and provides a plausible explanation for, the absence of cyclin D proteins and cyclin D-CDK complexes in cells lacking pRb [6,51,53]. A high level of p16 in cells lacking pRb function may lead to dissociation of cyclin D from CDK complexes and subsequent degradation. In addition, an increased level of *p16* mRNA in cells lacking p53 function (IMR90 cells expressing 16E6, Figure 2A) suggests that the expression of *p16* may also be regulated negatively by p53. Our results also provide a potential pathway by which the expression of *p16* is regulated by p53. An increased level of p21 activated by p53 inhibits the activity of various CDKs, preventing the phosphorylation of pRb and consequently leading to the repression of the *p16* promoter. This study, together with the discovery of the transcriptional regulation of *p21* by p53, dramatically exemplifies how the recently identified small CDK inhibitors link tumor suppressor gene function to cell cycle control.

CDK4 and CDK6 Associate with Many Small Cellular Proteins

Using the [^{35}S]-metabolic labeling-immunoprecipitation technique coupled with antigen competition, we have previously identified, mainly in human fibroblasts, a number of cellular proteins that are specifically associated with cyclins, CDKs and their complexes. These include the proliferating cell nuclear antigen PCNA, the p53-activated cyclin-CDK inhibitor p21, the CDK4 specific inhibitor p16, and an as yet uncharacterized cyclin A-associated polypeptide, p19 [70,71]. As many cyclin and CDK genes, in particular D-type cyclins, are expressed in a tissue and cell type-specific manner [e.g., [33,42,63,67]], we reasoned that additional cyclin or CDK associated proteins may exist and function in other tissues or cell types. Following this reasoning, the [^{35}S]-IP technique was then employed to search for proteins that associate with CDK4 and its closest relative CDK6, which shares 71% sequence identity.

[^{35}S]-methionine labeled lysates were prepared from a wide variety of human cell lines derived from different tissues and immunoprecipitated with antibodies specific to CDK4 and CDK6. In addition to the previously identified p21 and p16, this study revealed at least four other small cellular proteins that appear to associate with CDK4 and/or CDK6 in a specific manner. They include p14 and p15—present in a cell line of spontaneously immortalized human keratinocytes, HaCaT [8] (Figure 5A), and p18 and p20—present in an acute lymphoblastic leukemia cell line, CEM (Figure 5B). Each of these proteins represents a distinct polypeptide as determined by their different gel mobilities, partial V8 proteolysis patterns and antigenicities. The presence of each of these proteins in anti-CDK4 and/or anti-CDK6 immunocomplexes was effectively competed off by the pre-incubation of each antibody with a competing antigen peptide (lanes 2 and 4 of Figure 5A, lane 6 of Figure 5B), suggesting their specific associations. These results indicate that a potentially large number of small cyclin- and/or CDK-associated proteins are present in cells that have not yet been identified.

Cloning of Three p16-Related, CDK4- and CDK6-Specific Inhibitor Genes: *p14*, *p18* and *p20*

A genomic fragment located 10 kb upstream the *p16* locus that contains 93% DNA sequence identity to exon 2 of the *p16* gene (*MTS2*) was previously identified in a search for candidate tumor suppressor genes involved in melanoma [35]. It was not clear, however, whether this genomic fragment corresponded to a pseudogene of *p16* or encoded a functional gene distinct from *p16*. Oligonucleotide primers specific to *MTS2* were used to amplify cDNA templates prepared from a human HeLa cDNA library. A specific DNA fragment was amplified and used as probe to screen the same HeLa library for full length *MTS2* cDNA clones. Of five lambda cDNA clones isolated, the longest one, H2, was further analyzed by DNA sequencing. Comparison with the previously reported *MTS2* genomic sequence [35] indicates that cDNA clone H2 corresponds to *MTS2*. Conceptual translation of this clone revealed a 138 amino acid open reading frame starting from nucleotide 322. There are neither methionine nor in-frame stop codons 5′ to the putative initiating methionine. The predicted molecular weight of this protein is 14613 daltons (14.6 kDa, p14) and it contains 82% protein sequence identity to p16^{INK4} in the aligned region [[55], Figure 6A]. The sequence similarity between *MTS2* and *p16* is higher in exon 2 than in exon 1. In vitro translated MTS2 co-migrates with

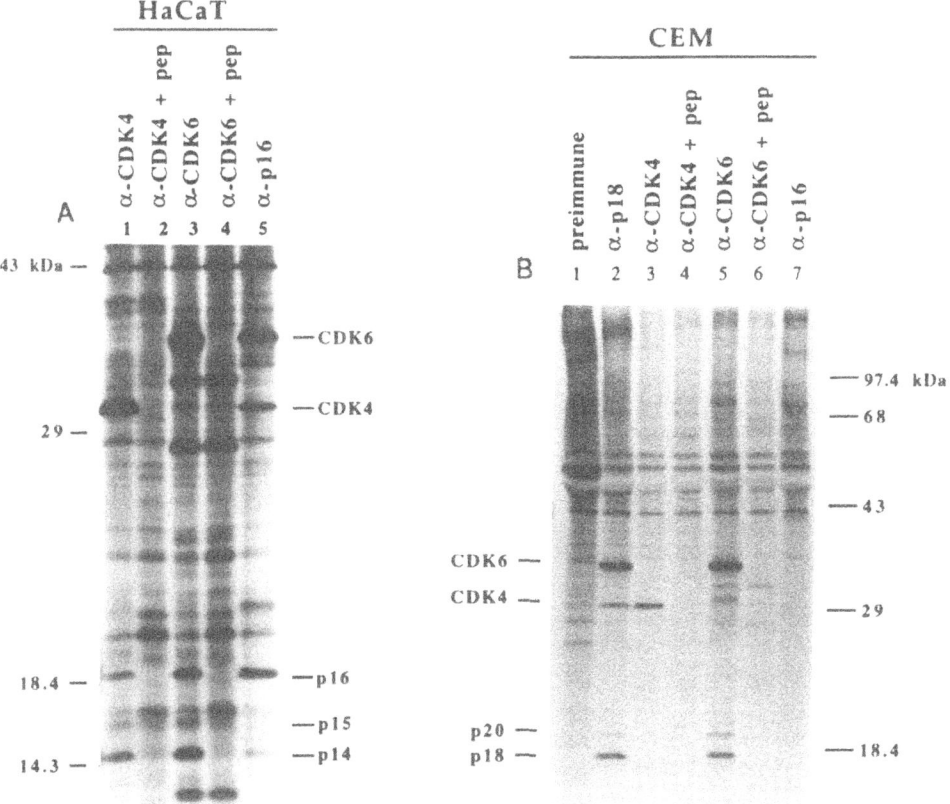

Figure 5. CDK4 and CDK6 associate with many small cellular proteins. [^{35}S]-methionine labeled lysates were prepared from a cell line of spontaneously immortalized human keratinocytes, HaCaT (A), and an acute lymphoblastic leukemia cell line, CEM (B). Lysates were immunoprecipitated with indicated antibody with or without pre-incubation with a competing antigen peptide as indicated at the top of each lane. The immunoprecipitated polypeptides were analyzed in each case by SDS-polyacrylamide gel electrophoresis. The mobility of protein molecular weight standards (Gibco-BRL) and relevant proteins are indicated.

the CDK4- and CDK6-associated p14 seen in HaCat cells (Figure 5A), and, like p14, also crossreacts with anti-p16 antibody (IVT data not shown). These results demonstrate that *MTS2* encodes a functional gene that corresponds to the CDK4- and CDK6-associated p14. p14 / *MTS2* has a DNA sequence that is almost identical to p15^{INK4B} [22,25]. p15^{INK4B} is stimulated by TGF-β treatment, suggesting that p14 / p15^{INK4B} may function as potential effector of TGF-β-induced cell cycle arrest [25].

We employed the yeast two-hybrid screening system to further identify proteins that interact with CDK6 [5]. The entire open reading frame of human *CDK6* [42] was fused to the *Gal4* DNA binding domain. Of an estimated 5 X 10^6 transformants screened, forty-two colonies were positive for His+ and β-galactosidase staining. Plasmid DNA was recovered from positive colonies and analyzed by sequencing. The majority of the forty-two clones corresponded to the previously reported p16^{INK4} [55]. One clone, 6H10, was found to contain sequences that are distantly related to p16^{INK4} and *MTS2* The cDNA insert from this clone was then used as probe to screen a human HeLa cDNA library to obtain full length se-

A

```
p20  (19p13.2)         MLLEEVRAGDRLSGAAAARGDVQEVRRLLHRELVHPDALNRFGKTALQVMM
p18  (1p32)            MAEPWGNELASAAAARGDLEQLTSLLQ-NNVNVNAQNGFGRTALQVMK
p16  (9p21)         MDPAAGSSMEPSADWLATAAAARGRVEEVRALLE-AGALPNAPNSYGRRPIQVMM
p14  (9p21)         MREENKGMPSGGGSDEGLASAAAARGLVEKVRQLLE-AGADPNGVNRFGRRAIQVMM


p20  FGSTAIALELLKQGASPNVQD-TSGTSPVHDAARTGFLDTLKVLVEHGADVNVPDGTGAL
p18  LGNPEIARRLLLRGANPDLKD-RTGFAVIHDAARAGFLDTLQTLLEFQADVNIEDNEGNL
p16  MGSARVAELLLLHGAEPNCADPATLTRPVHDAAREGFLDTLVVLHRAGARLDVRDAWGRL
p14  MGSARVAELLLLHGAEPNCADPATLTRPVHDAAREGFLDTLVVLHRAGARLDVRDAWGRL


p20  PIHLAVQEGHTAVVSFL--AAESDLHRRDARGLTPLELALQRGAQDLVDILQGHMVAPL 166
p18  PLHLAAKEGHLRVVEFLVKHTASNVGHRNHKGDTACDLARLYGRNEVVSLMQANGAGGATNLQ 168
p16  PVDLAEELGHRDVARYLRAAAGGTRG-SNHARIDAAEGPSDIPD 154
p14  PVDLAEERGHRDVAGYLRTATGD 138
```

B

```
p20          64  GASP-NVQDTSGTSPVHDAARTGFLDTLKVLVEHGADVNVPDGTGALPIHL
p18          60  GANP-DLKDRTGFAVIHDAARAGFLDTLQTLLEFQADVNIEDNEGNLPLHL
TAN 1-Hs   1918  GASLHNQTDRTGETALHLAARYSRSDAAKRLLEASADANIQDNMGRTPLHA
Motch-Mm   1907  GASLHNQTDRTGETALHLAARYSRSDRRKRL-EASADANIQDNMGRTPLHA
Xotch-Xl   1913  GAQLHNQTDRTGETALHLAARYARADAAKRLLESSADANVQDNMGRTPLHA
Notch-Br   1905  GANLHNQTDRTGETALHLAARYARSDAAKRLLESCADANVQDNMGRTPLHA
Notch-Dm   1940  GAELNATMDKTGETSLHLAARFARADAAKRLFHAGADANCQDNTCRTPLHA


p20              AVQEGHTAVVSFL--AAESDLHRRDARGLTPLELA-LQRGAQDLVDILQGHMVAPL
p18              AAKEGHLRVVEFLVKHTASNVGHRNHKGDTACDLA-RLYGRNEVVSLMQANGAGGA
TAN 1-Hs         AVSADAQGVFQILIRNRATDLDARMHDGTTPLILAARLAVEGMLEDLINSHADVNA
Motch-Mm         AVSADAQGVFQILLRNRATDLDARMHDGTTPLILAARLAVEGMLEDLINSHADVNA
Xotch-Xl         AVAADAQGVFQILIRNRATDLDARMFDGTTPLILAARLAVEGMLEDLINAHADVNA
Notch-Br         AVAADAQGVFQILIRNRATDLDARMHDGTTPLILATRLAVEGMVEELINCHADPNA
Notch-Dm         AVAADAMGVFQILLRNRATNLNARMHDGTTPLILAARLAIEGMVEDLITADADINA
```

Figure 6. Protein sequence comparison of p16 gene family. (A) Amino acid sequence comparison of four p16 related genes, p14/p15$^{MTS2/INK4b}$ [22,25], p16 [55], p18 [22] and p20 [23]. The complete coding regions of the four inhibitor proteins were aligned, and amino acid residues identical in all four sequences are in bold. Several small gaps were introduced as represented by hyphens. Chromosomal location of each gene is indicated in the parentheses preceding each sequence. (B) p16 genes are related to *Notch* proteins. 105 amino acid residues of the p18 and p20 sequence were compared with four members of the *Notch* gene family. Only residues that are identical to all five sequences are in bold. Two single residue gaps, represented by hyphens, were introduced in the p18 sequence. The number preceding each sequence indicates the position of the first amino acid residue in each gene. *TAN1*-Hs, the translocation-associated *Notch* homolog of humans [16]; *Xotch*-Xl, a Xenopus homologue of the Drosophila *notch* gene [11]; *Notch*-Br, a zebrafish homologue of Drosophila *notch* gene [7]; *Notch*-Dm, the Drosophila *notch* gene [66].

quences. One of the longest lambda cDNA clones, H18, was sequenced and found to contain an apparent full length coding region, as there is an in-frame stop codon located 6 base-pairs upstream of the putative ATG initiation codon [22]. Conceptual translation of this clone revealed an open reading frame with 168 amino acid residues starting at nucleotide 94 (Figure 6A). The predicted molecular weight of this protein is 18116 D (18 kDa, p18).

In our continuing attempts to identify *p16*-related genes, degenerate oligonucleotides were designed based on regions conserved among the p14, p16 and p18 sequences, and used as primers to amplify cDNA sequences from several different cell lines. One PCR fragment identified in cDNA prepared from human leukocytes encodes a potentially novel p16-related molecule and was used as a probe to screen a human spleen cDNA library to obtain the full length sequence. The longest lambda cDNA clone, S2, was completely sequenced and found to contain a 1254 bp insert and a short poly A tail preceded by a putative polyadenylation signal. Conceptual translation of this clone revealed an apparent full-length open reading frame with 166 amino acid residues starting at nucleotide 140 preceded by an in-frame termination codon present 54 bp 5' to the initiating methionine (Figure 6A). The predicted molecular weight of this protein is 17689 D, but its apparent molecular weight as seen in SDS-PAGE is 20 kDa (p20, see Figure 5B).

Among four p16-related genes isolated, p14 and p16 share the highest similarity (82%) and equal similarity to p18 and p20 (approximately 45% identity, Figure 6A). The sequence similarities are higher across the N-terminal two-thirds of the proteins than in the C-terminal regions. As first noticed in p16, other members of the family also contain tandem ankyrin repeats [55]. In addition, both p18 and p20 also shares significant protein sequence identity (37% and 35% respectively to human Notch homolog, TAN1) with the Notch genes which function in the developmental determination of embryonic cell fates [Figure 6B, see review in [20]]. Within this region, the shorter C-terminal ends of p16 (91 amino acids) and p14 (70 amino acid) also share considerably lower, but also potentially significant sequence similarities to the *Notch* genes (21% and 24% identity to TAN1 respectively). This region in p18/p20 and members of the Notch family of proteins also shows a limited sequence similarity to the previously identified cdc10/SWI6 ankyrin repeat [2,9,16,55]. As this region of p18 and p20 shows considerably higher similarity to the members of the Notch family than to any other ankyrin repeat containing proteins, it is not clear whether this region in p18 and Notch represents a distinct subset of ankyrin sequences, or defines an as yet uncharacterized functional relationship shared by p18 (and members of p16 family) and Notch.

p18 and p20 Are Specific Inhibitors of CDK4 and CDK6

We assessed the specificity of p18 and p20's interaction with known CDKs in a cell-free system. A fusion protein consisting of glutathione S-transferase and p18 or p20 (GST-p18 and GST-p20) was expressed in bacteria and purified GST-p18 and GST-p20 was mixed with equivalent amounts of the known CDK proteins that had been in vitro translated with [^{35}S]-methionine labeling. The GST-p18 and GST-p20 fusions were recovered from the different mixtures on glutathione-agarose beads, and proteins bound to GST-p18 or GST-p20 were resolved by SDS-PAGE. GST-p20 bound to CDK6 and CDK4 with equal affinity while GST-p18 bound strongly to CDK6, but weakly to CDK4. Neither p18 nor p20 interacts with any other CDKs (Figure 7A). The specificity of the interaction between p18 and p20 with CDK4 and CDK6 was also confirmed by yeast two-hybrid assay and reciprocal immunoprecipitation using anti-CDK antibodies [22,23].

To directly test whether p18 inhibits the kinase activity of CDK6 and CDK4, we assayed for its inhibition of cyclin D2 and CDK6 expressed in insect Sf9 cells. Human p18 protein was expressed in bacteria and purified to near homogeneity. Increasing amounts of purified p18 protein were incubated with equal amounts of Sf9 cell lysates prepared from insect cells infected with baculoviruses expressing both CDK6 and cyclin D2. p18 inhibits cyclin D2-CDK6 activity in a dose-dependent manner (Figure 7B). Similarly, p20 was also found to effectively inhibit the kinase activity of both CDK4 and CDK6 reconstituted using purified GST fusion proteins (Figure 7C). Consistent with in vitro binding assay, neither p18 nor p20 had any effect on the kinase activities of CDK2, CDC2, or cyclin A enzymes [[22,23], and data not shown].

Expression of p16 Gene Family

Northern blot analysis was carried out to determine the expression of *p16, p18* and *p20* mRNA in different human tissues. Under high stringency conditions, the *p18* probe corre-

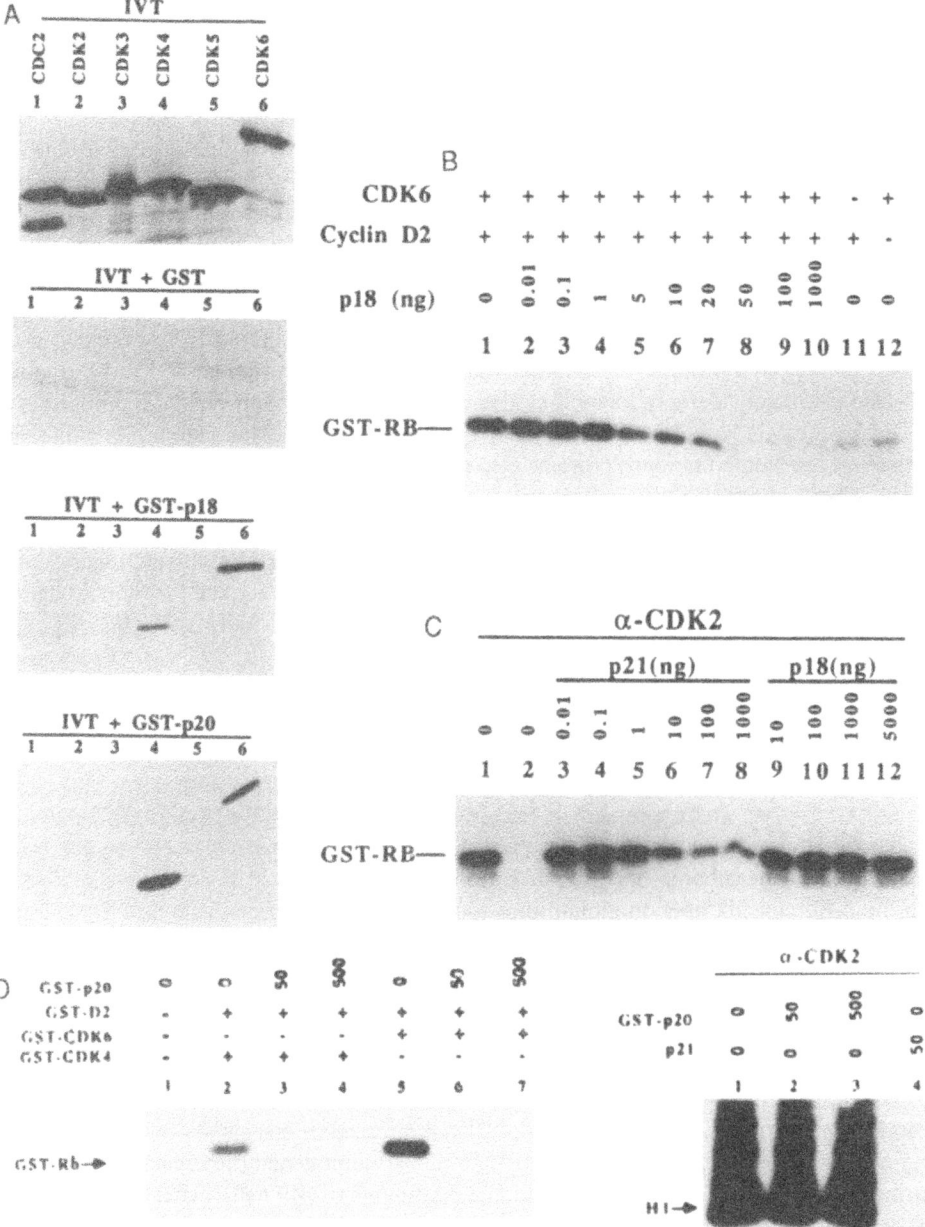

Figure 7. Interaction of p18 and p20 with CDKs. (A) Equal amounts of purified GST or GST-p18 fusion protein were incubated with equal amounts of each of the six [^{35}S]-methionine labeled, in vitro translated CDK proteins and recovered from the different mixtures on glutathione-agarose beads. Proteins bound to GST, GST-p18 or GST-p20 were resolved by SDS-PAGE. (B) Inhibition of CDK6-cyclin D2 kinase activity by p18. Increasing amounts (in nanograms) of purified p18 protein were added to a 25 μl kinase reaction containing the same amount of lysate derived from Sf9 insect cells that had been infected with baculovirus expressing cyclin D2 and CDK6 proteins as indicated. Phosphorylation of GST-Rb-Cterm fusion protein was analyzed by SDS-PAGE followed by autoradiography. (C) Inhibition of CDK4-cyclin D2 and CDK6-cyclin D2 kinase activity by p20. The purified recombinant GST-p20 fusion protein (in nanograms) was added to the activated CDK4 or CDK6 to assay for its inhibitory activity. Phosphorylated GST-Rb was indicated by an arrow. The kinase reaction was resolved on a 10% SDS gel, transferred to a nitrocellulose filter followed by a 20 minutes autoradiography.

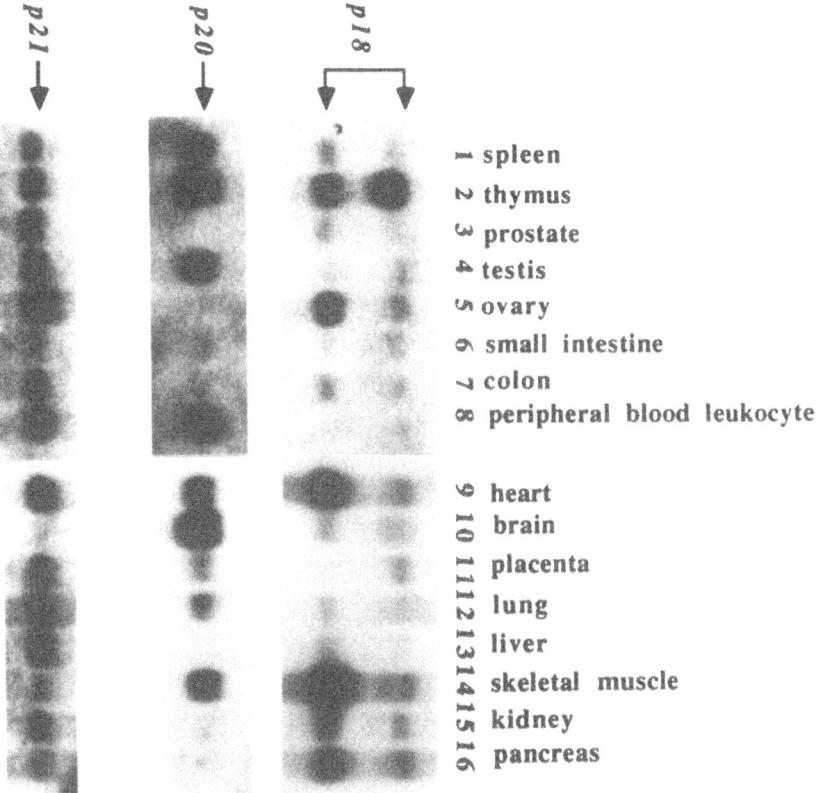

Figure 8. Expression of *p18* and *p20* mRNA. Expression of *p18* and *p20* mRNA in different human tissues. 2 µg of poly(A)⁺ RNA from sixteen different human tissues as indicated at the top of each lane were hybridized with a *p18* probe derived from the coding region of human *p18* that detects mainly two transcripts (top panel). The same blot was also hybridized with a probe derived from full length *p20* cDNA and a 1 4 kb discrete band was detected by this probe (middle panel). As comparison, the same blot was also hybridized with a p21 probe derived from the full length human p21 cDNA [69](bottom panel).

sponding to the coding region of human *p18* cDNA revealed two discrete bands, *p20* cDNA probe detected a single band of approximately 1.4 kb, and p16 and p14 mRNA were undetectable (Figure 8 and data not shown). The relative intensity of the *p18*-hybridizing bands appears to vary in different tissues. Two of these bands may result from different transcription initiations, since we have isolated from a cDNA library two classes of *p18* cDNA clones that differ in their 5′ ends. Sequence analysis revealed a class of two cDNA clones with an extension of approximately 500 nucleotides 5′ to the *p18* sequence [22], but it does not alter the coding capacity of *p18* (data not shown). Nevertheless, we cannot exclude the possibility that one of these discrete bands on the Northern blot may correspond to a yet unidentified gene related to *p18*. Whether the differential transcription initiation of *p18* plays a role in the regulation of *p18* function in vivo is not clear.

The level of both *p18* and *p20* mRNA varies dramatically between different human tissues (Figure 8). The highest level of *p18* mRNA was observed in human skeletal muscle, and moderate levels were present in thymus, ovary, heart, and pancreas. At the other end of the spectrum, *p18* mRNA was almost undetectable in peripheral blood leukocytes and placenta. Consistently, a drastic variation in the level of *p18* mRNA was also seen in different cell types (Y.L. and Y.X., unpublished). The level of *p20* mRNA also varied significantly between different human tissues. The highest level was observed in thymus, peripheral blood leukocytes, and brain. Moderate levels were present in spleen, testis, heart, and skeletal muscle, suggesting a preferential expression of *p20* mRNA in hematopoietic cells. Interestingly, the expression of *p20* and *p18* mRNAs were in startling contrast between the testis and ovary tissues. These results demonstrate a very different expression pattern for *p18* and *p20* mRNA than for two other cyclin-CDK kinase inhibitors, *p27* and *p21*, that appear to be expressed in most human tissues at a similar level [[52], Figure 8], indicating a tissue-specific regulation of *p18* gene expression and the possible involvement of *p18* function in cellular differentiation and development. Two critical aspects of cell differentiation are permanent withdrawal from the active cell division cycle and the prevention of terminally differentiated cells from re-entering the cell cycle. CDK4 and CDK6 are two major CDK enzymes that are activated during, and required for the G1 progression of the cell cycle, most likely by phosphorylating and thus down regulating the growth suppressing activity of pRb. Activation of a particular p16 family inhibitor's gene expression by a specific differentiation signal such as the activation of *p20* in hematopoietic cells or *p18* in muscle cells could effectively arrest G1 cell cycle progression to initiate differentiation. Alternatively, but not mutually exclusively, accumulation of a high level of a p16 family inhibitor may prevent terminally differentiated cells from re-entering the cell cycle through the same mechanism.

Growth Suppression by *p16* and *p18* Correlates with Wild-Type pRb Function

The biochemical analysis of *p16* and *p18* has demonstrated that they act as an inhibitor of CDK4 and CDK6. As such, one would predict that overexpression of *p16* or p18 in vivo may inhibit cell proliferation and growth—a property that has been previously shown for two other cyclin-CDK inhibitors, p21 [15,26,49,69] and p27 [52,64]. We employed a colony formation assay to directly test this prediction [73]. The full length coding region of *p16* or *p18* was placed under the control of a strong promoter of CMV that also carries a neomycin-resistance (*neo*) gene, and the resultant plasmid, pCMV-p16 and pCMV-p18, was transfected into human U-2OS osteosarcoma cells. The biological effect of ectopic expression of *p16* or *p18* was measured by scoring the number of G418-resistant colonies three weeks after culturing the transfected cells in a media supplemented with G418, and comparing with the number of G418-resistant colonies obtained from a parallel transfection with the parental vector plasmid pcDNA3 or a plasmid expressing antisense *p18* (pCMV-p16AS or pCMV-p18AS). Introduction of full length *p16* or *p18* into U-2OS cells significantly reduced their ability to grow as G418-resistant colonies (Table 1). These results provide evidence to support a function of *p18* and *p16* in negative regulation of cell growth, a notion that is consistent with its biochemical property of inhibiting the activity of cyclin-dependent kinases.

The function of pRb is known to be down-regulated by cell cycle-dependent phosphorylation and D-type cyclins and their associated kinases, primarily CDK4 and CDK6. The substrate specificity of CDK4 and CDK6 kinases and the specific interaction of p16, p18 and p20 with CDK6 and CDK4 provoked us to test whether cell growth suppression by *p18* is dependent on the existence of endogenous pRb. To test this possibility, another line of human osteosarcoma cells, Saos-2, was transfected with each of the four plasmid DNAs in parallel with the U-2OS cells as described above. U-2OS and Saos-2 cells ex-

Table 1. Inhibition of cell growth by *p18* correlates with pRb function. A colony formation assay was employed to test growth suppression by *p18*. The full length coding region of *p18*, as well as that of *p16*, was placed under the control of a strong promoter of CMV that also carries a neomycin-resistance (*neo*) gene in both sense and antisense orientations and the resultant plasmids, pCMV-p18, pCMV-p18AS, pCMV-p16 and pCMV-p16AS, were transfected into human U-2 OS and Saos-2 osteosarcoma cells. While an apparently normal p105^{pRb} protein was readily detectable in U-2 OS cells, it was not detected in Saos-2 cells—apparently due to a deletion in exons 21–27 of the *RB1* gene (Shew et al., 1990). The biological effect of ectopic expression of *p18* and *p16* was measured by scoring the number of G418-resistant colonies after three weeks of culturing the transfected cells in a media supplemented with G418, and comparing with the number of G418-resistant colonies obtained from a parallel transfection with parental vector plasmid (pcDNA3) or a plasmid expressing antisense *p18* (pCMV-p18AS) and *p16* (pCMV-p16AS). ND: not determined

Growth Suppression by p18 and p16

Recepient Cells	Transfected DNA	Average number of G418-Resistent Colonies		
		Exp. 1	Exp. 2	Exp. 3
U-2 OS (Rb+/+)	pCMV-p18	3	2	11
	pCMV-p18AS	41	68	62
	pCMV-p16	2	5	9
	pCMV-p16AS	45	36	44
	pcDNA3	ND	ND	54
Saos-2 (Rb-/-)	pCMV-p18	86	ND	71
	pCMV-p18AS	82	ND	74
	pCMV-p16	80	45	67
	pCMV-p16AS	83	39	74
	pcDNA3	ND	ND	69

press a similar level of CDK4 and CDK6 proteins as determined by immunoprecipitation (data not shown). However, unlike U-2OS cells, Saos-2 cells do not express endogenous wild-type pRb due to a deletion in exons 21–27 of the *RB1* gene [59], and our confirmatory results]. Strikingly, expression of the same pCMV-p18 and pCMV-p16 DNA that inhibited growth of U-2OS cells had no apparent effect on the growth of Saos-2 cells, as measured by scoring the number of G418-resistant colonies, and comparing with parallel transfections with vector pcDNA3 plasmid or plasmids expressing antisense *p18* and antisense *p16* (pCMV-p18AS and pCMV-p16AS) respectively. High level expression of p16 and p18 proteins and increased association with CDK4 and CDK6 in these stable transformants were verified by immunoprecipitations (data not shown). These results are in contrast to the previously reported growth suppression by p21 and p27, which inhibited the growth of Saos-2 as well as that of a number of additional tumor cell lines [15,26,49,64,69]. These results are the first example that growth suppression by a cyclin-CDK inhibitor is cell line specific and may be pRb dependent. They provide further in vivo support for the conclusion that p16 and p18 only specifically interact with CDK4 and CDK6, but not with

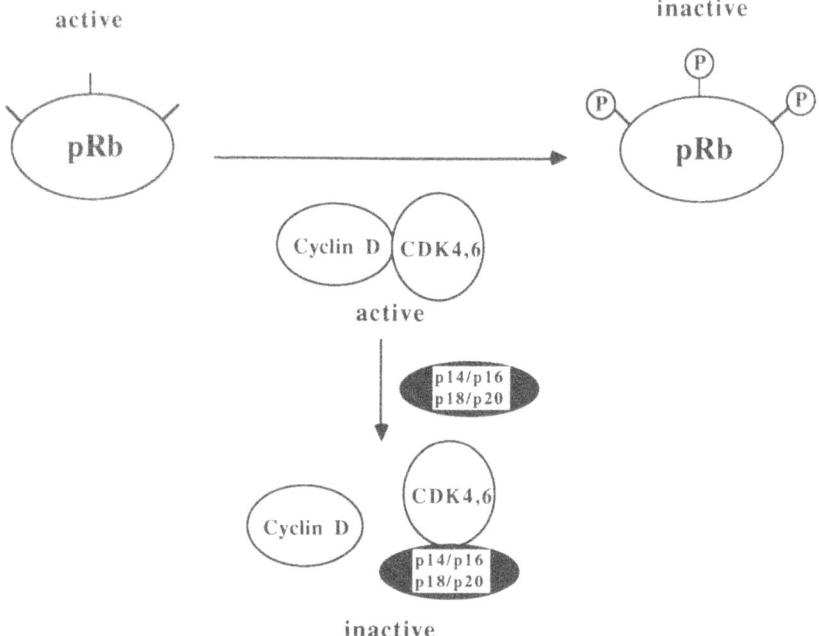

Figure 9. Mechanisms for growth suppression by p16 genes. Dependence on pRb for growth suppression by p16 and p18. Hypophosphorylated pRb actively suppresses cell cycle progression. pRb's growth suppressing activity may be inactivated in two ways: by mutation (as in Saos-2 cells) or by hyperphosphorylation. Inactivation of CDKs 4 and 6 by p14/p16/p18 prevents hyperphosphorylation of pRb, maintaining the active growth suppressing state.

other CDKs since no effect was observed even when they were overexpressed in pRb-deficient Saos-2 cells. Although other differences between these cell lines could also contribute to the observed differences in growth suppression by p18 and p16, our results can be most simply explained at this time by the difference in their pRb status. While a normal p105[pRb] protein was readily detectable in U-2OS cells, it was not detected in Saos-2 cells—apparently due to a deletion in exons 21–27 of the *RB1* gene [59]. Lacking functional pRb, and therefore being devoid of a functional target, overexpression of p16 or p18 and the resulting inhibition of CDK4 and CDK6 kinase activity is futile in Saos-2 cells (Table 1, Figure 9). This model is supported by the observation that high levels of p16 and p18 are expressed and tolerated in cells lacking functional pRb, and that p16 and p18 only interact with and inhibit the activity of CDK4 and CDK6 [55,71 and Figure 4]. The model is entirely consistent with the observations that DNA tumor virus oncoproteins or pRb mutations can relieve cells' requirements for cyclin D1 function in G1 [41,63]. It also suggests that pRb proteins are the critical, if not exclusive, in vivo targets of CDK4 and CDK6.

ACKNOWLEDGMENTS

We thank Drs. M.Serrano and D. Beach for providing anti-p16 antibody, M. Meyerson, E. Harlow, and G. Peters for providing anti-CDK6 antibody, P. Hinds for providing pCMV-pRb plasmid DNA, X.-F. Wang for helping with the luciferase assay, Charles

Sherr and Astar Winoto for communicating data prior to publication, Wade Harper and Zalin Yu for providing Sf9 cell lysates, Zhangying Guo for helping with the purification of the p20 protein, and B. Marzluff and T. Van Dyke for their encouragement and discussion during the course of this work. This study was supported by an American Cancer Society grant BE-171 and a National Institute of Health grant GM 51586 to K.G., by a start-up fund from the University of North Carolina at Chapel Hill and a National Institute of Health grant CA 65572 to Y.X.

REFERENCES

1. Afshari, C. A., M. A. Nichols, Y. Xiong, and M. Mudryj. The p21 protein interacts with multiple E2F complexes during the cell cycle. *submitted* (1994)

2. Andrews, B. J. and I. Herskowitz. The yeast SWI4 protein contains a motif present in developmental regulators and is part of a complex involved in cell-cycle dependent transcription. . *Nature* **342**:830–833(1989)

3. Aprelikova, O., Y. Xiong, and E. T. Liu. Both p16 and p21 families of CDK inhibitors block CDK phosphorylation bt the CDK activating kinase (CAK). *J. Biol. Chem.* **in press**:(1995)

4. Baker, S. J., E. R. Fearon, J. M. Nigro, S. R. Hamilton, A. C. Preisinger, J. M. Jessus, P. van Tuinen, D. H. Ledbetter, D. F. Barker, Y. Nakamura, R. White, and B. Vogelstein. Chromosome 17 deletions and p53 gene mutations in colorectal carcinoma. *Science* **244**:217–221(1989)

5. Bartel, P. L., C. -T. Chien, R. Sternglanz, and S. Fields. 1993. Using the two hybrid system to detect protein-protein interactions, p. 153–179. In D. A. Hartley (ed.), Cellular Interactions in Development: A Practical Approach. Oxford University Press, Oxford, UK.

6. Bates, S., D. Parry, L. Bonetta, K. Vousden, C. Dickson, and G. Peters. Absence of cyclin D / cdk complexes in cells lacking functional retinoblastoma protein. *Oncogene* **9**:1633–1640(1994)

7. Bierkamp, C. and J. A. Campos-Ortega. A zebrafish homologue of the Drosophila neurogenic gene Notch and its pattern of transcription during early embryogenesis. *Mech. Dev.* **43**:87–100(1993)

8. Boukamp, P., R. T. Petrussevska, D. Breitkreutz, J. Hornung, A. Markham, and N. E. Fusenig. Normal keratinization in a spontaneously immortalized aneuploid human keratinocyte cell line. *J. Cell Biol.* **106**:761–771(1988)

9. Breeden, L. and K. Nasmyth. Similarity between cell-cycle genes of budding yeast and fission yeast and the Notch gene of Drosophila. *Nature* **329**:651–654(1987)

10. Caldas, C., S. A. Hahn, L. T da Costa, M. S. Redston, M. Schutte, A. B. Seymour, C. L. Weinstein, R. H. Hruban, C. J. Yeo, and S. E. Kern. Frequent somatic mutations and homozygous deletions of the p16 (MTS1) gene in pancreatic adenocarcinoma. *Nature Genet.* **8**:27–32(1994)

11. Coffman, C., W. Harris, and C. Kintner. Xotch, the xenopus homolog of Drosophila notch. *Science* **249**:1438–1441(1990)

12. Datto, M. B., Y. Li, J. F. Panus, D. J. Howe, Y. Xiong, and X-F. Wang. TGF-β induces the cyclin-dependent kinase inhibitor, p21 through a p53 independent mechanism. *Proc. Natl. Acad. Sci. USA* **in press**:(1995)

13. Dulic, V., W. K. Kaufmann, S. J. Wilson, T. D. Tlsty, E. Lees, J. W. Harper, S. J. Elledge, and S. I. Reed. p53-dependent inhibtion of cyclin-dependent kinase activities in human fibroblasts during radiation-induced G1 arrest. *Cell* **76**:1013–1023(1994)

14. Dyson, N., P. M. Howley, K. Munger, and E. Harlow. The human papillomavirus-16 E7 oncoprotein is able to bind to the retinoblastoma gene product. *Science* **243**:934–937(1989)

15. El-Deiry, W. S., T. Tokino, V. E. Velculescu, D. B. Levy, R. Parsons, D. M Lin, W. E. Mercer, K. W. V Kinzler, and B. Vogelstein. WAF1, a potential mediator of p53 tumor suppression. *Cell* **75**:817–825(1993)

16. Ellisen, L. W., J. Bird, D. C. West, A. L. Soreng, T. C. Reynolds, S. D. Smith, and J. Sklar. TAN-1, the human homolog of the Drosophila Notch gene, is broken by chromosomal translocations in T lymphoblastic neoplasms. *Cell* **66**:649–661(1991)

17. Evans, T., E. T. Rosenthal, J. Youngblom, D. Distel, and T. Hunt. Cyclins: a protein specified by maternal mRNA in sea urchin eggs that is destroyed at each cleavage division. *Cell* **33**:389–396(1983)

18. Ewen, M. E. The cell cycle and the retinoblastoma protein family. *Cancer and Metastasis Rev.* **13**:45–66(1994)

19. Flores-Rozas, H., Z. Kelman, F. B. Dean, Z-Q. Pan, J. W. Harper, S. J. Elledge, M. O'Donell, and J. Hurwitz. Cdk-interacting protein directly binds with proliferating cell nuclear antigen and inhibits DNA replication catalyzed by the DNA polymerase d holoenzyme. *Proc. Natl. Acad. Sci. USA* **91**:8655–8659(1994)

20. Greenwald, I. S. and G. M. Rubin. Making a difference: the role of cell-cell interactions in establishing separate identities for equivalent cells. *Cell* **68**:271–281(1992)

21. Gu, Y., C. W. Turck, and D. O. Morgan. Inhibition of CDK2 activity in vivo by an associated 20K regulatory subunit. *Nature* **366**:707–710(1993)

22. Guan, K-L., C. W. Jenkins, Y. Li, M. A. Nichols, X. Wu, C. L. O'Keefe, A. G. Matera, and Y. Xiong. Growth suppression by p18, a p16$^{INK4/MTS1}$- and p14$^{INK4B/MTS2}$-related CDK6 inhibitor, correlates with wild-type pRb function. *Genes & Dev.* **8**:2939–2952(1994)

23. Guan, K. L., C. W. Jenkins, Y. Li, C. L. O'Keefe, S. Noh, X. Wu, M. Zariwala, A. G. Matera, and Y. Xiong. Isolation and characterization of *p20*, a p16-related inhibitor specific to CDK6 and CDK4. *submitted*(1995)

24. Halevy, O., B. G. Novitch, D. B. Spicer, S. X. Skapek, J. Rhee, G. J. Hannon, D. Beach, and A. B. Lassar. Terminal cell cycle arrest of skeletal muscle correlates with induction of p21 by MyoD. *Science* **267**:1018–1021(1995)

25. Hannon, G. J. and D. Beach. p15^{INK4B} is a potential effector of TGF-β-induced cell cycle arrest. *Nature* **371**:257–261(1994)

26. Harper, J. W., G. R. Adami, N. Wei, K. Keyomarsi, and S. J. Elledge. The p21 cdk-interacting protein cip1 is a potent inhibitor of G1 cyclin-dependent kinases. *Cell* **75**:805–816(1993)

27. Hartwell, L. Defects in a cell cycle checkpoint may be responsible for the genomic instability of cancer cells. *Cell* **71**:543–546(1992)

28. Hinds, P. W., S. Mittnacht, V. Dulic, A. Arnold, S. I. Reed, and R. A. Weinberg. Regulation of retinoblastoma protein functions by ectopic expression of human cyclins. *Cell* **70**:993–1006(1992)

29. Hollstein, M., D. Sidransky, B. Vogelstein, and C. C. Harris. p53 mutations in human cancers. *Science* **253**:49–53(1991)

30. Hu, Q. -J., C. Bautista, G. M. Edwards, J. D. Defeo, R. E. Jone, and E. Harlow. Antibodies specific for the human retinoblastoma protein identify a family of related polypeptides. *Mol. Cell Biol.* **11**:5792–5799(1994)

31. Hunter, T. and J. Pines. Cyclins and cancer II: cyclin D and CDK inhibitors come of age. *Cell* **79**:573–582(1994)

32. Hussussian, C. J., J. P. Struewing, A. M. Goldstein, P. A. T. Higgins, D. S. Ally, M. D. Sheahan, W. H. Clark, M. A. Tucker, and N. C. Dracopoli. Germline p16 mutations in familial melanoma. *Nature Genet.* **8**:15–21(1994)

33. Inaba, T., H. Matsushime, M. Valentine, M. F. Roussel, C. J. Sherr, and A. T. Look. Genomic organization, chromosomal localization, and independent expression of human cyclin D genes. *Genomics* **13**:565–574(1992)

34. Jiang, H., Z-Z. Su, F. Collart, E. Huberman, and P. Fisher. Induction of differentiation in human promyelocytic HL-60 leukemia cells activates p21, WAF1/CIP1, expression in the absence of p53. *Oncogene* **9**:3397–3406(1994)

35. Kamb, A., N. A. Gruis, J. Weaver-Feldhaus, Q. Liu, K. Harshman, S. V. Tavitgian, E. Stockert, R. S. Day, B. E. Johnson, and M. H. Skolnick. A cell cycle regulator potentially involved in genesis of many tumor types. *Science* **264**:436–440(1994)

36. Kamb, A., D. Shattuck-Eidens, R. Eeles, Q. Liu, N. A. Gruis, W. Ding, C. Hussey, T. Tran, Y. Miki, J. Weaver-Feldhaus, M. McClure, J. F. Aitken, D. E. Anderson, W. Bergman, R. Frants, D. E. Goldgar, A. Green, R. MacLennan, N. G. Martin, L. J. Meyer, P. Youl, J. J. Zone, M. H. Skolnick, and L. A. Cannon-Albright. Analysis of the p16 gene (CDKN2) as a candidate for the chromosome 9p melanoma susceptibility locus. *Nature Genet.* **8**:22–26(1994)

37. Kato, J., M. Matsuoka, K. Polyak, J. Massague, and C. J. Sherr. Cyclic AMP-induced G1 phase arrest mediated by an inhibitor (p27Kip1) of cyclin-dependent kinase 4 activation. *Cell* **79**:487–496(1994)

38. Lane, D. P. p53, guardian of the genome. *Nature* **358**:15–16(1992)

39. Li, Y., C. W. Jenkins, M. A. Nichols, and Y. Xiong. Cell cycle expression and p53 regulation of the cyclin-dependent kinase inhibitor p21. *Oncogene* **9**:2261–2268(1994)

40. Li, Y., M. A. Nichols, J. W. Shay, and Y. Xiong. Transcriptional repression of the D-type cyclin-dependent kinases inhibitor p16 by the retinoblastoma susceptibility gene product, pRb. *Cancer Res.* **54**:6078–6082(1994)

41. Lukas, J., H. Muller, J. Bartkova, D. Spitkovsky, A. A. Kjeruff, P. Jansen-Durr, M. Strauss, and J. Bartek. DNA tumor virus oncoproteins and retinoblastoma gene mutations share the ability to relieve the cell's requirement for cyclin D1 function in G1. *J. Cell Biol.* **125**:625–638(1994)

42. Meyerson, M., G. H. Enders, C-L. Wu, L-K. Su, C. Gorka, C. Neilson, E. Harlow, and L-H. Tsai. A family of human cdc2-related protein kinases. *EMBO J.* **11**:2909–2917(1992)

43. Meyerson, M. and E. Harlow. Identification of G1 kinase activity for cdk6, a novel cyclin D partner. *Mol. Cell Biol.* **14**:2077–2086(1994)

44. Michieli, P., M. Chedid, D. Lin, J. H. Pierce, E. Mercer, and D. Givol. Induction of WAF1/CIP1 by a p53-independent pathway. *Cancer Res.* **54**:3391–3395(1994)

45. Mori, T., K. Miura, T. Aoki, T. Nishihira, N. Shozo, and Y. Nakamura. Frequent somatic mutation of the MTS1/CDK4I (multiple tumor suppressor/cyclin-dependent kinase 4 inhibitor) gene in esophageal squamous cell carcinoma. *Cancer Res.* **54**:3396–3397(1994)

46. Nevins, J. R. E2F: a link between the Rb tumor suppressor protein and viral oncoproteins. *Science* **258**:424–429(1992)

47. Nigro, J. M., S. J. Baker, A. C. Preisinger, J. M. Jessup, R. Hostetter, K. Cleary, S. H. Bigner, N. Davison, S. Baylin, P. Devilee, T. Glover, F. Collins, A. Weston, R. Modali, C. C. Harris, and B. Vogelstein. Mutations in the p53 gene occur in diverse human tumor types. *Nature* **342**:705–708(1989)

48. Nobori, T., K. Mlura, D. J. Wu, A. Lois, K. Takabayashi, and D. A. Carson. Deletion of the cyclin-dependent kinase-4 inhibitor gene in multiple human cancers. *Nature* **368**:753–756(1994)

49. Noda, A., Y. Ning, S. F. Venable, O. M. Pereira-Smith, and J. R. Smith. Cloning of senescent cell-derived inhibitor of DNA synthesis using an expression screen. *Exp. Cell. Res.* **211**:90–98(1994)

50. Parker, S. B., G. Eichele, P. Zhang, A. Rawls, A. T. Sands, A. Bradley, E. N. Olson, J. W. Harper, and S. J. Elledge. p53-independent expression of p21^{Cip1} in muscle and other termnally differentiating cells. *Science* **267**:1024–1027(1995)

51. Parry, D., S. Bates, D. J. Mann, and G. Peters. Lack of cyclin D-Cdk complexes in Rb-negative cells correlates with high levels of p16$^{INK4/MTS1}$ tumour suppressor gene product. *EMBO J.* **14**:503–511(1995)

52. Polyak, K., M-H. Lee, H. Erdjument-Bromage, A. Koff, J. Roberts, P. Tempst, and J. Massague. Cloning of p27^{Kip1}, a cyclin-dependent kinase inhibitor and a potential mediator of extracellular antimitogenic signals. *Cell* **78**:59–66(1994)

53. Schauer, I. E., S. Siriwardana, T. A. Langan, and R. A. Sclafani. Cyclin D1 overexpression vs. retinoblastoma inactivation: implications for growth control evasion in non-small cell and small cell lung cancer. *Genes Chromosom Cancer* **91**:7827–7831(1994)

54. Scheffner, M., B. A. Werness, J. M. Huibregtse, A. J. Levine, and P. M. Howley. The E6 oncoprotein encoded by human papillomavirus types 16 and 18 promotes the degradation of p53. *Cell* **63**:1129–1136(1990)

55. Serrano, M., G. J. Hannon, and D. Beach. A new regulatory motif in cell cycle control causing specific inhibition of cyclin D/CDK4. *Nature* **366**:704–707(1993)

56. Shay, J. W., W. E. Wright, D. Brasiskyte, and B. A. Van Der Haegen. E6 of human papillomavirus type 16 can overcome the M1 stage of immortalization in human mammary epithelial cells but not in human fibroblasts. *Oncogene* **8**:1407–1413(1993)

57. Sherr, C. J. G1 phase progression: cycling on cue. *Cell* **79**:551–555(1994)

58. Sherr, C. J. and J. M. Roberts. Inhibitors of mammalian G1 cyclin-dependent kinases. *Genes & Dev.* **9**:1149–1163(1995)

59. Shew, J. Y., B. T. Lin, P. L. Chen, B. Y. Tseng, T. L. Yang-Feng, and W. H. Lee. C-terminal truncation of the retinoblastoma gene product leads to functional inactivation. *Proc. Natl. Acad. Sci. USA* **87**:6–10(1990)

60. Solomon, M. J. Activation of the various cyclin-cdc2 protein kinases. *Current Opin. Cell Biol.* **5**:180–186(1993)

61. Spruck III, C. H., M. Gonzalez-Zulueta, A. Shibata, A. R. Simoneau, M-F. Lin, F. Gonzales, Y. C. Tsai, and P. A. Jones. p16 gene in uncultured tumors. *Nature* **370**:183–184(1994)

62. Steinman, R. A., B. Hoffman, A. Iro, C. Guillouf, D. A. Liebermann, and M. E. El-houseini. Induction of p21 (WAF1/CIP1) during differentiation. *Oncogene* **9**:3389–3396(1994)

63. Tam, S. W., A. M. Theodoras, J. W. Shay, G. F. Draetta, and M. Pagano. Differential expression and regulation of Cyclin D1 protein in normal and tumor human cells: association with Cdk4 is required for Cyclin D1 function in G1 progression. *Oncogene* **9**:2663–2674(1994)

64. Toyoshima, H. and T. Hunter. p27, a novel inhibitor of G1 cyclin-Cdk proteins kinase activity, is related to p21. *Cell* **78**:67–74(1994)

65. Waga, S., G. J. Hannon, D. Beach, and B. Stillman. The p21 inhibitor of cyclin-dependent kinases controls DNA replication by interaction with PCNA. *Nature* **369**:574–578(1994)

66. Wharton, K. A., K. M. Johansen, T. Xu, and S. Artavanis-Tsakonas. Nucleotide sequence from the neurogenic locus notch implies a gene product that shares homology with proteins containing EGF-like repeats. *Cell* **43**:567–581(1985)

67. Won, K. A., Y. Xiong, D. Beach, and M. Z. Gilman. Growth-regulated expression of D-type cyclin genes in human diploid fibroblasts. *Proc. Natl. Acad. Sci. USA* **89**:9910–9914(1992)

68. Xiong, Y. and D. Beach. Population explosion in the cyclin family. *Current Biol.* **1**:362–364(1991)

69. Xiong, Y., G. Hannon, H. Zhang, D. Casso, R. Kobayashi, and D. Beach. p21 is a universal inhibitor of the cyclin kinases. *Nature* **366**:701–704(1993)

70. Xiong, Y., H. Zhang, and D. Beach. D-type cyclins associated with multiple protein kinases and the DNA replication and repair factor PCNA. *Cell* **71**:505–514(1992)
71. Xiong, Y., H. Zhang, and D. Beach. Subunit rearrangement of cyclin-dependent kinases is associated with cellular transformation. *Genes & Dev.* 7:1572–1583(1993)
72. Zhang, H., Y. Xiong, and D. Beach. Proliferating cell nuclear antigen and p21 are components of multiple cell cycle kinase complexes. *Mol. Biol. Cell* 4:897–906(1993)
73. Zhu, L., S. van den Heuvel, K. Helin, A. Fattaey, M. Ewen, D. Livingston, N. Dyson, and E. Harlow. Inhibition of cell proliferation by p107, a relative of the retinoblastoma protein. *Genes & Dev.* 7:1111–1125(1993)

DISCUSSION

M. Oren: Could you elaborate on the biochemical differences between the binary complexes of CDK/cyclin versus the ternary complex with one monomer of p21 both of which are active, in principle?

Y. Xiong: Yes and actually there have been quite a number of studies on that issue. The bottom line is that if we have one molecule of p21 per molecule of cyclin, CDK is still active. In other words, you need more than one molecule of p21, as well as p27 per molecule of CDK in order to inhibit. Whether it is two to one, or three to one is not very clear right now. And that even further indicates the possibility that p21 may actually play some kind of positive role, probably by stabilizing the cyclin CDK complex.

M. Oren: Is there evidence for that?

Y. Xiong: Not very directly. Not that I know about it.

M. Oren: Does the fact that PCNA is part of this quaternary complex have any significance in targeting, let us say, to the DNA replication machinery?

Y. Xiong: That is a good question. I mentioned that p21 can directly interact with PCNA and inhibit the PCNA-dependent DNA replication, but I must say that even though we have identified the quaternary complex containing cyclin, CDK, p21 in the PCNA we know absolutely nothing about what function p21 plays in those complexes.

M. Kulesz-Martin: You alluded to the idea that p21 may be coming up, at least at the MRNA level, in the G2 or G2/M transition - which of the cyclin-dependent kinase inhibitors do you think might have specific roles in G1 and which do you think have roles in G2 as well; could you speculate about their roles in G2?

Y. Xiong: Yes, but it is pretty misleading when people get CDK inhibitor proteins co-expressed with the CD20 marker. If I am right, in almost every case you can overexpress CDK inhibitors and invariably at also G1 arrest. And people intended to reach a conclusion that all those CDK inhibitors are G1 specific inhibitors. I frankly have difficulty accepting that conclusion. One possibility is that the G1 phase is more sensitive and this does not rule out the possibility of those CDK inhibitors also functioning in G2 phase. To answer your question, there is no direct evidence to link the function of any one CDK inhibitor with a G2 cell cycle check point. And we do have one piece of evidence that micro-injection of p20 proteins actually arrest cells in G2 as well as in G1. But at the moment we cannot say too much about it.

F. Rauscher: That is a really important point, that is, how are you going to experimentally test whether there is actually cell-cycle specificity in terms of a compartment for each of these particular kinase inhibitors. Since overexpression, as you said, is not sufficient at all. You are always going to get G1 expressed particularly in a heterogeneous population.

Y. Xiong: That is right. There are two ways to do that; one is to take a normal cell to determine what is a normal expression pattern during the cell cycle; or you can perform a cell cycle micro-injection experiment which allows you to pick up a cell at different stages and then look for the effect on DNA synthesis block or cell division.

D. Livingston: Two questions: first, regarding this very interesting model that suggests that Rb autoregulates the expression of the p16 gene, do you have any sense of what the transcription factor may be and have you tested any member of the E2F family to see whether it behaves in this way?

Y. Xiong: Yes, we did it and we have sequenced more than 3kb upstream of the p16 promoter. We did not detect any obvious E2F binding site. We also did a preliminary experiment to co-transfect E2F with p16 and we did not see any stimulation either. At the moment, we do not have any evidence that E2F is involved.

D. Livingston: If you E1A + Rb cotransfect an Rb-/- cell, like SAOS-2, can you activate the p16 locus?

Y. Xiong: That has not been done.

D. Livingston: Would you interpret your last set of experiments to imply that p18 has a specific role in linking cell cycle arrest to myogenesis?

Y. Xiong: Absolutely, and the most obvious question is, what is the upstream signal for the p18? We have no idea as to which factor activates p18 during myogenesis. We tested the myo D and it does not do it. It is not a myo D dependent.

E. Nigg: There is evidence from both David Morgan's lab and from my lab, that in order to form the CDK7/cyclin H complex, you do need a third component. Is there any evidence that you do need p21 to form a CDK4-cyclin D complex?

Y. Xiong: No. We actually tried hard at the beginning before we realized that the p21 can block CAK phosphorylation on CDK. Initially we tried very hard to detect the p21, either *in vitro* or *in vivo* in the CAK complex and the answer is that we cannot detect it.

E. Nigg: My question was whether there was evidence that p21 is actually needed to form, say a cyclin A-CDK2 or a cyclin D-CDK4 complex?

Y. Xiong: It does not need it for CDK-7-cyclin H.

E. Nigg: It does not need it?

Y. Xiong: It does not need it; perhaps it can stabilize it a little bit but it is not required. Cyclin A CDK can be assembled in the absence of p21 very nicely.

C. Goding: You said that low levels of p21 mixed with the cyclin CDK complex do not inhibit the cyclin CDK complex phosphorylation, is that right?

Y. Xiong: Yes, in low ratio, for example, one to one.

C. Goding: Is there any evidence that p21 or any of these other CDK inhibitors are activated, for example, by phosphorylation or by dephosphorylation?

Y. Xiong: There are studies from Beach lab published last year on Genes and Development that p21 is actually a phospho-protein, but there is not any data to say that that phosphorylation has anything to do with p21 functions. That is all I can tell.

D. Livingston: What is the evidence that allows one to say that a protein like p21 is not required physiologically *in vivo* to promote the formation of G1 cyclin CDK-2 complex?

Y. Xiong: Yes, I agree. First, there is no functional mutant of p21 available. Eventually you have to do the knock out experiment. But in cell lines the cyclin CDK complex can be assembled at the level of p21 that is almost undetectable. We sort of use that as indirect evidence to say that the p21 is not required for assembly, and that would be consistent with the *in vitro* data showing that you actually can assemble an active kinase complex without p21.

M. Fried: You get the impression that p21 activity is entirely dependent on p53, but can it be made in the absence of p53?

Y. Xiong: Right. But that is a very important question and I actually think I might have missed the point. Although p21 generated a lot of interest as a physiological target for p53, now it has been shown in several labs, including ours, that the p21 gene expression can be fully activated in the absence of wild type p53 function. For example, something I did not show you is that TGF-β can induce p21 expression. Those experiments were done in a cell line with mutant p53 and so yes, p21 can be induced or activated through a p53 independent pathway. I think that had been very nicely done in mouse p53 knock out cell lines and published just a few weeks ago by Tyler Jacks.

M. Fried: And the second question is that you showed that p18 might be cell specific but p16 is the one that is usually found deleted, is that also cell type specific?

Y. Xiong: Yes. That is a very good point. p16 functions in tumor growth suppression as it has been found deleted or mutated in several primary tumors. However, in normal human cells, we have examined more than fourteen different tissues, we can now detect p16 message using up to two micrograms poly-A plus RNA. In a sense, that would be consistent with the idea of expressing wild type Rb with a suppressed p16 expression. So, without being able to detect p16 in any of those tissues, we cannot really say what is the tissue specific pattern of p16 gene expression, at least not in human tissues.

G. Evan: Can I go back to this business about whether p21 might be required or essential during normal proliferation or some other aspect of cell behavior. I mean, is it a legitimate question to ask why is it that p21 is never lost in tumors? Given that there is clearly strong selection against p53 and one of the targets of p53 is p21, so why do we not lose p21 in any tumors that have been found?

Y. Xiong: The answer to that comment is two-fold. Number one, you do not need to mutate p21 if you already have in 50–60% of tumors loss of p53 function.

G. Evan: That is just saying that it is an alternative route. And you already said that there are other routes - other major routes - for expressing p21 anyway, so it would make sense to go downstream and exert stronger selection to lose p21 and p53, but it does not happen, why?

Y. Xiong: There are several pieces of data pointing to the possibility that p21 could promote cell cycle progression. When a cell comes out of G0 arrest, normally you would predict that the inhibitor proteins holding cells at G0 should decrease. Instead p21 goes up first, and that would be consistent with the idea that during the early G1, p21 might play some positive yet unidentified role. Mechanically, I have no idea what p21 might be doing. That is from speculation that p21 might be stabilizing cyclin CDK that would a positive role. Secondly, the induction of p21 during early G1 phase has been observed in a number of signaling pathways. And my suspicion is that the p21 might play a positive role in the early G1 phase when cells exit from G0. Right now I do not know of any good evidence to indicate that p21 is absolutely required for G1 progression.

G. Draetta: I wanted to comment on the p21 inhibition studies. There is a paper published by Wade Harper's group in which Cdk inhibition kinetics are reported. The p21 kI for cdc2/cyclin B complex was found by these authors to be at least 100-fold higher than the Ki for G1 cyclins and cyclin A complexes. At least *in vitro* therefore, there seem to be a clear preference of p21 for G1/S cyclin complexes, which might explain why, in response to p21 elevation cells arrest predominantly in the G1-phase of the cell cycle. I have a question for you. You had originally found that cyclin D1 can also associate with Cdk2 and with Cdk5. Have you done anything to show that those complexes have any role in the cell cycle?

Y. Xiong: Cyclin D1 is actually one of the most amazing cyclins among all those in the cyclin family. Although it has different affinities, Cyclin D1 can be detected easily *in vivo* associated with every CDK. Today, the only thing we know about D1 function is that it is active in CDK-4, CDK-6 toward Rb substrate. We do not have any idea what cyclin D1 is doing when it becomes associated with CDK-2, CDK-5 and CDC-2.

E. Nigg: I have a question about the presence of PCNA in all these complexes. I think all of us can make an intriguing link between PCNA and the cyclin A or cyclin D complexes, but I have trouble with the cyclin B part - why would PCNA be in cyclin B complexes? These are cytoplasmic and it is not at all clear if and how they are functionally related to replication.

Y. Xiong: Yes, I completely agree with you. As I said initially, we saw associations between cyclin D and PCNA and we were pretty excited for a few weeks, and we thought that PCNA was exactly what we had been looking for the function of cyclin D, so that must be how it does the job. And, as I said later, we realized that p21 and PCNA can be both detected in mitotic kinases such as cyclin B and the CDC-2. Apparently, that probably has nothing to do with DNA replication. I just have absolutely no idea what PCNA is doing in those associations. But those complexes are so stable and so easy to detect that you can reconstitute them *in vitro:* we just have to wait to find out what PCNA is doing in those complexes.

5

P53-MEDIATED APOPTOSIS

Regulatory and Mechanistic Aspects

Ygal Haupt,[1] Sheldon Rowan,[1] Eitan Shaulian,[1] Eyal Gottlieb,[1]
Elisheva Yonish-Rouach,[2] Karen Vousden,[3] and Moshe Oren[1]

[1] Department of Chemical Immunology
The Weizmann Institute of Science
Rehovot 76100, Israel
[2] Lab. Oncologie Moleculaire, IRSC
94891 Villejuif Cedex, France
[3] NCI-Frederick Research and Development Center
Frederick, Maryland 21702

INTRODUCTION

The p53 gene is an important tumor suppressor gene, whose inactivation appears to play a pivotal role in many types of cancer[1–3]. The p53 protein, encoded by this gene, is a potent sequence-specific transcriptional activator[4,5]. Binding of the p53 protein to genes which contain consensus p53 binding sites results in a pronounced increase in their transcription rates[6–11]. Transcriptional activation of relevant target genes, mediated through high affinity sequence-specific DNA binding, is believed to be responsible for many of the biological effects of the wild-type p53 (wt p53) protein. This is supported by the fact that the overwhelming majority of p53 mutations found in human tumors abrogate DNA binding, either by altering direct DNA contact residues or through destabilizing the structure of the DNA binding domain[12,13].

However, in addition to sequence-specific transactivation (SST), the p53 protein has been shown to possess a number of other, distinct biochemical activities. These include relatively non-specific transcriptional repression, DNA strand annealing, binding to single stranded DNA and RNA, and possibly also an ability to participate in translational regulation[3]. Whether, and to what extent, these other activities of p53 contribute to its biological effects and to its potential as a tumor suppressor, remains an open question.

In view of the strong indications that p53 is primarily a sequence-specific transcriptional activator, extensive efforts have been directed at identifying relevant target genes. Several very attractive candidates have already been identified, and their number is likely to grow. Among those described thus far, perhaps the most revealing is the Waf1/Cip1 gene. This gene encodes a polypeptide of 21 kDa (p21), which serves as a potent inhibitor of a wide array of cyclin/cyclin dependent kinase (cdk) complexes[14–17]. Induction of p21 expression typically follows the activation of p53 by a variety of signals and experimental manipulations [18,19]. When p21 accumulates to sufficiently high levels, it can block the kinase activity of cyclin/cdk complexes, thereby freezing the cell cycle machinery and forcing a growth arrest. In the case of p53, this arrest is most often in G1[20–24], although more recent studies demonstrate that under certain circumstances a p53-mediated G2 arrest can also occur[25–27]. In addition, p21 can form a physical association with PCNA, a co-factor of DNA polymerase δ, and block directly DNA replication[28–30]. Activation of p21 gene expression by p53 may therefore result in a coordinated block of the cell cycle machinery and of replicative DNA synthesis, thereby achieving a "balanced" growth arrest.

Other attractive p53 target genes include the Gadd45 gene[10], whose protein product also binds to PCNA, and can inhibit replicative DNA synthesis while at the same time enhancing repair DNA synthesis[31], the cyclin G gene[32,33], whose exact biochemical functions are presently unknown, and the mdm2 gene[34–36], whose major product probably functions within a negative feed-back loop to restrict the extent and duration of p53-mediated responses. Of particular interest is the Bax gene[37–39], overexpression of whose product can effectively induce apoptotic cell death[40]. Activation of Bax by p53 would appear to explain, at least in part, the propensity of wt p53 to elicit apoptosis under a variety of circumstances (see later). Other candidate p53 target genes, such as thrombospondin 1[41], may account for inhibitory effects of p53 during advanced stages of tumor progression in vivo.

In many cell types, overexpression of active wt p53 causes a viable growth arrest. Under physiological circumstances, this is believed to provide the cell with an opportunity to deal successfully with stress signals which operate through p53, and particularly to repair limited DNA damage so that faulty DNA is not replicated during the S phase of the cell cycle[24,42]. in addition, however, there are now many cases where p53 has been shown to induce cell death, through a process bearing the hallmarks of apoptosi[43].

The ability of wt p53 to trigger apoptosis has first been revealed in the murine myeloid leukemic cell line M1[44]. M1 cells express no detectable endogenous p53 mRNA or protein. They grow rapidly in culture in the presence of serum, without showing a requirement for specific hematopoietic growth factors. To study the effect of wt p53 on M1 cells, they were stably transfected with a temperature-sensitive p53 mutant, p53val135, to generate M1val135 clones. The p53val135 mutant is similar to typical tumor-derived p53 mutants when the cells are kept at 37.5°C, but regains wt p53 properties upon down-shift of the cells to 32°C[20]. When M1val135 cells are shifted to 32°C, the exogenous p53 protein is activated. This is followed by a rapid induction of p53 target gene expression, and a rapid repression of certain other genes such as c-myc[37,45,46]. Most remarkably, the induction of wt p53 activity at 32°C results in massive apoptotic cell death; at the level of the whole cell population, the process is usually evident within less than 10 hours, and is complete by 48 hours[44].

Subsequent studies have shown that overexpression of p53, achieved experimentally via the ts mutant p53val135 or through a variety of other means, can trigger apoptosis in a wide spectrum of cell types[47–54]. Importantly, the physiological relevance of these observations was enhanced by the finding that thymocytes of p53 null ("knock-out") mice are severely deficient in their ability to undergo apoptosis in response to irradiation[55,56], a treatment which normally results in a marked increase in p53 levels[24,57]. This fact may have important bearing on the response of cancer cells to DNA damage-based cancer therapy[58].

In addition, p53 has been shown to contribute, at least quantitatively, to the efficient apoptotic death of factor-dependent hematopoietic cells deprived of critical survival factors[60–63]. In this context p53 does not appear to be obligatory, as also suggested by the apparently normal development of the hematopoietic lineages in p53 null mice. Nevertheless, even a mild effect attained through the loss of p53 function may provide cells with a selective growth advantage, in an in vivo environment which imposes competition for limiting survival factors.

In view of the great potential clinical importance of this issue, there is a growing interest in trying to determine the factors which dictate whether a cell will respond to wt p53 activation by a viable growth arrest or by apoptotic death (it should be noted that a third option -no response at all- also exists, particularly in non-neoplastic cells). A recent study has shown that the outcome can depend on the presence of appropriate survival factors[64], which is in line with the above-mentioned effect of p53 on death following factor deprivation. It is conceivable, however, that there may be many additional factors which modulate the cellular response to p53. The experiments described below were undertaken to address this important question, as well as to probe some of the biochemical pathways that underlie p53-mediated apoptosis.

OVEREXPRESSION OF WILD-TYPE P53 FAILS TO INDUCE A GROWTH ARREST IN M1 CELLS, BUT COOPERATES WITH IL-6 TO INDUCE A VIABLE G_0-LIKE ARREST

We wished to find out whether the apoptotic effect of excess wt p53 activity in M1 cells is coupled with a cell cycle arrest. To that end, M1val135 cells were shifted to 32°C, resulting in the induction of wt p53 activity and the eventual apoptotic elimination of the cells. Cell cycle progression was monitored by FACS analysis of cells stained with propidium iodide, to allow the quantification of total cellular DNA content as a measure of cell cycle distribution. In parallel, the incorporation of bromodeoxy-uridine (BrdU) was determined as a measure of the rate of S phase DNA synthesis.

This analysis revealed that the activation of wt p53 failed to alter significantly the cell cycle distribution of M1val135 cells[45]. The cells continued to exhibit a substantial S phase sub-population, and there was no increase in the proportion of cells in G_1. This was in striking contrast to the effect that the same ts p53val135 protein exerted on ras-transformed fibroblasts, where a very prominent growth arrest was easily discernible[20,45,65,66] Moreover, M1 cells exposed to high levels of wt p53 activity continued to replicate their DNA in S phase, as reflected by extensive BrdU incorporation. In contrast, wt p53-overexpressing fibroblasts practically ceased completely to incorporate BrdU when maintained for 24 hours at 32°C[45].

A very different picture was revealed when M1val135 cells were shifted down to 32°C in the presence of interleukin-6 (IL-6). IL-6 is capable of offering M1val135 cells substantial protection against p53-mediated apoptosis[44]. This is in keeping with its role as a potent survival factor for hematopoietic cells[67]. When a cell cycle analysis was performed at 32°C in the presence of IL-6, it was easily evident that the M1val135 cells now underwent a very pronounced growth arrest. This was reflected both by the accumulation of the vast majority of the population in a G_0-like state, as well as by a dramatic reduction in the rate of BrdU incorporation into cellular DNA[46,62]. It is of note that, at least within the first 24 hours after its addition, IL-6 alone did not cause a significant alteration in the

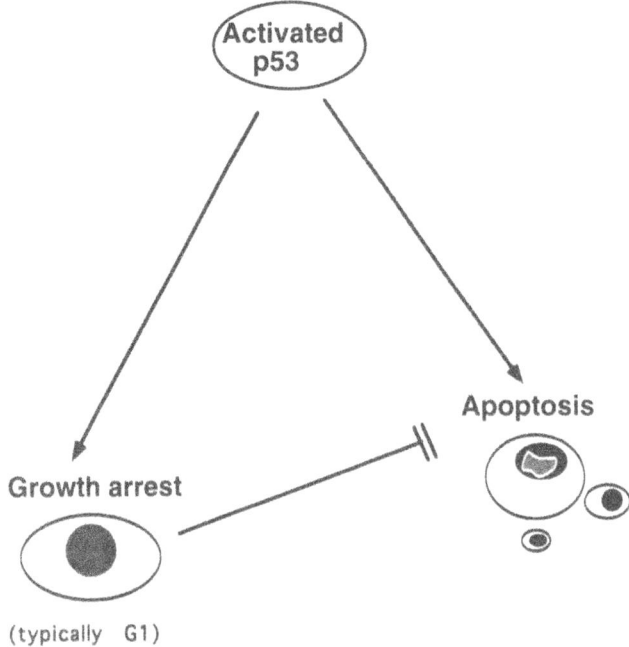

Figure 1. Simplified dual-signal model for the effect of p53 activation on cell fate. See text for further details.

cell cycle of M1val135 cells at 37.5°C, when wt p53 activity was absent[62]. Hence, the ability of IL-6 to rescue M1 cells from p53-mediated apoptosis is coupled with an ability to convert an ongoing cell cycle into a tight growth arrest.

IL-6 has multiple effects on M1 cells[67]. Nevertheless, one very attractive interpretation of our observations could be that the effective growth arrest induced by IL-6 is causally related to the ability of this cytokine to act as an inhibitor of p53-mediated apoptosis. One could propose that p53, when activated, gives rise to a dual signal (fig. 1). On the one hand, it triggers events which will normally culminate in a tight growth arrest. In parallel, it activates an apoptotic response. The model depicted in fig. 1 proposes that if a proper growth arrest is established, it will protect cells from p53-mediated apoptosis. Conversely, if for any reason the cell fails to undergo a "well balanced" growth arrest, the apoptotic option will be executed. The prediction is therefore that conditions, physiological or pathological, which interfere with the ability of p53 to enforce a "well balanced" growth arrest, will predispose the cell to undergo apoptosis in response to the activation of wt p53.

OVEREXPRESSION OF FUNCTIONAL pRB PROTECTS FROM p53-MEDIATED APOPTOSIS

What is the nature of the p53-dependent "well balanced" growth arrest, proposed in fig. 1? Many recent studies have suggested that p53 arrests cell proliferation primarily through the transcriptional activation of the Waf1 gene. The consequent production of the p21 polypeptide is then expected to block the kinase activity of a variety of cyclin/cdk

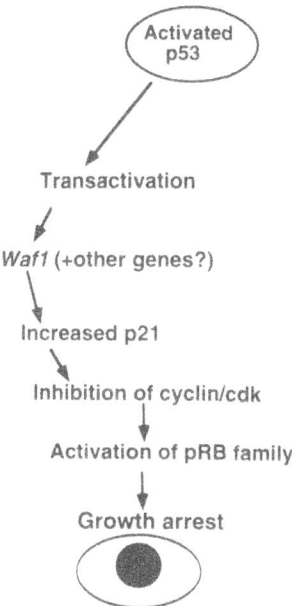

Figure 2. chematic model for the induction of a p53-mediated "well balanced" growth arrest. See text for further details.

complexes, and particularly that of the G1 cyclin-associated kinases. These kinases are believed to be responsible for the cell cycle-regulated phosphorylation of the pRB protein encoded by the retinoblastoma susceptibility tumor suppressor gene, as well as of the related p107 and p130 proteins (the "RB family"). Hence, induction of p21 by p53 will eventually lead to the accumulation of underphosphorylated pRB family members (fig. 2), which constitute the growth-inhibitory forms of these proteins. The end result is proposed to be the "well balanced" growth arrest.

The schematic model shown in fig. 2 identifies the pRB family as a critical component of the pathway leading to a "well balanced" p53-mediated growth arrest. A further prediction from this model, along with the one shown in fig. 1, is that cells deficient in normal pRB family function will be poised to apoptose when confronted with excess wt p53 activity. We sought to subject this prediction to an experimental test. To that end, use was made of HeLa cells. HeLa cells are derived from a human cervical carcinoma, and express the E6 and E7 proteins of human papilloma virus (HPV). The E6 protein inactivates the cellular p53 function, by targeting the endogenous HeLa wt p53 for rapid ubiquitin-dependent degradation, as well as by interfering with the transcriptional activity of the residual protein[68]. Similarly, the E7 protein eliminates endogenous pRB family protein function, in this case by binding to the latter proteins and preventing their interaction with their normal cellular targets[68].

HeLa cells can thus be viewed as being highly deficient in both p53 and pRB family function. According to the rationale outlined above, they should fail to undergo a "well balanced" growth arrest in response to wt p53 activation. Instead, they will be expected to exhibit an apoptotic response. Moreover, if the model is correct, re-introduction of high levels of wt pRB into HeLa cells, enough to overcome the inhibitory effect of HPV E7, should now restore the proper arrest pathway and rescue the cells from p53-mediated apoptosis.

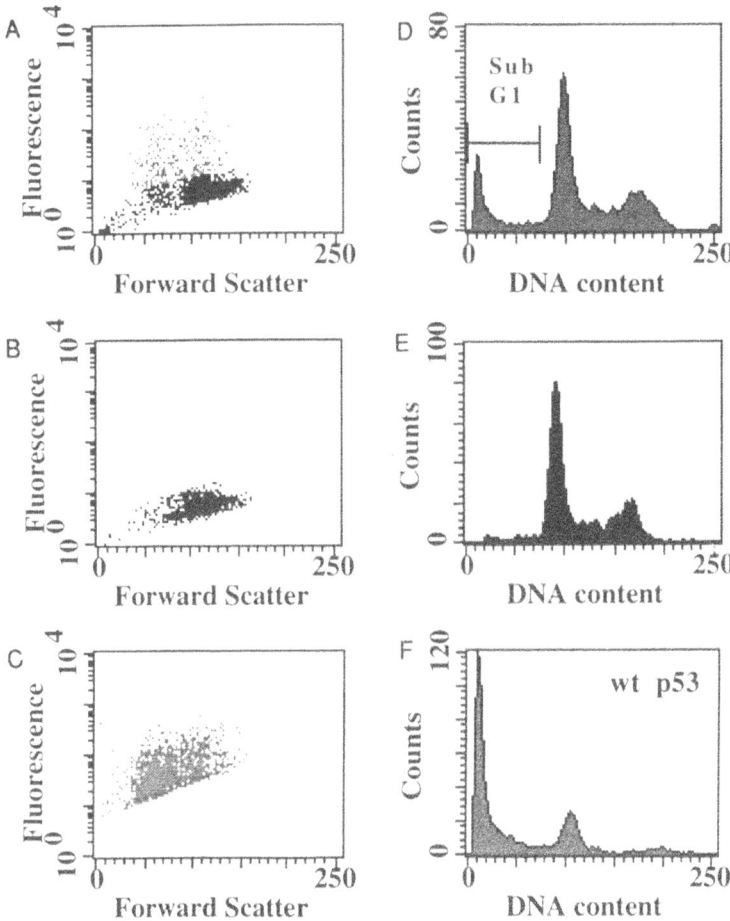

Figure 3. Induction of apoptosis by overexpression of wt p53 in HeLa cells. HeLa cells were transiently transfected, by the calcium phosphate method, with an expression plasmid encoding mouse wt p53. Cells were fixed 56
hours later, and stained with monoclonal antibody PAb248 to monitor mouse p53 expression, and with propidium
iodide to monitor DNA content. Cells were then analysed in the FACS (FACSCAN, Becton-Dickinson). Panel A
depicts p53 content as a function of cell size in the total population. Panel D depicts the corresponding DNA content distribution. Panels B and C are similar to A, except that cells were gated to resolve high p53 expressors (C)
from non-expressors (B). The corresponding DNA content distributions are shown in panels F and E, respectively.

These predictions were tested in a transient transfection-based apoptosis assay.
Briefly, HeLa cells are transfected by the calcium phosphate method, and 48–72 hours
were subjected to FACS analysis. Two parameters are monitored in parallel- level of p53
expression (assayed by a specific monoclonal antibody), and DNA content (assayed by
propidium iodide staining). The latter serves as an indication of the position of a given cell
within the cell cycle.

The results of such an analysis are shown in fig. 3. Panel A depicts the distribution
of p53 fluorescence intensity, plotted against cell size (forward scatter). It is obvious that
the majority of cells in the transfected culture exhibit only background staining, suggesting that they don't express significant amounts of the exogenous wt p53. In addition,

though, there are some cells (typically a few percent of the total) which exhibit highly elevated p53 levels; note that p53 fluorescence is depicted on a log scale. These p53 overexpressors are absent in mock-transfected cultures (data not shown), and therefore must represent the successfully transfected cells which express the exogenous wt p53.

Analysis of the DNA content in the total transfected culture revealed that the majority of cells displayed a normal cell cycle distribution (fig. 3D). In addition, however, there was also a small fraction of cells with sub-G1 DNA content. Such reduced DNA content is the result of the loss of DNA, and is characteristic of apoptotic cells. The data therefore imply the presence of some apoptotic cells within the total population of the HeLa culture.

As p53-overexpressing cells represented a small minority in the culture, they were resolved from the bulk population of non-transfected cells by setting an appropriate gate in the FACS for p53 expression level. Fig. 3C and fig. 3B show the p53-positive sub-population and the bulk p53-negative sub-population, respectively. Each panel contains an equal number (2000) of cells; in the case of panel C, many more cells had to be sorted in order to obtain the required number of p53-positive cells.

The DNA content patterns of each sub-population are shown in panels E and F. A very striking difference is immediately obvious. Whereas the bulk, p53-negative fraction exhibits a perfectly normal cell cycle distribution, with very little apoptosis (panel E), the p53-positive cells (panel F) are predominantly in the sub-G1 catergory, implying that they are highly apoptotic. In fact, they practically account for all the apoptotic events seen in the non-gated population (panel D). This experiment demonstrates very clearly that overexpression of wt p53 in HeLa cells is correlated with a massive induction of apoptosis, in keeping with the above model. It is of note that, unlike wt p53, a variety of tumor-derived murine and human p53 mutants were essentially devoid of any apoptotic activity in the same assay[54,69].

We next wished to find out whether excess pRB can reverse the apoptotic effect of p53 in HeLa cells, presumably the correcting the growth arrest defect. Cells were therefore transiently transfected as in fig. 3, except that this time some of the transfection mixtures included also expression plasmids encoding either functional, wt pRB, or a non-functional mutant thereof (pRBD22). The results of such an analysis are shown in fig. 4. As expected, transfection with wt p53 plus a control plasmid resulted in a substantial fraction of cells with sub-G1 DNA content, implying extensive apoptosis (panel A, right). Cells co-transfected with wt p53 plus wt pRB, on the other hand, exhibited a much smaller proportion of sub-G1 cells (tRB; panel B, right). This was in contrast to the picture obtained when mutant pRB was used; in this case (mRB; panel C, right), the extent of apoptosis was practically indistinguishable from that seen in the absence of a pRB plasmid. Thus, the overexpression of functional pRB, but not of a defective pRB mutant, can greatly reduce the ability of p53 to elicit apoptosis in HeLa cells. Similar observations, in a different cell system, were also reported by Qin et al[70]. This finding lends strong support to the model outlined in figures 1 and 2.

TRANSACTIVATION-DEFICIENT MUTANTS OF p53 CAN ELICIT APOPTOSIS IN HELA CELLS

Most, if not all, existing data suggest that p53 functions primarily as a sequence-specific transcriptional activator. It was of great interest to find out whether sequence-specific transcriptional activation of target genes could also account for all the apoptotic effects of wt p53. To that end, a series of deletion mutants was constructed, removing various portions of the C-terminal region of p53. These mutants are schematically drawn in figure 5.

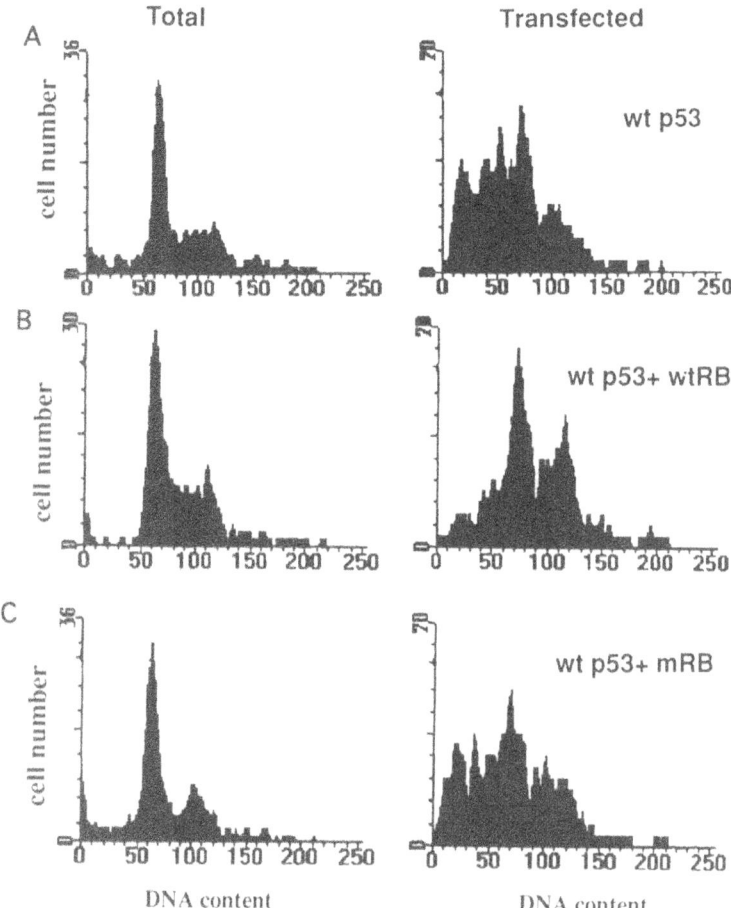

Figure 4. Excess pRB protects HeLa cells from p53-mediated apoptosis. Experimental details are as in figure 3 except that, in addition to a wt mouse p53 expression plasmid, the transfection mixtures also included plasmids encoding wt pRB (panels B), mutant pRB (pRBΔ22, panels C), or an empty vector control (panels A). In each case, the left and right panels depict the non-expressing and the p53-overexpressing subpopulation, respectively. Reproduced, with permission, from Haupt et al. [69]

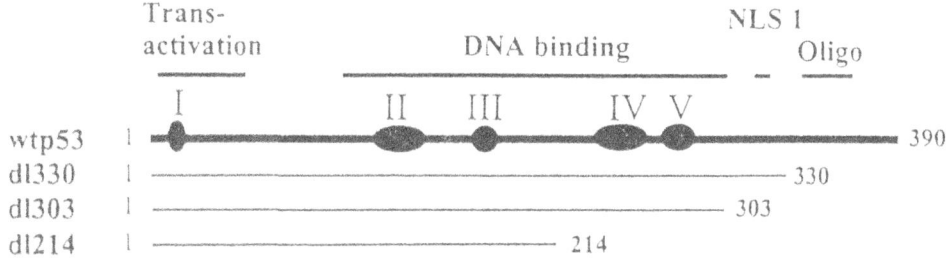

Figure 5. Schematic map of the p53 C-terminal deletion mutants employed in this study. The top line indicates some hallmarks of wt p53; these include the transcriptonal transactivation domain, the sequence-specific DNA binding domain.

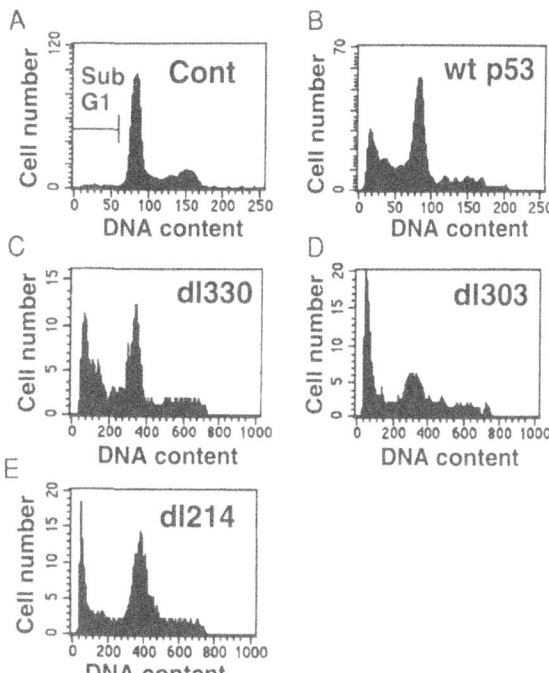

Figure 6. Induction of apoptosis by various p53 deletion mutants. The mutants are schematically described in fig. 5. Analysis was as in fig. 3; only the p53-overexpressing sub-population is shown in each case. Panel A depicts the analysis of cells which do not overexpress exogenous p53.

Each of the mutants, along with appropriate controls, was subjected to a transient transfection assay for apoptosis in HeLa cells. The results are shown in figure 6.

As expected, full length wt p53 was an effective inducer of apoptosis (panel B). Two mutants which delete relatively small portions of the C terminus, p53dl330 (panel C) and p53dl303 (panel D), also elicited an apoptotic response. Both these mutants, although missing the oligomerization domain of p53, have previously been shown to activate p53-responsive target genes when expressed at sufficiently high concentrations[71]. More surprisingly, however, a remarkable fraction of apoptotic cells was also present following transfection with the p53dl214 mutant, which retains only the first 214 residues of mouse p53 (panel E). This mutant lacks a major portion of the sequence-specific DNA binding domain[72], and is thus not expected to recognize target genes bearing p53 consensus binding sites. Since such recognition is required for SST of p53 target genes, p53dl214 is unlikely to retain the ability to activate p53-responsive promoters. As shown in figure 7, this was indeed found to be the case. Thus, under the conditions used for the apoptosis assay, wt p53 could induce the expression of the RGC-luciferase promoter, containing 17 tandem synthetic p53 binding sites. In contrast, p53dl214 failed to activate this p53-responsive promoter (fig. 7), or another p53-responsive promoter, containing the natural mdm2 gene intronic promoter (data not shown). In agreement with earlier findings[71], p53dl330 retained a partial potential for SST in HeLa cells.

Taken together, the data imply that p53dl214 can induce apoptosis in transiently transfected HeLa cells, despite being unable to stimulate the SST of p53-responsive promoters. Essentially similar observations were made with a human p53 mutant bearing 2 point mutations at positions 22 and 23 of its transactivation domain. This mutant is markedly compromised for SST[73], and is rather ineffective in the activation of natural p53-responsive promoters in HeLa cells (data not shown). Nevertheless, it is a potent inducer of

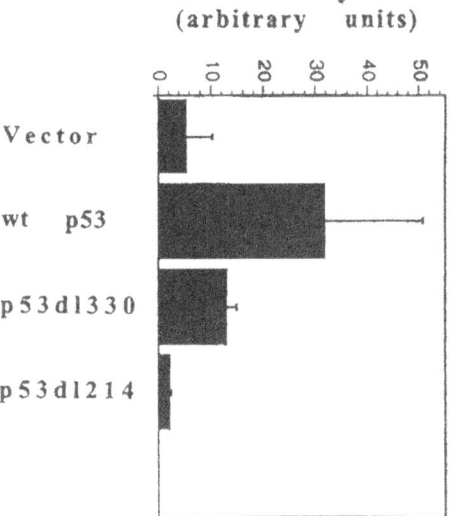

Activity
(arbitrary units)

Vector

wt p53

p53dl330

p53dl214

Figure 7. Activation of a p53-responsive reporter gene by p53 variants. HeLa cells were transfected with CMV-driven expression plasmids encoding the indicated p53 variants, along with a reporter plasmid (RGC-luciferase) containing 17 copies of a synthetic p53 binding site (derived from the ribosomal gene cluster) in front of the firefly luciferase gene. CMV- vector control. Extracts were prepared and luciferase activity determined 18 hours later. The analysis was carried out early after transfection, to minimize secondary effects of the cell death processes.

apoptosis in these cells (data not shown). On the assumption that a failure to transactivate a transfected p53-responsive reporter is a faithful reflection of an inability to induce endogenous p53-responsive genes, the data argue that p53-mediated apoptosis can be achieved, at least in some cell types, through a pathway which does not rely on the SST of typical p53 target genes.

The ability to induce apoptosis in the absence of detectable SST does not imply that SST is normally dispensable for this process. In fact, the opposite is most likely to be the case. This is also suggested by the data in fig. 8. In the analysis shown in this figure, the fraction of apoptotic (sub-G1 DNA content) cells was assessed at various times following transfection of HeLa cells with either wt p53 (black bars), p53dl214 (dashed bars), or a tumor-derived murine p53 mutant, p53phe132 (gray bars). It can be clearly seen that the onset of wt p53-mediated apoptosis is faster than that achieved by p53dl214. In the case of p53dl214, massive accumulation of apoptotic cells is seen only at later time points. This is not due to differences in the amount of protein; p53dl214 is actually expressed very efficiently in HeLa cells (data not shown). Hence, wt p53 appears to possess an additional activity, lacking in p53dl214, which enhances apoptosis. Our data do not specify the nature of this activity. Nevertheless, SST is a most likely candidate. If that is indeed the case, then these observations would argue that, even in cell types where high enough levels of SST-deficient p53 are sufficient for apoptosis, SST is still required for optimal apoptotic activity of p53.

Discussion

The data described above delineate two distinct aspects of p53-mediated apoptosis. First, the decision of a cell whether or not to respond to the activation of wt p53 by undergoing apoptosis is dependent, at least in part, on the functional state of the pRB family. Second, at least in some cell types, overexpression of an SST-deficient p53 molecule suffices to drive the cell into apoptosis. A comprehensive model, which attempts to fit together these and other published observations, is presented in figure 9.

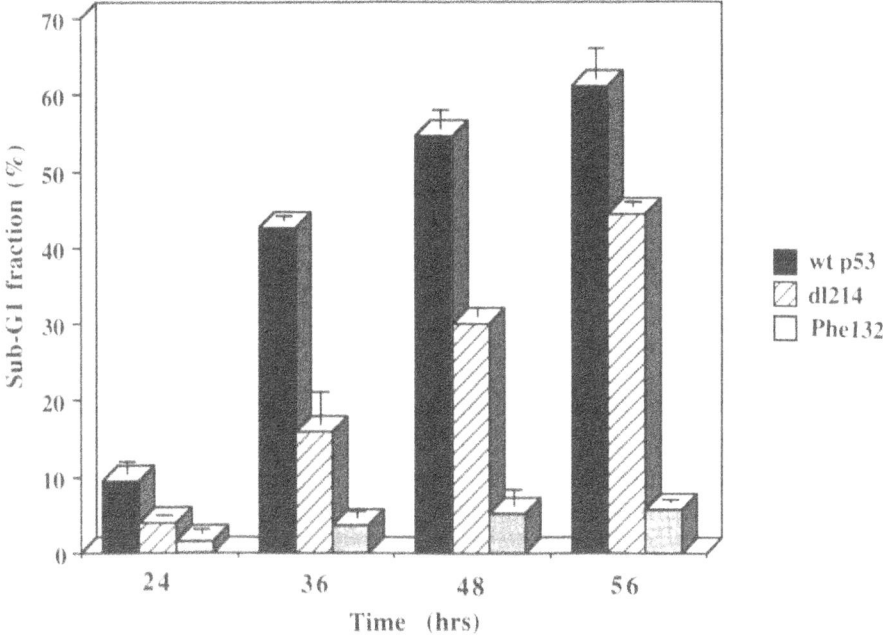

Figure 8. Kintetic analysis of p53-mediated apoptosis in HeLa cells. Cells were transfected with the indicated p53 expression plasmids and analysed for the induction of apoptosis, as described in fig. 3, at the indicated time points.

The findings reported in the first part of the paper are consistent with many earlier studies. A variety of conditions, including also the presence of certain viral oncoproteins, can disrupt the functional integrity of the pRB family. The model shown in fig. 9 predicts that such conditions should abrogate the ability of wt p53 to effectively arrest cell proliferation. Numerous reports, utilizing the adenovirus E1a proteins, the HPV E7 protein and the N-terminal region of the SV40 large T antigen, all of which inactivate the pRB family, support this contention[52,74–82]. Moreover, many of these studies also demonstrate that blocking the pRB pathway triggers p53-mediated apoptosis. The apoptotic effect of pRB

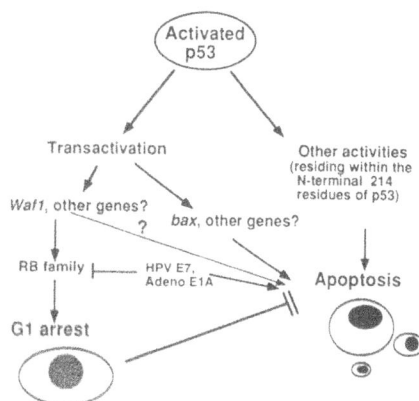

Figure 9. Comprehensive model of regulatory and mechanistic aspects of p53-mediated cellular responses. See text for further details.

inactivation is likely to operate through members of the E2F family of transcription factors[53,70].

The interplay between p53 and pRB in the induction of apoptosis could have a variety of implications. Very importantly, it may underlie a mechanism through which cells can monitor the integrity of their growth regulatory pathways. If these pathways become defective, owing either to pRB family gene mutations or to activation of certain dominant oncogenes (e.g. c-myc), the cells may lose the ability to growth arrest in response to p53 activation, resulting in the apoptotic elimination of these potentially hazardous cells. Increased accumulation of p53 appears to be coupled, at least post-translationally, with some of these aberrations[83]. This coupling may be important in ensuring that a p53-dependent response will indeed be initiated in such cells. It is also of note that recent reports indicate an involvement of p53 in myc-induced apoptosis[84,85]; this will be in keeping with the above model.

In addition to these pathological situations, there may also be situations where normal cells down regulate the activity of their pRB family members, for instance by maintaining constitutively high levels of cyclin-dependent kinase activity. Such cells may be predisposed to undergo apoptosis, rather than growth arrest, whenever p53 is activated. This could explain the propensity of some types of normal cells to apoptose in response to DNA damage.

The other major conclusion of this study, namely the ability of p53 to induce apoptosis even in the absence of SST, is perhaps more surprising. However, it is in line with earlier reports showing that p53-dependent apoptosis can occur in the presence of RNA and protein synthesis inhibitors[84,85]. Furthermore, a possible uncoupling between SST and at least some inhibitory effects of p53 may be related to the existence of certain tumor-derived mutants which retain an apparently normal SST activity[86,87].

It should be kept in mind, though, that SST is still most likely to play a key role in many p53-mediated apoptotic processes. The transcriptional activation by p53 of death related genes, such as Bax, is likely to be of consequence. The data presented above would argue, though, that optimal induction of apoptosis by p53 may depend on the combined action of two parallel mechanisms, one operating through SST and the other through a distinct function of the N terminal part of p53. This combined effect, perhaps synergistic, might underlie the very vigorous apoptotic response achieved by the relatively modest levels of p53 encountered physiologically.

REFERENCES

1. A.J. Levine. 1993. The tumor suppressor genes. *Ann. Rev Biochem.* **62**: 623–651.
2. L.A. Donehower and A. Bradley. 1993. The tumor suppressor p53. *Biochim Biophys Acta* . **1155**: 181–205.
3. R. Haffner and M. Oren. 1995. Biochemical properties and biological effects of p53. *Curr. Op. Genet. Develop.* . **5**: 84–90.
4. C. Prives and J.J. Manfredi. 1993. The p53 tumor suppressor protein - meeting review. *Genes Dev* . **7**: 529–534.
5. B. Vogelstein and K.W. Kinzler. 1992. p53 function and dysfunction. *Cell* . **70**: 523–526.
6. G. Farmer, J. Bargonetti, H. Zhu, P. Friedman, R. Prywes and C. Prives. 1992. Wild-type p53 activates transcription in vitro. *Nature* . **358**: 83–86.
7. S.E. Kern, J.A. Pietenpol, S. Thiagalingam, A. Seymour, K.W. Kinzler and B. Vogelstein. 1992. Oncogenic forms of p53 inhibit p53-regulated gene expression. *Science* . **256**: 827–830.
8. G.P. Zambetti, J. Bargonetti, K. Walker, C. Prives and A.J. Levine. 1992. Wild-type p53 mediates positive regulation of gene expression through a specific DNA sequence element. *Genes Dev* . **6**: 1143–1152.

9. W.D. Funk, D.T. Pak, R.H. Karas, W.E. Wright and J.W. Shay. 1992. A transcriptionally active dna-binding site for human p53 protein complexes. *Mol Cell Biol* . **12**: 2866–2871.

10. M.B. Kastan, Q.M. Zhan, W.S. Eldeiry, F. Carrier, T. Jacks, W.V. Walsh, B.S. Plunkett, B. Vogelstein and A.J. Fornace. 1992. A mammalian cell cycle checkpoint pathway utilizing p53 and GADD45 is defective in Ataxia-Telangiectasia. *Cell* . **71**: 587–597.

11. A. Zauberman, Y. Barak, N. Ragimov, N. Levy and M. Oren. 1993. Sequence-specific DNA binding by p53 - identification of target sites and lack of binding to p53-MDM2 complexes. *EMBO J* . **12**: 2799–2808.

12. C. Prives. 1994. How loops, beta sheets, and alpha helices help us to understand p53. *Cell* . **78**: 543–546.

13. S. Friend. 1994. p53: a glimpse at the puppet behind the shadow play. *Science* . **265**: 334–335.

14. W.S. El-Deiry, T. Tokino, V.E. Valculescu, D.B. Levy, R. Parsons, J.M. Trent, D. Lin, W.E. Mercer, K.W. Kinzler and B. Vogelstein. 1993. WAF1, a potential mediator of p53 tumor suppressor. *Cell* . **75**: 817–825.

15. J.W. Harper, G.R. Adami, N. Wei, K. Keyomarsi and S.J. Elledge. 1993. The p21 CDK-Interacting protein cip1 is a potent inhibitor of g1 cyclin-dependent kinases. *Cell* . **75**: 805–816.

16. Y. Xiong, G.J. Hannon, H. Zhang, D. Casso, R. Kobayashi and D. Beach. 1993. p21 is a universal inhibitor of cyclin kinases. *Science* . **366**: 701–704.

17. A. Noda, Y. Ning, S.F. Venable, O.M. Pereira-Smith, and J.R. Smith. 1994. Cloning of senescent cell-derived inhibitors of DNA synthesis using an expression screen. *Exp. Cell Res*. 211: 90–98.

18. V. Dulic, W.K. Kauffmann, S.J. Wilson, T.D. Tlsty, E. Lees, J.W. Harper, S.J. Elledge, and S.I. Reed. 1994. p53-dependent inhibition of cyclin-dependent kinase activities in human fibroblasts during radiation-induced G1 arrest. *Cell* 76: 1013–1023.

19. W.S. El-Deiry, J.W. Harper, P.M. O'Connor, V.E. Verculescu, C.E. Canman, J. Jackson, J.A. Pietenpol, M. Burrell, D.E. Hill, Y. Wang, W.K. Wiman, W.E. Mercer, M.B. Kastan, K.W. Kohn, S.J. Elledge, K.W. Kinzler, and B. Vogelstein. 1994. WAF1/CIP1 is induced in p53-mediated G1 arrest and apoptosis. *Cancer Res*. **54**: 1169–1174.

20. D. Michalovitz, O. Halevy, and M. Oren. 1990. Conditional inhibition of transformation and of cell proliferation by temperature-sensitive mutant of p53. *Cell* 62: 671–680.

21. W.E. Mercer, M.T. Shields, M. Amin, G.J. Sauve, E. Appella, S.J. Ullrich and J.W. Romano. 1990. Negative growth regulation in a glioblastoma tumor cell line that conditionally expresses human wild-type p53. *Proc. Natl. Acad. Sci. USA* . **87**: 6166–6170.

22. S.J. Baker, S. Markowitz, E.R. Fearon, K.V. Willson and B. Vogelstein. 1990. Suppression of human colorectal carcinoma cell growth by wild-type p53. *Science* . **249**: 912–915.

23. L. Diller, J. Kassel, C.E. Nelson, M.A. Gryka, G. Litwak, M. Gebhardt, B. Bressac, M. Ozturk, S.J. Baker, B. Vogelstein and S.H. Friend. 1990. p53 functions as a cell cycle control protein in osteosarcoma. *Mol. Cell. Biol.* . **10**: 5772–5781.

24. M.B. Kastan, O. Onyekwere, D. Sidransky, B. Vogelstein and R.W. Craig. 1991. Participation of p53 protein in the cellular response to DNA damage. *Cancer Res.* . **51**: 6304–6311.

25. N. Stewart, G.G. Hicks, F. Paraskevas and M. Mowat. 1995. Evidence for a second cell cycle block at G2/M by p53. *Oncogene* . **10**: 109–115.

26. R. Aloni-Grinstein, D. Schwartz and V. Rotter. 1995. Accumulation of wild-type p53 protein upon gamma irradiation induces a G2 arrest-dependent immunoglobulin kappa light chain gene expression. *EMBO J.* . **14**: 1392–1401.

27. S.M. Cross, C.A. Sanchez, C.A. Morgan, M.K. Schimke, R. S., R. Idzerda, W.H. Raskind and B.J. Reid. 1995. A p53-dependent mouse spindle checkpoint. *Science* . **267**: 1353–1356.

28. S. Waga, G.J. Hannon, D. Beach and B. Stillman. 1994. The p21 inhibitor of cyclin-dependent kinases controls DNA replication by interaction with PCNA. *Nature* . **369**: 574–578.

29. Y. Luo, J. Hurwitz and J. Massague. 1995. Cell-cycle inhibition by independent CDK and PCNA binding domains in p21^{Cip1}. *Nature* . **375**: 159–161.

30. J. Chen, P. Jackson, M.W. Kirschner and A. Dutta. 1995. Separate domains of p21 involved in the inhibition of Cdk kinase and PCNA. *Nature* . **374**: 386–388.

31. M.L. Smith, I.T. Chen, Q. Zhan, I. Bae, C.Y. Chen, T. Gilmer, M.B. Kastan, P.M. O'Connor and A.J.J. Fornace. 1994. Interaction of the p53-regulated protein Gadd45 with proliferating cell nuclear antigen. *Science* . **266**: 1376–1380.

32. K. Okamoto and D. Beach. 1994. Gyclin G is a transcriptional target of the p53 tumor suppressor protein. *EMBO J* . **13**: 4816–4822.

33. A. Zauberman, A. Lupo and M. Oren. 1995. Identification of p53 target genes through immune selection of genomic DNA: the cyclin G gene contains two distinct p53 binding sites. *Oncogene* . **10**: (in press).

34. X.W. Wu, J.H. Bayle, D. Olson and A.J. Levine. 1993. The p53-mdm-2 autoregulatory feedback loop. *Genes Dev* . **7**: 1126–1132.

35. Y. Barak, E. Gottlieb, T. Juven-Gershon and M. Oren. 1994. Regulation of mdm2 expression by p53: alternative promoters produce transcripts with nonidentical translation potential. *Genes Dev* . **8**: 1739–1749.

36. Y. Barak, T. Juven, R. Haffner and M. Oren. 1993. mdm2 expression is induced by wild type-p53 activity. *EMBO J* . **12**: 461–468.

37. M. Selvakumaran, H.K. Lin, T. Miyashita, H.G. Wang, S. Karajewski, J.C. Reed, B. Hoffman and D. Lieberman. 1994. Immediate early up-regulation of bax expression by p53 but not TGF beta 1: a paradigm for distinct apoptotic pathways. *Oncogene* . **9**: 1791–1798.

38. Q.M. Zhan, S.J. Fan, I. Bae, C. Guillouf, D.A. Liebermann, P.M. O'Connor and A.J. Fornace. 1994. Induction of bax by genotoxic stress in human cells correlates with normal p53 status and apoptosis. *Oncogene* . **9**: 3743–3751.

39. T. Miyashita and J.C. Reed. 1995. Tumor suppressor p53 is a direct transcriptional activator of the human bax gene. *Cell* . **80**: 293–299.

40. Z.N. Oltvai, C.L. Milliman and S.J. Korsmeyer. 1993. bcl-2 heterodimerizes in vivo with a conserved homolog, bax, that accelerates programed cell death. *Cell* . **74**: 609–619.

41. K.M. Dameron, O.V. Volpert, M.A. Tainsky and N. Bouck. 1994. Control of angiogenesis in fibroblasts by p53 regulation of thrombospondin-1. *Science* . **265**: 1582–1584.

42. D.P. Lane. 1992. p53, guardian of the genome. *Nature* . **358**: 15–16.

43. M. Oren. 1994. Relationship of p53 to the control of apoptotic cell death. *Seminars Cancer Biol* . **5**: 221–227.

44. E. Yonish-Rouach, D. Resnitzky, J. Lotem, L. Sachs, A. Kimchi and M. Oren. 1991. Wild-type p53 induces apoptosis of myeloid leukaemic cells that is inhibited by Interleukin-6. *Nature* . **352**: 345–347.

45. E. Yonish-Rouach, D. Grunwald, S. Wilder, A. Kimchi, E. May, J.J. Lawrence, P. May and M. Oren. 1993. p53-mediated cell death - relationship to cell cycle control. *Mol Cell Biol* . **13**: 1415–1423.

46. N. Levy, E. Yonish-Rouach, M. Oren and A. Kimchi. 1993. Complementation by wild-type p53 of interleukin-6 effects on M1 cells - induction of cell cycle exit and cooperativity with c-myc suppression. *Mol. Cell.Biol* . **13**: 7942–7952.

47. P. Shaw, R. Bovey, S. Tardy, R. Sahli, B. Sordat and J. Costa. 1992. Induction of apoptosis by wild-type p53 in a human colon tumor-derived cell line. *Proc Natl Acad Sci USA* . **89**: 4495–4499.

48. T. Ramqvist, K.P. Magnusson, Y.S. Wang, L. Szekely, G. Klein and K.G. Wiman. 1993. Wild-type p53 induced apoptosis in a Burkitt lymphoma (BL) line that carries mutant p53. *Oncogene* . **8**: 1495–1500.

49. Y.S. Wang, T. Ramqvist, L. Szekely, H. Axelson, G. Klein and K.G. Wiman. 1993. Reconstitution of wild-type p53 expression triggers apoptosis in a p53-negative v-myc retrovirus-induced T-cell lymphoma line. *Cell Growth Differ* . **4**: 467–473.

50. J.J. Ryan, R. Danish, C.A. Gottlieb and M.F. Clarke. 1993. Cell cycle analysis of p53-induced cell death in murine erythroleukemia cells. *Mol Cell Biol* . **13**: 711–719.

51. P. Johnson, S. Chung and S. Benchimol. 1993. Growth suppression of Friend virus-transformed erythroleukemia cells by p53 protein is accompanied by hemoglobin production and is sensitive to erythropoietin. *Mol Cell Biol* . **13**: 1456–1463.

52. M. Debbas and E. White. 1993. Wild-Type p53 mediates apoptosis by E1A, which is inhibited by E1B. *Genes Dev* **7**: 546–554.

53. X.W. Wu and A.J. Levine. 1994. p53 and E2F-1 cooperate to mediate apoptosis. *Proc Natl Acad Sci USA* . **91**: 3602–3606.

54. E. Yonish-Rouach, J. Borde, M. Gotteland, Z. Mishal, A. Viron and E. May. 1994. Induction of apoptosis by transiently transfected metabolically stable wtp53 in transformed cell lines. *Cell Death Diff.* . **1**: 39–47.

55. S.W. Lowe, E.M. Schmitt, S.W. Smith, B.A. Osborne and T. Jacks. 1993. p53 is required for radiation-induced apoptosis in mouse thymocytes. *Nature* . **362**: 847–849.

56. A.R. Clarke, C.A. Purdie, D.J. Harrison, R.G. Morris, C.C. Bird, M.L. Hooper and A.H. Wyllie. 1993. Thymocyte apoptosis induced by p53-dependent and independent pathways. *Nature* . **362**: 849–852.

57. W. Maltzman and L. Czyzyk. 1984. UV-irradiation stimulates levels of p53 cellular tumor antigen in nontransformed mouse cells. *Mol. Cell. Biol.* . **4**: 1689–1694.

58. S.W. Lowe, H.E. Ruley, T. Jacks and D.E. Housman. 1993. p53-dependent apoptosis modulates the cytotoxicity of anticancer agents. *Cell* . **74**: 957–967.

60. J. Lotem and L. Sachs. 1993. Hematopoietic cells from mice deficient in wild-type p53 are more resistant to induction of apoptosis by some agents. *Blood* . **82**: 1092–1096.

61. E. Gottlieb, R. Haffner, T. Von Ruden, E.F. Wagner and M. Oren. 1994. Down-regulation of wild-type p53 activity interferes with apoptosis of IL-3-dependent hematopoietic cells following IL-3 withdrawal. *EMBO J* . **13**: 1368–1374.

62. E. Gottlieb, R. Haffner, E. Yonish-Rouach, T. von Ruden, E. Wagner and M. Oren. 1994. Wild type p53 activity contributes to dependence on hematopoietic survival factors. *Apoptosis (E. Mihich and R.T. Schimke, eds.)* . pp. 31–45. Plenum, New York.

63. Y.M. Zhu, D.A. Bradbury and N.H. Russell. 1994. Wild-type p53 is required for apoptosis induced by growth factor deprivation in factor-dependent leukaemic cells. *Br J Cancer* **69**: 468–472.

64. C.E. Canman, T.M. Gilmer, S.B. Coutts and M.B. Kastan. 1995. Growth factor modulation of p53-mediated growth arrest versus apoptosis. *Genes Dev.* . **9**: 600–611.

65. J. Martinez, I. Georgoff, J. Martinez and A.J. Levine. 1991. Cellular localization and cell cycle regulation by a temperature-sensitive p53-protein. *Genes Dev.* **5**: 151–159.

66. J.V. Gannon and D.P. Lane. 1991. Protein synthesis required to anchor a mutant p53 protein which is temperature-sensitive for nuclear transport. *Nature* . **349**: 802–806.

67. L. Sachs. 1990. The control of growth and differentiation in normal and leukemic blood cells. *Cancer* . **65**: 2196–2206.

68. K. Vousden. 1993. Interactions of human papillomavirus transforming proteins with the products of tumor suppressor genes. *FASEB J.* **7**: 872–879.

69. Y. Haupt, S. Rowan and M. Oren. 1995. p53-mediated apoptosis in HeLa cells can be overcome by excess pRB. *Oncogene* . **10**: 1563–1571.

70. X.-Q. Qin, D.M. Livingston, W.J. Kaelin and P.D. Adams. 1994. Deregulated transcription factor E2F-1 expression leads to S-phase entry and p53-mediated apoptosis. *Proc. Natl. Acad. Sci. USA* . **91**: 10918–10922.

71. E. Shaulian, I. Haviv, Y. Shaul and M. Oren. 1995. Transcriptional repression by the C-terminal domain of p53. *Oncogene* . **10**: 671–680.

72. Y.J. Cho, S. Gorina, P.D. Jeffrey and N.P. Pavletich. 1994. Crystal structure of a p53 tumor suppressor-DNA complex: understanding tumorigenic mutations. *Science* . **265**: 346–355.

73. J.Y. Lin, J.D. Chen, B. Elenbaas and A.J. Levine. 1994. Several hydrophobic amino acids in the p53 amino-terminal domain are required for transcriptional activation, binding to mdm-2 and the adenovirus 5 E1B 55-kD protein. *Genes Dev.* **8**: 1235–1246.

74. D. Michael-Michalovitz, F. Yehiely, E. Gottlieb and M. Oren. 1991. Simian virus-40 can overcome the antiproliferative effect of wild-type-p53 in the absence of stable large t-antigen-p53 binding. *J.Virol.* **65**: 4160–4168.

75. R.S. Quartin, C.N. Cole, J.M. Pipas and A.J. Levine. 1994. The amino-terminal functions of the simian virus 40 large T antigen are required to overcome wild-type p53-mediated growth arrest of cells. *J Virol* . **68**: 1334–1341.

76. R.J.C. Slebos, M.H. Lee, B.S. Plunkett, T.D. Kessis, B.O. Williams, T. Jacks, L. Hedrick, M.B. Kastan and K.R. Cho. 1994. p53-dependent G1 arrest involves pRB-related proteins and is disrupted by the human papillomavirus 16 E7 oncoprotein. *Proc Natl Acad Sci USA* . **91**: 5320–5324.

77. H. Pan and A.E. Griep. 1994. Altered cell cycle regulation in the lens of HPV-16 E6 or E7 transgenic mice: implications for umor suppressor gene funciton in development. *Genes Dev.* **8**: 1285–1299.

78. A.E. White, E.M. Livanos and T.D. Tlsty. 1994. Differential disruption of genomic integrity and cell cycle regulation in normal human fibroblasts by the HPV oncoproteins. *Genes Dev.* **8**: 666–677.

79. G.W. Demers, S.A. Foster, C.L. Halbert and D.A. Galloway. 1994. Growth arrest by induction of p53 in DNA damaged keratinocytes is bypassed by human papillomavirus 16 E7. *Proc Natl Acad Sci USA* . **91**: 4382–4386.

80. E.S. Hickman, S.M. Picksley and K.H. Vousden. 1994. Cells expressing HPV16 E7 continue cell cycle progression following DNA damage induced p53 activation. *Oncogene* . **9**: 2177–2181.

81. S.D. Morgenbesser, B.O. Williams, T. Jacks and R.A. Depinho. 1994. p53-dependent apoptosis produced by Rb-deficiency in the developing mouse lens. *Nature* . **371**: 72–74.

82. M.L. Smith, Q.M. Zhan, I.S. Bae and A.J. Fornace. 1994. Role of retinoblastoma gene product in p53-mediated DNA damage response. *Exp Cell Res* . **215**: 386–389.

83. S.W. Lowe and H.E. Ruley. 1993. Stabilization of the p53 tumor suppressor is induced by adenovirus-5 E1A and accompanies apoptosis. *Genes Dev.* **7**: 535-

84. H. Hermeking and D. Eick. 1994. Mediation of c-myc-induced apoptosis by p53. *Science* . **265**: 2091–2093.

85. A.J. Wagner, J.M. Kokontis and N. Hay. 1994. Myc-mediated apoptosis requires wild-type p53 in a manner independent of cell cycle arrest and the ability of p53 to induce p21$^{waf1/cip1}$. *Genes Dev.* **8**: 2817–2830.

85. C. Caelles, A. Helmberg and M. Karin. 1994. p53-dependent apoptosis in the absence of transcriptional activation of p53 target genes. *Nature* . **370**: 220–223.

86. T. Crook, N.J. Marston, E.A. Sara and K.H. Vousden. 1994. Transcriptional activation by p53 correlates with growth suppression but does not preclude the acquisition of transforming function. *Cell* . **79**: 817–827.

87. K. Ory, Y. Legros, C. Auguin and T. Soussi. 1994. Analysis of the most representative tumour-derived p53
     mutants reveals that changes in protein conformation are not correlated with loss of transactivation or inhi-
     bition of cell proliferation. *EMBO J.* . **13**: 3496–3504.

DISCUSSION

F. Rauscher: So, what is the model then; you are excluding essentially most of p53's known biochemical functions by the mutants you are making. Do you have a model?

M. Oren: I will try to answer that. There are two models: One model, which I tried to make, is that normally p53 would signal apoptosis by more than one biochemical mechanism. I would suggest that, it in order to get an efficient cellular response to the activation of p53 with the amounts of p53 that are physiologically present, you may need a synergistic effect of both those two activities together. Now, that would make a prediction that, if in some cases only one thing works and the other does not work, cells will not respond biologically to p53, and maybe that explains some cases where we can activate p53, see induction of target genes, yet nothing happens to the cells and they keep on going happily. The other question is: What is the function of the N-terminal half of p53 which is important, if it is not transactivation? The obvious candidate is transcriptional repression, which p53 does in a variety of ways. It has been suggested, both by Tom Shenk and by Eilene White, that transcriptional repression may have something to do with the induction of apoptosis. There are at least some good correlations between ability of Bcl-2 to rescue cells from p53-mediated apoptosis and the ability of Bcl-2 to alleviate a transcriptional repression by p53.

F. Rauscher: But you are saying transcriptional repression mediated by p53 in the absence of DNA binding?

M. Oren: Yes, right. Transcriptional repression through some protein-protein interactions. Our data so far are not fully consistent with this notion, but we suspect that we may not be looking at the right targets of transcriptional repression, and this is something that we are working on.

F. Rauscher: Is this effect MDM-2 dependent as well?

M. Oren: Not from our work. The ability of the dl214 induced apoptosis to be rescued by MDM-2 still has to be determined, and that is being done now.

M. Kulesz-Martin: The N-terminus of p53 is also binding TBP. Have you looked into associations of p53 with other proteins, other transcription factors, whereby you get an indirect effect on transcription, and do you think the transcriptional repression effect of p53 is somewhat specific or do you think it is global on quite a number of genes through tying up necessary transcription factors?

M. Oren: The short answer is that we do not know--we are trying to figure that out. There is a long list of proteins that we have to go through.

M. Fried: Do you think HeLa are good cells to deal with, because they contain E6. Is it possible that 214 actually binds E6 and inactivates it and then allows the endogenous p53 to be activated and that is why you see apoptosis.

M. Oren: Supposedly, at least according to the mapping of the p53-E6 interaction site to the C terminus of p53, this does not seem to be a serious concern.

M. Fried: But E7 is still there, so if you inactivate the E6 you might then induce the endogenous p53 to become active. Have you looked at endogenous p53 under those circumstances?

M. Oren: We looked at endogenous p53 by Western blot. We are transfecting mouse p53 into human cells, so that gives us an advantage because we can use species-specific antibodies. So we looked at human endogenous p53 by Western in the presence of dl214, and under standard Western conditions we cannot see human endogenous p53 in those HeLa cells, either before or after transfection with dl214, This does not mean that is not increased, but it does not increase to any level we can detect. Further on that, if that endogenous p53 would have been increased to a high enough level to transactivate p53 responsive genes, dl214 should have increased the activity of the reporter genes, albeit indirectly. What we see, if anything, is a reduction. So, if anything, it represses rather than transactivates. That would argue against transcriptional activation of the endogenous p53. It may be doing something else which we can not measure; there is always this possibility.

D. Livingston: Have you tried to fuse a foreign DNA binding domain like BPV or GAL-4 to dl214 versus wild type? What is the transcription regulating activity of such a chimera?

M. Oren: These are all good points. We have done only part of that, and got very partial results so far. The only thing which is meaningful is that if we take the GAL-4 VP16 fusion or the GAL-4 dl214 fusion, GAL-4 VP16 transactivates strongly the GAL-4 target and does not induce apoptosis. This, in fact, was surprising to us. GAL-4-dl214 transactivates less efficiently than GAL-4 VP16, much less efficiently, but induces apoptosis, although less efficiently than dl214. So the experiments are indicating some specificity, but more has to be done. Now TBP, TATA--we have not done tested it yet.

Y. Xiong: Compared to the Rb rescue of p53 induced apoptosis, have you done, or would you predict over-expression of CDK inhibitor would rescue the p53 induced apoptosis as they can activate the Rb function by blocking CDK kinase activity?

M. Oren: Well, it depends. To begin with, in HeLa you do not have Rb function, so CDK inhibitors would be upstream to the defect, and should not make a difference. Presumably those cells have constitutively E2F and as long as you do not touch Rb they stay in cycle. In HeLa cells, upstream to Rb is not something we want to look at.

T. Graf: My perception is that mutated p53 on top of being dominant-negative has a function in cell transformation which is more than just inactivating wild-type p53. Could this be related to the internal function which you seem to have discovered?

M. Oren: OK, that is a whole new issue. There are indications that mutant forms of p53, of the type that you find in cancer, have a gain of function. This is not relevant to what we see here, because the same mutants do not induce apoptosis. So, whatever dl214 is doing has nothing to do with what tumor derived mutants are doing, and is a different story. We would argue that it is part of what wild type p53 is doing.

M. Kulesz-Martin: I know that you do not think that there is any transcriptional activation going on with the dl214, but did you actually measure the p21 levels?

M. Oren: It is not easy in this kind of assay, not the way we do it. This is something that still has to be done properly.

G. Evan: Even if you synchronize cells and activate p53 damage you get a synchronous apoptosis. So, here we must distinguish presumably between the act of death and any genetic event that lead up to the death. Do you have any thoughts about how those two might be related, because clearly the Karin data suggest formally that there is a non-transcriptional induction of cell death which seem to be more associated with the actual action of death itself: what he shows is that cells can go from alive to dead state without any new protein synthesis or gene expression, which our Myc data would fully agree with, but when they do it is not clear why some take a long time and some take a shorter time. Have you got any thoughts about that.

M. Oren: First of all I want to thank you for reminding me to mention the work of Michael Karin, which was the first indication that p53 can induce apoptosis in a transcription independent manner. transcription. Now to your question, perhaps we do not really have a simple answer. We do not even have an explanation why some cells will respond quickly to activation of p53 and die with kinetics of twelve hours or less, and in other systems with the same amount of p53 it takes forty-eight hours. So, there are other determinants which probably have to do with the readiness of the cell to start the death process. Those things might be totally random, a critical level of something.

G. Evan: Does it depend on how much p53 you express, have you done those experiments?

M. Oren: Partially yes. Up to a certain limit it depends on how much p53 you express. If you have more p53 the population dies faster but then again it might just mean that since these are viability counts, the chances of any given cell to die within the first cell cycle are increased, but the death process itself is the same.

G. Evan: Do you have any information on where in the cycle they are when they die?

M. Oren: On the HeLa cells we do not really have any good information. In the M1/p53 system they seem to be in S-phase.

G. Evan: So that is beyond the normal G1 checkpoint?

M. Oren: The commitment seems to be in G1, if you do experiments with elutriated cells. Those experiments tell you that cells which are in G1 at the time of activation of p53 are the first to die. But when they actually die, which is a few hours later, they are already in S. Remember that these cells do not growth arrest.

M. Kulesz-Martin: David Lane just published a paper in which he looked at a truncated form of p53 losing, I guess, the last fifty amino acids and the subject of the paper was a direct effect of the truncated form which may be like the alternatively spliced form that we have been studying on arrest of DNA synthesis using *in vitro* xenopus systems to look at DNA replication. What do you think about the possibility that the one which contains the N-terminus and part of the DNA binding domain plays a role for one of the pathways? If you think there are multiple pathways as to how apoptosis might be induced by the p53 that you are studying?

M. Oren: This is an interesting possibility. As far as our HeLa experiments go, we do not really know what happens to DNA replication. I cannot tell whether or not that is relevant. In the M1 system that does not seem to be the explanation, because there we see no arrest of DNA replication, yet the cells die suggestibly in S phase. So it is not that the cell is trying to arrest replication is S and therefore the cells die. Since, I do not know whether dl214 in the Lane assay will, or will not arrest replication, the easiest way would be to test it. If it still does, then you have to consider it seriously. If it does not, then this concern is irrelevant.

M. Kulesz-Martin: Because of all the mapping studies that you have done, in terms of the C terminus and now these studies that you have just talked about, can you tell us where you think the activity maps that you have been studying?

M. Oren: Partially we know that it maps to the transactivation domain. If you delete the bulk of the transactivation domain there is no more induction of apoptosis, so definitely something there, presumably some protein-protein interactions, are required.

M. Kulesz-Martin: So you do not know whether the partial DNA binding domain that you have in dl214 is important?

M. Oren: The answer is that we still do not know.

F. Rauscher: Your dl214 protein does not contain the classic nuclear localization signal right? Yet the immunofluorescence showed p53 to be nuclear! So is MDM-2 shuttling it into there? Does this affect require nuclear localization?

M. Oren: When you look at dl214 staining, very often what we see is quite a significant amount of protein making it into the nucleus. So we reason that the protein is probably small enough to go in and out. If MDM-2 may help carry it in, I do not know. Our guess is that those cells would not have much MDM-2 because the mdm-2 gene is not transactivated by that protein.

D. Livingston: You could fuse some junk to the C terminal end of dl214, make it big enough so that it cannot leak into the nucleus. Then you could ask if it can still promote apoptosis. If not, I think you would be on your way to getting an answer.

6

THE MOLECULAR GENETICS OF WILMS TUMOR

Jerry Pelletier,[1] Hitoshi Nakagama,[2] and David E. Housman[3*]

[1] Department of Biochemistry and McGill Cancer Center,
McGill University
Montreal, Quebec, Canada, H3G 1Y6
[2] National Cancer Research Institute
5–1–1 Tsukiji Chuo-ku, Tokyo 104, Japan
[3] Center for Cancer Research
Massachusetts Institute of Technology
Cambridge, Massachusetts 02139

Wilms' tumor (WT), a malignancy of embryonal kidney cells, posesses several significant opportunities and challenges to the understanding of the molecular basis of tumorigenesis and treatment response. First, from the perspective of the genetic basis of tumorigenesis, WT provides one of the most clear cut circumstances under which the underlying genetic contributions to tumorigenesis can be analyzed. Second, from the perspective of molecular biology, the isolation of the WT1 tumor suppressor gene provides a critical initiation point for developing an understanding of the relationship between normal differentiation and tumorigenesis. Third, from the perspective of treatment response, WT provides a critical challenge to investigators concerned with extending the high success rate for treatment of WT to other forms of cancer.

GENETICS OF WT

Although most cases of WTs are sporadic and unilateral, ~5–10% of WTs are bilateral, and have an earlier age of onset than unilateral cases (Matsunaga, 1981). The analysis by Knudson and Strong of the relationship between age of onset and occurrence of WT has led to the view that like retinoblastoma, the occurrence of WT is governed by a small number of rate limiting steps (Knudson and Strong, 1972). In individuals with a genetic predisposition to WT, this analysis suggests that there is a single rate limiting step to tu-

---

* Address for Correspondence: Dr. David Housman, Center for Cancer Research, 40 Ames St., Massachusetts Institute of Technology, Cambridge, MA 02139 Fax: (617) 253–5202.

Cancer Genes, edited by Mihich and Housman
Plenum Press, New York, 1996

morigenesis. In sporadic WT, analysis of age of onset data are most compatible with two
rate limiting steps of approximately equal frequency. Unlike retinoblastoma, however, hereditary predisposition to WT can not be attributed to a single genetic locus.

The most definitive analysis identifying a genetic locus predisposing to WT derives
from the epidemiological analysis of Miller, Fraumeni and Manning who in 1964 defined
the WAGR (WT, aniridia, genitourinary anomalies, mental retardation) constellation
(Miller et al, 1964). In this analysis WT, which occurs in approximately 1 in 10,000 children, was found to be associated with bilateral aniridia, a condition which affects approximately 1 in 50,000 children, far more frequently than might be expected by chance.
Approximately 2% of children with WT also have bilateral aniridia. Conversely, the risk
of WT to children with bilateral aniridia is approximately one third. When aniridia is present in conjunction with WT, the tumors are much more likely to be bilateral indicating
multiple independent tumorigenic events and suggesting hereditary predisposition to WT.
These two infrequent conditions, are associated in the WAGR syndrome with two other
more common conditions, genitourinary malformations and mental retardation. Karyotypic analysis has identified hemizygous deletions of chromosome 11 band p13 associated
with WAGR syndrome (Riccardi et al., 1978). These observations provided the framework which led to the identification of the WT1 tumor suppressor gene.

Denys-Drash syndrome (DDS) is a second WT associated developmental disorder
comprising of WT, intersex disorders, and renal nephropathy (Denys et al., 1969; Drash et
al., 1970). This range of anomalies clearly indicates an underlying defect in the normal
process of differentiation and development of the genital system more severe than observed in individuals with WAGR syndrome. Germline lesions within the WT1 tumor suppressor gene are associated with DDS, having been identified in almost all cases analyzed
to date (for a review, see Bruening and Pelletier, 1994).

A second site on chromosome 11p which appears to harbor a WT suppressor gene is
band 11p15.5. This region is the site to which family studies and karyotypic rearrangements have mapped the gene for Beckwith-Weidemann syndrome (Turleau et al., 1984;
Joy Ping et al., 1989; Koufos et al., 1989). This syndrome is characterized by umbilical
hernia, macroglossia, neonatal hypoglycemia, gigantism, and increased risk for development of certain childhood cancers (Beckwith, 1963; Wiedemann, 1964). The prevalence
of BWS is ~ 7 per 100,000 births and ~5–10% of these individuals will develop WTs, ad-
renocortical carcinoma, or hepatoblastoma (Sotelo-Avila et al., 1980). Patients with this
overgrowth disorder show an 80 fold increase over the normal population in incidence of
WT. In addition, this chromosomal region shows an extremely high frequency of loss of
heterozygosity in WTs (~50%) supporting the location of a tumor suppressor gene in this
chromosomal segment (Reeve et al., 1989; Mannens et al., 1988).

The existence of a third predisposing WT locus has been postulated in familial WT
cases lacking linkage to DNA markers on the short arm of chromosome 11p (Grundy et
al., 1988; Huff et al., 1988; Schwartz et al., 1991). These results raise the interesting possibility that different loci may be implicated in the pathogenesis of different WTs. They
may be involved in various steps of the same regulatory pathway, the abrogation of any of
which could lead to the malignant state. Alternatively, inactivation of several of these loci
may be required for tumor initiation. Allelic loss at 16q24 in 20% (Maw et al., 1992) and
at 11q23.3-qter in 37% (Radice et al., 1995) of informative tumors indicates additional
loci involved in tumor progression. The 16q region has been excluded by linkage analysis
from being involved in five WT families (Huff et al., 1992). WT thus contrasts with retinoblastoma, in which a single genetic locus, the RB-1 locus on chromosome 13q14 is the
major locus associated with sporadic and familial retinoblastoma. To date only the WT1

predisposing locus has been molecularly cloned from WT and characterized. The discussion which follows focuses on the WT1 locus.

MOLECULAR BIOLOGY OF THE WT1 TUMOR SUPPRESSOR GENE

Unlike the ubiquitously expressed tumor suppressor genes p53 and RB, WT1 gene expression is restricted to a small set of tissues. The expression pattern has been studied in mouse, human, and rat, and is very similar in all three species (Pritchard-Jones et al., 1990; Pelletier et al., 1991; Armstrong et al., 1992; Sharma et al., 1992). During embryogenesis WT1 expression is highest in three situations—differentiation of the metanephric mesenchyme into nephrons, formation of mesothelium from the mesenchyme lining the coelomic cavity, and production of the sex cords from the mesenchyme of the primitive gonad. During nephrogenesis, the highest level of WT1 mRNA expression is in the glomerular epithelium during formation of the S-shaped bodies (Pritchard-Jones et al., 1990; Pelletier et al., 1991). As the nephron matures, WT1 mRNA expression becomes extinguished. In the adult, highest WT1 mRNA levels are observed in the granulosa and epithelial cells of the ovary, Sertoli cells of the testis, the uterus, and the spleen (Pritchard-Jones et al., 1990; Pelletier et al., 1991; Armstrong et al., 1992; Sharma et al., 1992).

WT1 encodes a polypeptide composed of two functional domains: a proline/glutamine rich amino terminus and four zinc fingers of the Cys_2-His_2 variety at the carboxyl terminus (Call et al., 1990). The predicted protein product is very similar among humans, mice, and rats (> 95% at the amino acid level), indicating an evolutionarily conserved function for this polypeptide product (Fig. 1)(Call et al., 1990; Buckler et al., 1991; Sharma et al., 1992). The structure of the WT1 gene zinc fingers most closely resembles those of the early growth response gene, EGR-1 (also known as Zif 268). EGR-1 contains three zinc fingers of the Cys_2-His_2 variety and activates transcription in a sequence specific manner (Christy et al., 1988). Crystallization of a Zif 268 zinc finger-DNA ($^{5'}GCGTGGGCG^{3'}$) complex has permitted the determination of a structure in which three key three amino acids in each zinc finger interact directly through hydrogen bond contacts with three nucleotides in the major groove of the target DNA sequence (Pavletich and Pabo, 1991) (Fig. 2). The structural analysis of EGR-1/Zif 268 has been a key to the understanding of the mechanism of DNA binding by WT1.

However, the WT1 DNA binding domain differs from that of EGR1 in a number of key structural features suggesting significant differences exist between the specificity of DNA binding. WT1 has four zinc fingers, while EGR1 has only three. While the second, third and fourth zinc fingers of WT1 most closely resemble fingers one, two and three of EGR1 (64% identity at the amino acid level); the first WT1 zinc finger does not share significant homology with any of the three EGR-1 zinc fingers (Call et al., 1990). Alternative splice site selection within the WT1 coding region leads to the production of four isoforms (Haber et al., 1990; Haber et al., 1991). The second alternative splice inserts, or removes three amino acids (KTS) between zinc fingers III and IV—a change which alters the DNA binding specificity of the protein (Rauscher et al., 1990). Amino acid conservation between EGR1 and WT1 is restricted to the zinc fingers with significant differences outside these structure possibly affecting ancillary functions in DNA binding.

Determining the identity of genes controlled by WT1 is a crucial element in understanding its role in controlling differentiation and cell growth. Rauscher et al. (1990) have identified sequences containing a GC rich motif with the conserved feature,

```
Human:  MetGlySerAspValArgAspLeuAsnAlaLeuLeuProAlaValProSerLeuGlyGlyGlyGly    22
Mouse:  -  -  -  -  -  -  -  -  -  -  -  -  -  -  -  - Ser  -  -  -  -  -
Rat:    -  -  -  -  -  -  -  -  -  -  -  -  -  -  -  - Ser  -  -  -  -  -

        Gly...CysAlaLeuProValSerGlyAlaAlaGlnTrpAlaProValLeuAspPheAlaProPro    43
        - Gly - Gly -  -  -  -  - Arg -  -  -  -  -  -  -  -  -  -  -
        - ... - Gly -  -  -  -  - Arg -  -  -  -  -  -  -  -  -  -  -

        GlyAlaSerAlaTyrGlySerLeuGlyGlyProAlaProProProAlaProProProProProPro    65
        -  -  -  -  -  -  -  -  -  -  -  -  -  -  -  -  -  -  -  -  -
        -  -  -  -  -  -  -  -  -  -  -  -  -  -  -  -  -  -  -  -  -

        ProProProHisSerPheIleLysGlnGluProSerTrpGlyGlyAlaGluProHisGluGluGln    87
        -  -  ...  -  -  -  -  -  -  -  -  -  -  -  -  -  -  -  -  -  -
        -  -  ...  -  -  -  -  -  -  -  -  -  -  -  -  -  -  -  -  -  -

        CysLeuSerAlaPheThrValHisPheSerGlyGlnPheThrGlyThrAlaGlyAlaCysArgTyr   109
        -  -  -  -  -  - Leu -  -  -  -  -  -  -  -  -  -  -  -  -  -
        -  -  -  -  -  - Leu -  -  -  -  -  -  -  -  -  -  -  -  -  -

        GlyProPheGlyProProProSerGlnAlaSerSerGlyGlnAlaArgMetPheProAsnAla      131
        -  -  -  -  -  -  -  -  -  -  -  -  -  -  -  -  -  -  -  -  -
        -  -  -  -  -  -  -  -  -  -  -  -  -  -  -  -  -  -  -  -  -

        ProTyrLeuProSerCysLeuGluSerGlnProAlaIleArgAsnGlnGlyTyrSerThrValThr   153
        -  -  -  -  -  -  -  -  -  -  -  - Thr -  -  -  -  -  -  -  -
        -  -  -  -  -  -  -  -  -  -  -  - Ser -  -  -  -  -  -  -  -

        PheAspGlyThrProSerTyrGlyHisThrProSerHisHisAlaAlaGlnPheProAsnHisSer   175
        -  -  - Ala -  -  -  -  -  -  -  -  -  -  -  -  -  -  -  -  -
        -  -  - Ala -  -  -  -  -  -  -  -  -  -  -  -  -  -  -  -  -

        PheLysHisGluAspProMetGlyGlnGlnGlySerLeuGlyGluGlnGlnTyrSerValProPro   197
        -  -  -  -  -  -  -  -  -  -  -  -  -  -  -  -  -  -  -  -  -
        -  -  -  -  -  -  -  -  -  -  -  -  -  -  -  -  -  -  -  -  -

        ProValTyrGlyCysHisThrProThrAspSerCysThrGlySerGlnAlaLeuLeuLeuArgThr   219
        -  -  -  -  -  -  -  -  -  -  -  -  -  -  -  -  -  -  -  -  -
        -  -  -  -  -  -  -  -  -  -  -  -  -  -  -  -  -  -  -  -  -

        ProTyrSerSerAspAsnLeuTyrGlnMetThrSerGl..LeuGluCysMetThrTrpAsnGlnMet  241
        -  -  -  -  -  -  -  -  -  -  -  -  -  -  -  -  -  -  -  -  -
        -  -  -  -  -  -  -  -  -  -  -  -  -  -  -  -  -  -  -  -  -

        AsnLeuGlyAlaThrLeuLysGly_ValAlaAlaAlaGlySerSerSerSerValLysTrpThrGluGly  263
        -  -  -  -  -  -  -  - Met -  -  -  -  -  -  -  -  -  -  -
        -  -  -  -  -  -  -  - Met -  -  -  -  -  -  -  -  -  -  -

        GlnSerAsnHisSerThrGlyTyrGluSerAspAsnHisThrThrProIleLeuCysGlyAlaGln   285
        -  -  -  - Gly -  -  -  - Glu -  -  - Ala -  -  -  -  -  -
        -  -  -  - Gly -  -  -  - Glu -  -  - Thr -  -  -  -  -  -

        TyrArgIleHisThrHisGlyValPheArgGlyIleGlnAspValArgArgValProGlyValAla   307
        -  -  -  -  -  -  -  -  -  -  -  -  -  -  -  - Ser -  -  -
        -  -  -  -  -  -  -  -  -  -  -  -  -  -  -  - Ser -  -  -

        ProThrLeuValArgSerAlaSerGluThrSerGluLysArgProPheMet_CysAlaTyrProGly   329
        -  -  -  -  -  -  -  -  -  -  -  -  -  -  -  -  -  -  -  -  -
        -  -  -  -  -  -  -  -  -  -  -  -  -  -  -  -  -  -  -  -  -

        CysAsnLysArgTyrPheLysLeuSerHisLeuGlnMetHisSerArgLysHisThrGlyGluLys   351
        -  -  -  -  -  -  -  -  -  -  -  -  -  -  -  -  -  -  -  -  -
        -  -  -  -  -  -  -  -  -  -  -  -  -  -  -  -  -  -  -  -  -

        ProTyrGlnCysAspPheLysAspCysGluArgArgPheSerArgSerAspGlnLeuLysArgHis   373
        -  -  -  -  -  -  -  -  -  -  -  -  -  -  -  -  -  -  -  -  -
        -  -  -  -  -  -  -  -  -  -  -  -  -  -  -  -  -  -  -  -  -

        GlnArgArgHisThrGlyValLysProPheGlnCysLysThrCysGlnArgLysPheSerArgSer   395
        -  -  -  -  -  -  -  -  -  -  -  -  -  -  -  -  -  -  -  -  -
        -  -  -  -  -  -  -  -  -  -  -  -  -  -  -  -  -  -  -  -  -

        AspHisLeuLysThrHisThrArgThrHisThrGlyLysThrSerGluLysProPheSerCysArg   417
        -  -  -  -  -  -  -  -  -  -  -  -  -  -  -  -  -  -  -  -  -
        -  -  -  -  -  -  -  -  -  -  -  -  -  -  -  -  -  -  -  -  -

        TrpProSerCysGlnLysLysPheAlaArgSerAspGluLeuValArgHisHisAsnMetHisGln   439
        - His -  -  -  -  -  -  -  -  -  -  -  -  -  -  -  -  -  -  -
        - Tyr -  -  -  -  -  -  -  -  -  -  -  -  -  - Lys -  -  -

        ArgAsnMetThrLysLeuGlnLeuAlaLeu                                       449
        -  -  -  -  -  - HisVal -  -
        -  -  -  -  -  - HisVal -  -
```

Figure 1. Amino acid comparison of the WT1 gene from humans, mouse, and rats. The sequence of the mouse (Buckler et al., 1991), rat (Sharma et al., 1992), and are compared to the human (Call et al., 1990) amino acid sequence and only differences in sequence are indicated. The two alternatively spliced exons are double underlined and the zinc finger domains are singly underlined.

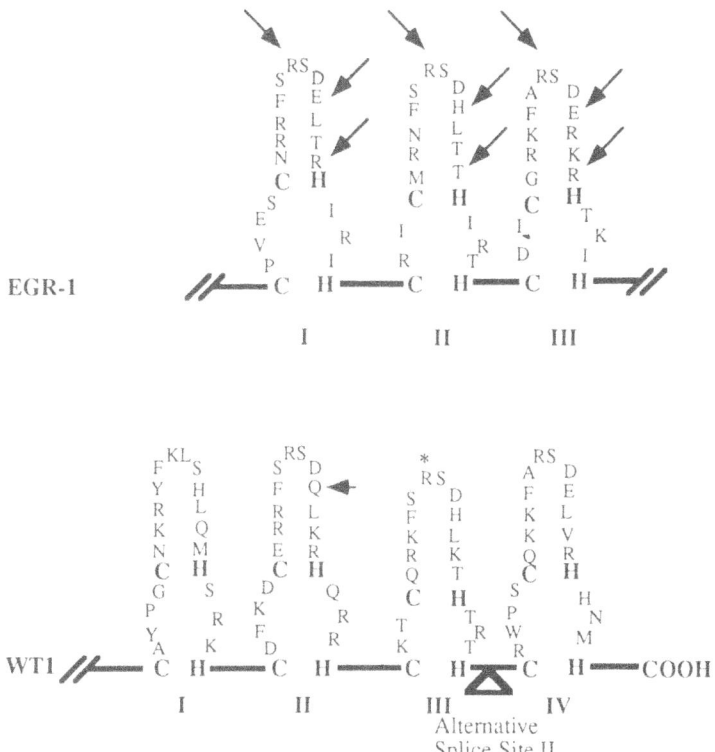

Figure 2. EGR-1 and WT1 zinc fingers. Amino acids within the EGR-1 zinc fingers predicted to directly interact with DNA have been indicated by arrows. The most common amino acid found altered in Denys-Drash syndrome is indicated by an asterisks. See text for more details.

$5'G^G/_\gamma GGGGGA^G/_C 3'$, similar to the EGR-1 binding site, $5'GCGGGGGCG^{3'}$, as being capable of forming specific complexes with the WT1 protein. WT1 was shown to directly interact with this motif by mobility shift assays and was able to repress transcription of reporter genes under control of promoters containing several EGR-1 binding sites. Based on this data, WT1 and EGR-1 have been proposed to form a binary on/off system of transcriptional control by competing for the same binding sites (Sukhatme, 1991). WT1 has also been shown to mediate transcriptional control through another DNA site consisting of $(TCC)_n$ repeats (Wang et al., 1993). More recently, whole genome based PCR has identified a high affinity wt1 binding site, called WTE: $5'GAGT\textbf{GCGTGGGAGT}AGAA^{3'}$ (Nakagama et al., 1995). This sequence, although similar to the EGR-1 recognition site (particularly the core motif highlighted in bold), binds to WT1 with 20- to 30-fold higher affinity than the EGR-1 site (Nakagama et al., 1995). Footprinting experiments revealed partial protection of a thymine residue in the tenth nucleotide position of the WTE site (Nakagama et al., 1995). DNA probes differing in identity of this residue were analyzed by mobility shifts and indicated that the nature of the last thymine nucleotide within the WTE motif has a significant influence on binding affinity.

Data from Nakagama et al. (1995) demonstrates a clear role for the first zinc finger of WT1 in sequence recognition. Deletion of this finger, or site-directed mutagenesis affecting residues predicted to chelate zinc, decrease the efficiency of DNA-protein complex formation (~10-fold). The importance of this finger to WT1 biology is underscored by the identification of a germline missense mutation affecting a cysteine residue (and presumably Zn++ binding) associated with Denys-Drash syndrome (Bruening et al., 1992). If WT1 zinc finger I is also involved directly in DNA recognition, then one would predict that the contiguous triplet next to the WTE site should be protected by footprinting analysis yielding a 12 bp, rather than 10 bp protected fragment (Nakagama et al., 1995). Surprisingly, only one additional nucleotide, a thymine, was found to be partially protected by DNA footprinting. The lack of a clear footprint at this nucleotide may indicate that the interaction between zinc finger I and the 3' most T in WTE may not be tight enough to be recognized in such an analysis. Alternatively, this finger may not directly interact with DNA. Experiments assaying DNA binding in WT1 mutants with alterations within finger I demonstrate the same base pair requirement as with the wild type WT protein and are not consistent with a direct role of finger I in DNA binding. One possibility stems from a recent model described in GLI-DNA complexes by Pavletich and Pabo (1993). In this model, they described the involvement of a hydrogen bond contact in the zinc finger-DNA complex made by Asp residues at position 2 in the zinc finger helices. According to this model, the Asp (D) residues in Zif268-fingers interact with adenine (A) or cytosine (C) residues on the opposite strand. If we apply this model to the wt1-WTE interaction, wt1 zinc fingers II, III and IV contain Asp (D) residues in position 2 of the α-helices which may interact with adenine or cytosine residues (^{10}A, ^{7}C and ^{4}A) on the opposite strand of WTE respectively: $^{5'}$GCG**T**GG**G**AG**T**$^{3'}$ (Fig. 2). Currently, we do not understand the physical properties of wt1 zinc finger I which mediates sequence specificity. Like the first finger of the GLI-DNA complex, wt1 finger I may play a key role in stabilizing nucleotide recognition by finger II through protein-protein interactions or structural stabilization of the entire DNA binding domain (Pavletich and Pabo, 1993).

Genetic studies of individuals with Denys-Drash syndrome have revealed that germline mutations within the wt1 DNA binding domain serve to deregulate normal differentiation of the urogenital system (Pelletier et al., 1991; Bruening et al., 1992). The most common WT1 lesion associated with this syndrome is a missense ^{1180}C to T transition within zinc finger 3, converting ^{394}Arg to Trp (Fig. 2). By analogy to EGR-1, ^{394}Arg of WT1 is predicted to contact a guanine residue in the DNA target sequence. Converting ^{394}Arg to Trp abolishes this interaction, and the mutant version of wt1 can no longer bind to the EGR consensus sequence (Pelletier et al., 1991). At the germline level, these mutations are always heterozygous and are predicted to act in a dominant-negative fashion, with the mutant protein behaving *trans*-dominantly to inhibit activity of the normal wt1 protein. Consistent with this interpretation is the recent demostration that wt1 can homodimerize and that mutants can functionally antagonize the activity of wild-type protein (Reddy et al., 1995; Mofett et al., 1995). These studies demonstrate that WT1 occupies a unique role as both a tumor suppressor gene and transcription factor essential for development of the urogenital system. This conclusion is supported by experiments in which the murine WT1 gene was ablated and homozygous mice failed to develop a urogenital system (Kriedberg et al., 1993).

To date, several studies have directed their efforts towards the identification of downstream targets of WT1 by scanning known promoter regions for the EGR-1 like consensus sequences. Using this approach several potential targets have been identified and include insulin-like growth factor II (Drummond et al., 1992), insulin-like growth factor 1 receptor (Werner et al., 1993), platelet-derived growth factor A-chain (Gashler et al., 1992; Wang et al., 1992), colony stimulating factor-1 (Harrington et al., 1993), transforming growth factor-β1 (Dey et al., 1994), retinoic acid receptor-α (Goodyer et al. 1995),

Pax-2 (Ryan et al., 1995), c-myb (McCann et al., 1995), epidermal growth factor receptor (Englert et al., 1995), and the WT1 gene itself (Rupprecht et al. 1994). Reporter constructs harboring minimal promoters from these genes can be negatively or positively regulated by wt1 in transient transfection systems. However, a more detailed and precise analysis is required to determine if the EGR-1 consensus site is involved in the biology of wt1. The ability to achieve trans-repression in transient transfection assays is not quantitative and will not discriminate between low- and high affinity sites, particularly in the presence of excess effector protein. The results of Nakagama et al. (1995) question the physiological significance of analyzing EGR-1 core motifs in promoter elements as a means of identifying downstream genes under the regulation of wt1, since these sites may have binding affinities quite low relative to other motifs not yet identified. Clearly, more general and less biased screening methods need to be adopted to identify downstream targets.

A small set of WTs having cytogenetically visible deletions at 11p13 were invaluable in identifying the WT1 gene. Deletions within the WT1 gene, detectable by Southern blotting analysis, are observed in ~10% of WTs (for a review, see Bruening et al., 1995). More subtle mutations are detected at a frequency of ~6% in WTs and have yielded important insight into the functional domains of WT1 (Little et al., 1992; Copppes et al., 1993; Varanasi et al., 1994). These mutations include missense alterations within the wt1 zinc fingers, predicted to disrupt DNA binding activity, or nonsense or frameshift mutations. Two missense mutations have been described which convert wt1 from a transcriptional repressor to an activator (Park et al., 1993b; 1993c). Recently, Park et al. (1993a) have found WT1 to be mutated in two of twenty nephrogenic rests analyzed. These results indicate that inactivation of WT1 appears to be an early genetic event which can lead to nephrogenic rest formation, and that additional genetic lesions are required for tumor formation. The majority of alterations occur within the zinc finger domains, indicating this is a "hotspot" for mutations. In some tumors, inactivation of both WT1 alleles has occurred, whereas in others, one wild-type allele remains, suggesting that in these cases the mutations behave in a dominant-negative fashion.

WT AS A MODEL FOR UNDERSTANDING TUMOR TREATMENT RESPONSE

The prognosis for a child diagnosed with WT today is quite good. WT is a highly curable pediatric malignancy in which chemotherapeutic regimens, in combination with surgical resection, have produced survival rates approaching >85% for stage I and stage II (favorable histology) tumors. However, patients harboring the aggressive anaplastic subtype of WT (which represents ~5% of the total cases) have a considerably worse prognosis. In order to determine the role of *p53* inactivation in the etiology of WT, a large series of tumors were analyzed for the presence of *p53* mutations. The presence of point mutations was determined by analyzing individual p53 exons by single strand conformational polymorphism analysis and confirmed by direct sequencing. In addition, tumors were classified by their clinical grade (i.e. non-anaplastic or anaplastic).

Results were obtained from the analysis of 134 tumors of known histology. *p53* mutations were uncommon in WTs and occurred in ~12% of the tumors analyzed. However, there was a striking correlation between *p53* mutation and anaplasia—70% of anaplastic tumors contained detectable p53 mutations, but no mutations were observed in non-anaplastic tumors (Bardeesy et al., 1994). Subsequent studies indicated that anaplastic WT harboring *p53* mutations have a substantial decrease in spontaneous apoptosis compared to non-anaplastic tumors (Bardeesy et al., 1995). These data link *p53* mutations and attenuated apoptosis with tumor progression to anaplasia, and hence, poor prognosis. The prospects of understanding tumor treatment response in WT provide a framework for better understanding the molecular basis of tumor response to chemotherapy. Insight into strategies which may lead to treatment response rates comparable to those observed in WT for other cancer types would clearly be of great interest. Our data suggests that anaplastic WTs are part of a group of malignancies whose p53 gene status correlates with a lack of response to cytotoxic agents (Lowe et al., 1993). The detection of p53 mutations in WTs may be useful in supporting histological diagnosis and provide a prognostic indicator for tumor progression.

The characterization of WT-associated syndromes has been greatly aided by genetic studies, and for WAGR and DDS, there is now a molecular definition of each syndrome that can be more readily applied than a subjective examination of phenotype. The information generated by studying WTs has provided a broad base for diagnoses at the molecular level of some of the phenotypes associated with this disease and sets the stage for the identification of genetic events involved in progression of this malignancy.

ACKNOWLEDGMENTS

J.P. is a Medical Research Council Scientist. Work in the authors lab. are supported by grants from the Medical Research Council (J.P.), Kidney Foundation (J.P.), National Cancer Institute of Canada (J.P.), NIH R01-HG00299 (D.H.), and NIH P01-CA42063 (D.H.).

REFERENCES

Armstrong, J.F., Pritchard-Jones, K., Bickmore, W.A., Hastie, N.D., and Bard, J.B.L. (1992). The expression of the Wilms' tumour gene WT1 in the developing mammalian embryo. *Mech. Develop.* **40**, 85–97.

Bardeesy, N., Falkoff, D., Petruzzi, M.-J., Nowak, N., Zabel, B., Adam, M., Aquiar, M.C., Grundy, P., Shows, T., and Pelletier, J. (1994). Anaplastic Wilms' tumor, a subtype displaying poor prognosis, harbours p53 gene Mutations. *Nature Genetics* **7**, 91–97.

Bardeesy, N., Beckwith, J.B., and Pelletier, J. (1995). Clonal expansion and attenuated apoptosis in Wilms' tumors are associated with p53 gene mutations. *Cancer Res.* **55**, 215–219.

Beckwith, J.B. (1963). Extreme cytomegaly of the fetal adrenal cortex, omphalocoele, hyperplasia of kidneys and pancreas, and Leydig-cell hyperplasia. Another syndrome? Presented at the Annual Meeting of Western Society for Pediatric Research, Los Angeles, California, Nov. 11.

Bruening, W., Bardeesy, N., Silverman, B.L., Cohn., R.A., Machin, G.A., Aronson, A.J., Housman, D., and Pelletier, J. (1992). Germline intronic and exonic mutations in the Wilms' tumour gene (WT1) affecting urogenital development. *Nature Genet.* **1**, 144–148.

Bruening, W., and Pelletier, J. (1994). Denys-Drash syndrome: a role for the WT1 tumour suppressor gene in urogenital development. *Seminars in Developmental Biology* **5**, 333–343.

Bruening, W., Winnett, E., and Pelletier, J. (1995) Wilms' tumor: a paradigm for insights into development and cancer. *Cancer Investigation* **13**, 431–443.

Buckler, A., Pelletier, J., Haber, D.A., Glaser, T., and Housman, D.E. (1991). Isolation, characterization and expression of the murine Willms' tumor gene (WT1) during kidney development. *Mol. Cell. Biol.* **11**, 1707–1712.

Call, K. M., Glaser, T., Ito, C.Y., Buckler, A.J., Pelletier, J., Haber, D.A., Rose, E.A., Kral, A.,Yeger, H., Lewis, W.H., Jones, C., and Housman, D.E. (1990). Isolation and characterization of a zinc finger polypeptide gene at the human chromosome 11 Wilms' tumor locus. *Cell* **60**, 509–520.

Christy, B., Lau, L. F., and Nathans, D. (1988). A gene activated in mouse 3T3 cells by serum growth factors encodes a protein with zinc finger sequences. *Proc. Natl. Acad. Sci. USA.* **85**, 7857–7861.

Coppes, M. J., Liefers, G.J., Paul, P., Yeger, H., and Williams, B.R.G. (1993). Homozygous somatic WT1 point mutations in sporadic unilateral Wilms tumor. *Proc. Natl. Acad. Sci. USA.* **90**, 1416–1419.

Denys, P., Malvaux, P., van den Berghe, H., Tanghe, W., and Proesmans, W. (1967). Association d'un syndrôme anatomo-pathologique de pseudohermaphrodisme masculin, d'une tumeur de Wilms', d'une nephropathie parenchymateuse et d'un mosaïcism XX/XY. *Arch. Fr. Pediatr.* **24**, 729–739.

Dey, B.R., Sukhatme, V.P., Roberts, A.B., Sporn, M.B., Rauscher III, F.J., and Kim, S.-J. (1994). Repression of the transforming growth factor-β1 gene by the Wilms' tumor suppressor WT1 gene product. *Mol. Endocrin.*, **8**, 595–602.

Drash, A., Sherman, F., Hartmann, W.H., and Blizzard, R.M. (1970). A syndrome of pseudohermaphroditism, Wilms' tumor, hypertension, and degenerative renal disease. *J. Pediatr.* **76**, 585–593.

Drummond, I.A., Madden, S.L., Rohwer-Nutter, P., Bell, G.L., Sukhatme, V.P., and Rauscher III, F.J. (1992). Repression of the insulin-like growth factor II gene by the Wilms' tumor suppressor gene WT1. *Science* **257**, 674–678.

Englert, C., Hou, X., Maheswaran, S., Bennett, P., Ngwu, C., Re, G.G., Julian, Garvin, A., Rosner, M.R., and Haber, D.A. (1995). WT1 suppresses synthesis of the epidermal growth factor receptor and induces apoptosis. *EMBO J.*, **14**, 4662- 4675.

Gashler, A.L., Bonthron, D.T., Madden, S.L., Rauscher III, F.J., Collins, T., and Sukhatme, V.P. (1992). Human platelet-derived growth factor A chain is transcriptionally repressed by the Wilms' tumor suppressor WT1. *Proc. Natl. Acad. Sci. USA* **89**, 10984–10988.

Goodyer, P., Dehbi, M., Torban, E., Bruening, W., and Pelletier, J. (1995). Repression of the retinoic acid receptor-α gene by the Wilms' tumor suppressor gene product, wt1.*Oncogene* **10**, 1125–1129.

Grundy, P., Koufos, A., Morgan, K., Li, F.P., Meadows, A.T., and Cavenee, W.K. (1988). Familial predisposition to Wilms' tumour does not map to the short arm of chromosome 11. *Nature* **336**, 374–378.

Haber, D. A., Buckler, A.J., Glaser, T., Call, K.M., Pelletier, J., Sohn, R.L., Douglass, E.C., and Housman, D.E. (1990). An internal deletion within an 11p13 zinc finger gene contributes to the development of Wilms' tumor. *Cell* **61**, 1257–1269.

Haber, D. A., Sohn, R.L., Buckler, A.J., Pelletier, J., Call, K.M., and Housman, D.E. (1991). Alternative splicing and genomic structure of the Wilms tumor gene WT1. *Proc. Natl. Acad. Sci. USA.* **88**, 9618–9622.

Harrington, M.A., Konicek, B., Song, A., Xia, X., Fredericks, W.J., and Rauscher III, F.J. (1993). Inhibition of colony-stimulating factor-1 promoter activity by the product of the Wilms' tumor locus. *J. Biol. Chem.* **268**, 21271–21275.

Huff, V., Compton, D.A., Chao, L.-Y., Strong, L.C., Geiser, C.F., and Saunders, G.F. (1988). Lack of linkage of familial Wilms' tumour to chromosome band 11p13. *Nature* **336**, 377–378.

Huff, V., Reeve, A.E., Leppert, M., Strong, L.C., Douglass, E.C., Geiser, C.F., Li, F.P., Meadows, A., Callen, D.F., Lenoir, G., and Saunders, G.F. (1992). Nonlinkage of 16q markers to familial predisposition to Wilms' tumor. *Cancer Res* **52**, 6117–6120.

Joy Ping, A., Reeve, A.E., Law, D.J., Young, M.R., Boehnke, M., and Feinberg, A.P. (1989). Genetic linkage of Beckwith-Wiedemann syndrome to 11p15. *Am. J. Hum. Genet.* **44**, 720–723.

Knudson Jr., A.G. and Strong, L.C. (1972). Mutation and cancer: A model for Wilms' tumor of the kidney. *J. Natl. Cancer Inst.* **48**, 313 -324.

Koufos, A., Grundy, P., Morgan, K., Aleck, K.A., Hadro, T., Lampkin, B.C., and Cavenee, W.K. (1989). Familial Wiedemann-Beckwith syndrome and a second Wilms' tumor locus both map to 11p15.5. *Am. J. Hum. Genet.* **44**, 711–719.

Kreidberg, J. A., Sariola, H., Loring, J.M., Maeda, M., Pelletier, J., Housman, and Jaenisch, R. (1993). WT-1 is required for early kidney development. *Cell* **74**, 679–691.

Little, M. H., Prosser, J., Condie, A., Smith, P.J., van Heyningen, V., and Hastie, N.D. (1992). Zinc finger point mutations within the WT1 gene in Wilms tumor patients. *Proc. Natl. Acad. Sci. USA.* **89**, 4791–4795.

Lowe, S.W., Ruley, H.E., Jacks, T., and Housman, D.E. (1993). p53-Dependent apoptosis modulates the cytotoxicity of anticancer agents. *Cell* **74**, 957–967.

Mannens, M., Slater, R.M., Heyting, C., Bliek, J., de Kraker, J., Coad, N., de Pagter- Holthuizen, P., and Pearson, P.L. (1988). Molecular nature of genetic changes resulting in loss of heterozygosity of chromosome 11 in Wilms' tumours. *Hum. Genet.* **81**, 41–48.

Matsunaga, E. (1981). Genetics of Wilms' tumor. *Hum. Genet.* **57**, 231–246.

Maw, M.A., Grundy, P.E., Millow, L.J., Eccles, M.R., Dunn, R.S., Smith, P.J., Feinberg, A.P., Law, D.J., Paterson, M.C., Telzerow, P.E., Callen, D.F., Thompson, A.D., Richards, R.I., and Reeve, A.E. (1992). A third Wilms' tumor locus on chromosome 16q. *Cancer Res.* **52**, 3094–3098.

McCann, S., Sullivan, J., Guerra, J., Arcinas, M., and Boxer, L.M. (1995). Repression of the *c-myb* gene by WT1 protein in T and B cell lines. *J. Biol. Chem.* **270**, 23785- 23789.

Miller, R.W., Fraumeni, J.F., and Manning, M.D. (1964). Association of Wilms' tumor with aniridia, hemihypertrophy and other congenital malformations. *N. Eng. J. Med.* **270**, 922–927.

Nakagama, H., Heinrich, G., Pelletier, J., and Housman, D. (1995). Sequence and structural requirements for high-affinity DNA binding by the WT1 gene product. *Mol. Cel.l Biol.* **15,** 1489–1498.

Park, S., Bernard, A., Bove, K.E.,Sens, S.A., Hazen-Martin, D.-J., Julian Garvin, A., Haber, D.A. (1993a) Inactivation of WT1 in nephrogenic rests, genetic precursors to Wilms' tumour. *Nature Genetics* **5,** 363–367.

Park, S., Schalling, M., Bernard, A.,Maheswaran, S., Shipley, G.C., Roberts, D., Fletcher, J., Shipman, R., Rheinwold, J., Demetri, G., Griffin, J., Minden, M., Housman, D.E., and Haber, D.A. (1993b). The Wilms' tumour gene WT1 is expressed in murine mesoderm-derived tissues and mutated in a human mesothelioma. *Nature Genetics* **4,** 415–420.

Park, S., Tomlinson, G., Nisen, P., Haber, D.A. (1993c). Altered trans-activational properties of a mutated WT1 gene product in a WAGR-associated Wilms' tumor. *Cancer Res* **53,** 4757–4760.

Pavletich, N.P., and Pabo, C.O. (1991). Zinc finger-DNA recognition: Crystal structure of a Zif268-DNA complex at 2.1A. *Science* **252,** 809–817.

Pavletich, N.P., and Pabo, C.O. (1993). Crystal structure of a five-finger GLI-DNA complex: New perspectives on zinc fingers. *Science* **261,** 1701–1707

Pelletier, J., Bruening, W., Kashtan, C.E., Mauer, S.M., Manivel, J.C., Striegel, J.E., Houghton, D.C., Junien, C., Habib, R., Fouser, L., Fine, R.N., Silverman, B.L., Haber, D.A., and Housman, D.E. (1991). Germline mutations in the Wilms' tumor suppressor gene are associated with abnormal urogenital development in Denys- Drash syndrome. *Cell* **67,** 437–447.

Pelletier, J., Schalling, M., Buckler, A.J., Rogers, A., Haber, D.A., and Housman, D. (1991). Expression of the Wilms' tumor gene WT1 in the murine urogenital system. *Genes & Develop.* **5,** 1345–1356.

Pritchard-Jones, K., Fleming, S., Davidson, D., Bickmore, W., Porteous, D., Gosden, C., Bard, J., Buckler, A., Pelletier, D., Housman, D., van Heyningen, V., and Hastie, N. (1990). The candidate Wilms' tumour gene is involved in genitourinary development. *Nature* **346,** 194–197.

Radice, P., Perotti, D., de Benedetti, V., Mondini, P., Radice, M.T., Pilotti, S., Luksch, R., Bellani, F.F., and Pierotti, M.A. (1995) Allelotyping in Wilms' tumors identifies a putative third tumor suppressor gene on chromosome 11. *Genomics* **27,** 497–501.

Rauscher III, F. J., Morris, J.F., Tournay, O.E., Cook, D.M., and Curran, T. (1990). Binding of the Wilms' tumor locus zinc finger protein to the EGR-1 consensus sequence. *Science* **250,** 1259–1262.

Reeve, A.E., Sih, S.A., Raizis, A.M., and Feinberg, A.P. (1989). Loss of allelic heterozygosity at a second locus on chromosome 11 in sporadic Wilms' tumor cells. *Mol. Cell. Biol.* **9,** 1799–1803.

Riccardi, V.M., Sujansky, E., Smith, A.C., and Francke, U. (1978). Chromosomal imbalance in the aniridia/Wilms' tumor association: 11p interstitial deletion. *J. Pediatr.* **61,** 604–610.

Rupprecht, H.D., Drummond, I.A., Madden, S.L., Rauscher III, F.J., and Sukhatme, V.P. (1994). The Wilms' tumor suppressor gene WT1 is negatively autoregulated. *J. Biol. Chem.* **269,** 6198–6206.

Ryan, G., Steele-Perkins, V., Morris, J.F., Rauscher III, F.J., and Dressler, G.R. (1995). Repression of Pax-2 by WT1 during normal kidney development. *Develop.,* **121,** 867–875.

Schwartz, C.E., Haber, D.A., Stanton, V.P., Strong, L.C., Skolnick, M.H., and Housman, D.E. (1991). Familial predisposition to Wilms' tumor does not segregate with the WT1 gene. *Genomics* **10,** 927–930.

Sharma, P.M., Yang, X., Bowman, M., Roberts, V., and Sukumar, S. (1992) Molecular cloning of rat Wilms' tumor complementary DNA and a study of messenger RNA expression in the urogenital system and the brain. *Cancer Res.* **52,** 6407–6412.

Sotelo-Avila, C., Gonzalez-Crussi, F., and Fowler, J.W. (1980). Complete and incomplete forms of Beckwith-Wiedemann syndrome: Their oncogenic potential. *J. Pediatr* **96,** 47–50, 1980.

Sukhatme, V.P. (1991). Proliferation of renal tubular cells and growth factors: The EGR family of nuclear signal transducers. *Am. J. Kidney Dis.* **17,** 615–618.

Turleau, C., de Grouchy, J., Chavin-Colin, F., Martelli, H., Voyer, M., and Charlas, R. (1984). Trisomy 11p15 and Beckwith-Wiedemann syndrome: A report of two cases. *Hum. Genet.* **67,** 219–221.

Varanasi, R., Bardeesy, N., Ghahremani, M., Petruzzi, M.-J., Nowak, N., Adam, M.A., Grundy, P., Shows, T., and Pelletier, J. (1994). Fine structure analysis of the WT1 gene in sporadic Wilms' tumors. *Proc. Natl. Acad. Sci. USA* **91,** 3554–3558.

Wang, Z.Y., Madden, S.L., Deuel, T.F., and Rauscher III, F.J. (1992). The Wilms' tumor gene product, WT1, represses transcription of the platelet-derived growth factor A-chain gene. *J. Biol. Chem.* **267,** 21999–22002.

Wang, Z.-Y., Qiu, Q.-Q., Enger, K.T., and Deuel, T.F. (1993). A second transcriptionally active DNA-binding site for the Wilms' tumor gene product, WT1. *Proc. Natl. Acad. Sci. USA* **90,** 8896–8900.

Werner, H., Re, G.G., Drummond, I.A., Sukhatme, V.P., Rauscher III, F.J., Sens, D.A., Garvin, A.J., LeRoith, D., and Roberts Jr, C.T. (1993) Increased expression of the insulin-like growth factor 1 receptor gene, IGF1R, in Wilms' tumor is correlated with modulation of IGF1R promoter activity by the WT1 Wilms' tumor gene product. *Proc. Natl. Acad. Sci. USA* **90,** 5828–5832.

Wiedemann, H.R. (1964). Complexe malformatif familial avec hernie ombilicale et macroglossie-Un syndrome noveau? *J. Genet. Hum.* **13**, 223–232.

DISCUSSION

M. Fried: Maybe I missed it, what is the treatment for Wilm's tumor?

D. Housman: Generally kids get various forms of chemotherapy, adriamycin is part of it, radiation used to be used alone with a cure of about 40%—with a combination of chemo it is up to about 90%.

M. Oren: In the anaplastic Wilm's you could assume that perhaps those subsets arose through not only a loss of the Wilm's tumor function, but also through activation of an E1A-like oncogene, which put those cells under constitutive selection against p53-mediated apoptosis. Therefore, also when you irradiate them you get the same resistant phenotype. The question is: have people looked at anaplastic Wilm's and is there any indication that things like myc or myc-related functions might be up-regulated?

D. Housman: Well let me take you back two spaces because that actually brings up an issue I think I did not emphasize as well as I should have, and that is that no matter how hard you look, only about 10–15% of Wilm's tumors show legions in WT1 and it is a confusing situation because, in fact, there are even occasional cases where you have a WAGR case and you look and look, and you cannot find the mutation. Which makes you think, well maybe in that case it has to be there, so maybe we do not know at least one place to look. Nevertheless, I think it is clear, as I tried to say at the beginning of the talk, there are other Wilms tumor genes so now the question becomes to get back to the original question—looking at myc up-regulation, one of the problems you run into, I think, is that these are complex mixtures of cells—they are essentially not a single cell type and the question becomes, what do you use as your baseline? In fact, just with WT1 expression alone, which you would think would be a key indicator of what is going on in the tumor, you can see dramatic variations hundreds of fold variations in levels of expression of the tumor suppressor genes and I am not sure what you can get out of making the myc measurement without having a clear idea of what the control population ought to be. So, people have looked but I am not sure what it means, is the view that I would have.

M. Oren: Pursuing this argument, if I understand correctly, anaplastic tumors would be those which are less differentiated, right?

D. Housman: Yes.

M. Oren: That would tie in at least nicely with lots of indications that myc function in excess would prevent differentiation. If you inactivate things like RB or have excess E2F activity, you might also block differentiation. So maybe the fact that those cells are anaplastic is already indicating that something there got turned on genetically, and, at the same, time also programmed the cells to p53 mediated death?

D. Housman: Yes, the good experiment to do, I think, would be to take tumors like the one you saw and do a direct comparison between the anaplastic focus and the adjacent non-anaplastic area. That would be a comparison I would be a little more comfortable with. But it is a very good thought and I think it is an important one.

D. Livingston: Two questions: First of all, do you know whether the anaplastics respond as well to chemo and radiation therapy as the non-anaplastic legions?

D. Housman: Well, the anaplastics fail almost all the time.

D. Livingston: So that leaves open the possibility that there is a defect in some death mechanism?

D. Housman: Sure.

D. Livingston: But there is also the possibility that the p53 mutation is driving some other feature of those tumor cells, as was originally shown by Varda Rotter when she put back a mutant p53 into an Abelson tumor and acquired potent tumor formation. Arnie Levine has shown that p53 mutations drive tumor cells to be more professional tumor cells than they might otherwise. So mutant p53 might cancel p53 mediated death. It is also possible that a mutant p53 allele drives tumor growth independent of the death phenomenon.

D. Housman: Undoubtedly. Anaplasia is certainly more that just the cancellation of apoptosis—no question about it. Dr. Jerry Pelletier has done some work to suggest that in fact there is a major difference in the apoptotic response of the standard versus the anaplastic tumors, but that may not sort of address the issue that you are raising. Which is that the difficulties that one has in treating the anaplastic tumor may derive in fact from more than just its apoptotic response.

D. Livingston: One other question: Is there a role for dominant negative WT-1 mutants as biological perturbants in the mouse?

D. Housman: Experiments are ongoing but to address this question, we are not doing it with transgenes. It sort of depends on how you want to think about the experiment. Basically what is going on is Jordan Kriedberg at Children's Hospital in Boston, and Dr. Julia Alberta in my lab are putting different versions of WT1 back in under the control of its own promoter hoping to see either restoration of normal function with one of the four splice forms, or same trouble in the mice that you get in humans. One way or the other you should win, because if you can manage to correct the defect in the knockout then you can start to make any mutant you want. Alternatively, if putting in one of the four splice forms causes the same difficulty as the Denys Drash patients get, then you study that, and you figure out where it takes you. So those experiments that are going on now. But you know what the time frame on those things are.

F. Rauscher: That is a really good point and that brings up the whole aspect of really Wilm's tumor genetics and what is going on with the tumor and other mutations. Wilm's essentially presented just like retinalblastoma did genetically, and in fact, was used by Knudson in his early articles in the 70's to predict the recessive oncogene hypothesis and for retinalblastoma that has been completely borne out. You inherit a bad gene, you get a homozygous change in the tumor and with Wilm's this is completely not the case. In fact, there are probably five patients in the world, excluding the Drash patients, that have either inherited or have a homozygous loss in the tumor. And the real question is: Is there hap-lainsufficiency going on here? Is it a dosage effect? What David Livingston is pointing out is that genetically it looks like a transdominant. There is no biochemical evidence at all that there is transdominance. These proteins bind DNA as monomers essentially. So the question is are you looking really at two independent defects at independent loci so it is still two hit genetics at the genetic level? Or is one hit in WT1 predisposing to some other event that we do not know? Maybe you want to expand on that, David, because it is puzzling everybody and you have thought about the genetics a lot longer than we have.

D. Housman: Let me make comments on both sides of the question. First, haplainsuffi-ciency may be adequate to explain at least a part of the occurrence of Wilm's tumors in both WAGR patients and other patients who suffer germline legions, point mutations to the gene. And the thought is that, in fact, when you survey the kidney of the WAGR pa-tients you see proto-legions, if you will, they are called Wilm's tumor, nephregenic rests, they would increase the population of target cells for the next mutation down the road, if you go back to Gerard's talk this morning. Perhaps up to a point where the next set of events that have to occur to lead to the full-fledged tumor are made much more likely. On the other side of the coin it is certainly the case that there is plenty of loss of heterozygo-city even in 11—p13, there are certainly patients like T.S. out there, and that is not the only example where the lesion is passed from one generation to the next and both T.S.—in T.S.'s tumor I did not show you the slide for that is homozygous there is no normal band, so, haploinsufficiency was at least in the end stage not adequate to drive tumor genesis in that patient. So, again, the question arises how sharp is the knife with which we are cut-ting and finding mutations in WT1 that are responsible for some of the cases that we know must have WT1 in mutations? So, if taking both sides of the question but if that has not helped the audience, I apologize but I will do the best I can.

M. Fried: Did I hear you say that WT1 binds to p53?

D. Housman: Well, Frank can expand on this point more than I can. Dan Haber is origi-nally the person who did that work after he left my lab and the significance of the interac-tion and exactly what its functional relationship is to the story I just told you.

M. Fried: That is just what I was going to ask you, if that complex is important to the sur-vival of the cell than you might retain a wild type p53.

F. Rauscher: This is something that is quite unclear at the moment, at least biochemi-cally, although the observation was real and it was first made by Dan Haber as David cor-rectly pointed out. If you overexpress WT1 or even mutants of WT1 in baby rat kidney cells and then immunoprecipitate these proteins you can find a complex that contains WT1 and p53 when you make a relatively mild cell extract. You can also in-vivo cross-link those proteins with chemical cross linkers in the live cell, so this does occur and it is not just occurring when you lyse the cells. Dan Haber and I together mapped this interac-tion and it seems to be a metal-dependent interaction; that is, we know that p53 binds zinc and WT1 does as well. And, in fact, only the DNA binding regions of p53 are required to stick to the DNA binding region of WT1 which can be as small as two zinc fingers. So both of them do not have to bind DNA sequence specifically but they must both chelate zinc. If you strip zinc from these molecules they do not interact anymore. This has also been seen for EGR-1 and p53 and SP1 and p53 too. So the question is: Is there a physiologically relevant metal-dependent p53 interaction! If you go into a normal developing kidney where WT1 and p53 are expressed and are wild type you can also find this interaction by co-immuno precipitation. So something is going on there and that is the summary of the story as we know it now. And we are following it up. It is quite interesting.

Maybe we could talk about DNA binding a little bit? We have tried this WTE site which is quite interesting and I should point out that, and, as you pointed out as well, too, the G residues are completely conserved and those are the contact residues in the crystal structure for EGR-1. So every G that is there is a contact residue for the arginines in WT1 and, in fact, the wobble positions, those nucleotides in the binding site that are not contacted are what are making a difference in your binding site. And so it may be a little unfair to call it a non-EGR site simply because the contact residues are there, however, they certainly do make a difference. And let me point out that they do make a difference depending on the type of gel shift assay utilized. As you know, often DNA binding assays are performed with short, synthetic oligos anneal label and then you use in a gel shift. However, and in that assay you can certainly find a good difference between a classic EGR site and a WTE site, however, if you put that alago in the context of a longer stranded DNA, that is, something that has more secondary structure like a 200 base pair thing, you greatly diminish what you are seeing in terms of a difference between WTE. So it may be a context dependent thing that is less flexible than the DNA. And the final issue is really whether a WTE site or an EGR site is a better reporter in-vivo. And when we have done those experiments with synthetic binding sites we can see no difference in the ability of a WTE or EGR site to really report to a WTE expression vector.

D. Housman: Yes, we can really get into this in fairly significant depth because the flip side of this is we certainly see context dependent binding if we switch the sequences which surround the binding site, be it WTE or EGR1 there is clearly an effect of that as well.

F. Rauscher: Absolutely, I think the flexibility of the flanking DNA is going to be really important for these proteins that really wrap around the major groove and make contacts all along one strand of the DNA.

D. Housman: I think we could both agree that the most frustrating thing is that what we would rally like to have is a set of genes *in vivo* where you can put WT1 in, turn it on, turn if off and see the direct readout of an endogeneous gene and that is really the missing link in this problem and it is a frustrating one.

F. Rauscher: Absolutely, I agree.

M. Oren: Back to the p53 and the anaplastic Wilm's. If those anaplastic tumors are continuously exposed to an apoptotic signal which is p53 dependent, and that is why they mutate, you would predict that if you reconstitute p53 function there, they would go into apoptosis without any added DNA damage signal. Now, are there any experimental systems, cell lines presumably, which recapitulate that anaplastic Wilm's phenotype, which you can test this model in?

D. Housman: Not that I know of, maybe Frank can comment on this.

F. Rauscher: This is a really difficult field in the Wilm's tumor field. Essentially there are no cell lines at all that recapitulate the normal histology of a tumor. Again it is a very mesenchymal tumor usually has stromal and epitheleal elements it is very difficult to grow those. Dan Haber has one Wilm's tumor cell line where he has done the "add back" experiment, where you can transfect the wild type WT1 gene and see a down regulation of cell growth. This is essentially the most stringent assay for the function of a tumor suppressor gene. Moreover, these are not anaplastic—anaplastic tumors do not grow.

D. Housman: Yes, anaplastic tumors are rare to begin with. So, the chances of both getting lucky and hitting a cell line are diminished significantly by that. It is unfortunate, and let me say, someday if we ever figure out how to make the mice, or some other experimental animal produce both nephroblastoma and perhaps anaplasia, there from, then I think the kind of experiment you are talking about may become feasible.

G. Evan: I have just got a quick question. Do they not grow or do they not survive?

D. Housman: The Wilm's tumors when you try to put them in culture?

G. Evan: That is right.

D. Housman: Well, both. They are sort of, I think, a typical unpleasant tissue culture experience. You put them down and some of the time, essentially nothing much happens, if you are really nice to them, stuff starts to grow, and even the best of circumstances it is a nursing home type relationship between you and the cells.

M. Kulesz-Martin: I wonder if there are any parallels in the mouse skin model. It has been found, in our lab, that altered expression of the wild type p53 gene occurs right at the point where preneoplastic cells become neoplastic. And yet in Klein-Szanto's lab and Alan Balmain's lab, it is known that mutations in p53 occur in 40% or so of the tumors, and they occur right at the point where the cells become metastatic or when they become spindle cell tumors where they have lost their differentiation markers. Now, do you know whether the anaplastic Wilm's tumors are a later progression of the more differentiated or non-anaplastic ones? And you mentioned also that there were really one hundred fold differences in the expression of wild type WT1 gene in various tumors. Do you think it is possible that some earlier stages have altered expressions of the wild type gene and that it is in the later point when they are becoming less differentiated that now you select for the mutations?

D. Housman: The WT1 mutations of the p53 mutations?

M. Kulesz-Martin: I was asking whether p53 changes, first in expression of the wild type genes and then by mutations, may be responsible for progress from more differentiated to anaplastic tumors? Maybe, I am suggesting there may be parallels between the mouse epidermal progression model and the WT1 gene and the Wilm's tumor situation with respect to defects in p53 gene function? I guess in the human tumor samples that you get it is difficult to demonstrate what influences progression from one stage to another.

D. Housman: That is one of the issues. It seems like you can give the same answer to half the questions which is: if we had better control of the development of tumors in animals then I think we could start to address that kind of question because you could take cells out at various stages. It is very frustrating. You get one shot at it. You got a large lump of tissues that there is a lot of it but what happens before and what would have happened after if you allowed it to grow is completely opaque so it is really hard to know.

F. Rauscher: That experiment has been done by Jerry Pelletier. He has been able to take archival specimens where there are slides there and he can micro-dissect the non-anaplastic from anaplastic tumor.

D. Housman: Yes, that is what I showed you.

F. Rauscher: Yes and you find a p53 mutation in the anaplastic but not the non-anaplastic tumor. I think that is the question you are asking. It is that it is evolving in that particular tumor and the anaplastic thing that is histologically anaplastic has a p53 mutation whereas the non-anaplastic Wilm's does not.

D. Housman: Yes, the challenging issue is whether the p53 mutation is the one and only step between the non-anaplastic and anaplastic portion of the tumor, or is something else happening that essentially makes the cells permissive to p53 mutation and then there is a tremendous drive—selective drive—to lose p53 function and that happens at high frequency.

M. Kulesz-Martin: You said that the ratios of the four alternative splice forms of WT1 did not seem to change much in development or in different tissues—is that based on studies of a whole organ? In other words, if you took the mesenchyme dissected from the epitheleum, do you know whether there might be changes in WT1 splice forms?

D. Housman: Well, essentially if you do *in situ* hybridization on the mesenchyme as it is interacting the the ureteric bud but the mesenchymal cells are blazing the uruteric bud is blank. It is another striking contrast to retinoblastoma in that the gene is expressed in a very, very tissue specific manner and then again in the sertoli cells there is tremendous expression whereas in the granulosa cells—surrounding cells—have none. So, I think there is pretty strong evidence that would say that you are going to see the gene on in the cells that you are concerned with, with respect to tumor formation and what surrounding cells are essentially going to be off.

D. Livingston: Did I understand before, that you and Tyler Jacks have done the following experiment: you have taken double knockout ES cells and generated chimeric animals?

D. Housman: This was not Tyler that was Jordan Kriedberg from Children's Hospital in Boston.

D. Livingston: You have taken plus-plus ES and minus-minus ES made a mélange and isolated chimeric animals?

D. Housman: Correct.

D. Livingston: And those animals are perfectly healthy?

D. Housman: Those animals are perfectly healthy, we do not know if they are completely fertile, nobody has bred particularly well, but they show high ES cell contribution by coat color.

D. Livingston: In the kidney as well?

D. Housman: We have not killed them. We are waiting for some tumor to show up but pretty soon we are going to start killing them.

D. Livingston: Because that is a fairly important piece of data?

D. Housman: Yes, it is a trade off, obviously, because on the one hand you keep hoping next week we are going to have our tumor and you think so I will not kill the animal. But if you kill the animal, and you eventually want to kill the animal, do a careful dissection of the kidney. We are particularly interested in the genital systems since they have not bred either which, as you know, sometimes chimeras do not breed. But these guys are consistently doing poorly in this.

D. Livingston: Because there is a window in time during which an individual is at risk, and I assume that is a very short time during gestation.

D. Housman: In terms of kids and age of diagnosis, in general, you are diagnosed before age five. If you have a germ-line mutation, you are diagnosed, on average, a year or more earlier than if you have a sporadic case. But presumably what is going on is that the events that lead to tumorogenesis occurred either in utero or shortly after birth when all the stuff is going on with developing kidneys.

D. Livingston: Small window, because you do not see second and third recurrences arising after the original treatment.

D. Housman: And then he comes back and he is the dad of a patient now.

D. Livingston: That is right. Healthy, no second line neoplasms, not like retinoblastoma?

D. Housman: That is a controversial or perhaps less that statistically significant but noticable trend. There is a trend towards leukemias.

D. Livingston: But not like RB, no?

D. Housman: It is not like RB, but if you talk to physicians who deal with Wilm's tumor kids, they will swear by the fact that there is a significant but not statistically significant leukemia rise which may be iatrogenic or may be due to the WT1 germ line lesion. It is always tough, I think, with the particular leukemias to call that one, one way or the other. But other than that, there is not much.

A. Nordheim: Is there any progress in identifying target genes of WT1?

D. Housman: Well, it depends on what you call progress. You want to comment on this Frank?

F. Rauscher: No, I'd rather just sigh as well.

D. Housman: Certainly, IGF-2 is as good a guess as is out there. But what you really want, again, is the *prima facie* evidence *in vivo* that you put WT1 into a cell which is WT1 deprived and off goes IGF-2. That experiment is really harder to do than one would like it to be, and I think that is the frustration in the field because we really do not have that.

F. Rauscher: We have looked in non-Wilm's tumor cells that express IGF-2 from its proper promoter, that is the p3 promoter (there are about six promoters in the IGF-2 locus). By and large, if you transfect WT1 wild type it does not repress the endogenous gene very well, however, there is some effect. Yet in a transient assay, and all assays, you can look and it is a very good target gene.

D. Housman: Yes, maybe we should go back a space. In general, the thinking is in transient assay systems WT1 is acting as a repressor rather than an activator.

T. Beerman: I wanted to change the topic a little bit. I am curious about the relationship between DNA damage and apoptosis because it appears to be talked about that the DNA damage is kind of a passive event; that is, you take any kind of DNA damaging agent and that is going to lead to apoptosis. Has anybody looked at it in terms of first just quantitatively how much DNA damage does it take, and also qualitatively what kinds of DNA legions would lead to apoptosis, are they all just the same in the end?

D. Housman: Does not have to be genotoxic drugs; in fact, we have done experiments, and others have as well, where you use microtubular agents, we have actually done protein synthesis inhibitors. When Scott was doing the first run of experiments, we wanted a treatment which would give necrosis rather than apoptosis and so I suggested using ouabain because I figured that has got to kill them fast—no, that gave apoptosis. Sodium azide gave necrosis. So, it looks like it is somewhere beyond genotoxic agents and, I guess going back to the original question, has anyone quantitated how much damage you got to do in order to get so much response—I am sure somebody has. Maybe Moshe can say more about it than I can, but we have not done quite that systematically.

T. Beerman: I mean, the second part, I would think if you put some kind of binding agent on DNA and you cannot replicate—but that is lethal and so whether it goes through apoptosis or not—would that always matter?

D. Housman: But how do you deal with a drug like ouabain or a drug like hygromycin, both of which actually—I mean, you can always say there is a secondary effect on the genome and the actual lethal event is something to do with a damage to genome and p53 picks that up but that gets tougher to quantitate it must be fairly sensitive. Actually, thinking back to data from other folks, it does not take a lot of DNA damage to activate p53, as I recall.

G. Evan: Are those EGR-1 transgenics and do they look in anyway like the Wilm's tumor?

D. Housman: There are EGR-1 knockouts, they do not look like the Wilm's tumor knockouts.

G. Evan: Right, but EGR-1 is a transactivator so is it the flip side of WT?

F. Rauscher: That was the original thought, it would have been nice, essentially the EGR-1 and its cohorts which are EGR-2, 3 and 4 all having the exact same DNA binding domain are expressed relatively ubiquitously a lot and all activators when you measure them, as we do, and transient assays. The thought originally was that it might be exactly as you say, it would compete for EGR binding sites, however, EGR-1 is very poorly expressed in the kidney anyway.

G. Evan: You cannot transgenically target it to the kidney then ask what happens?

7 in top right corner

HTLV-I TAX

A Paradigm for How a Single Auxiliary Factor Can Regulate the Expression of Viral and Cellular Genes

Giovanni Perini and Michael R. Green

Howard Hughes Medical Institute
Program in Molecular Medicine
University of Massachusetts Medical Center
Worcester, Massachusetts 01605

1. INTRODUCTION

Human T-cell Leukemia Virus type I (HTLV-I) is a human retrovirus that causes disease mainly in the Mediterranean and south tropical areas such as Southern Europe, Middle East, Japan, Philippines, South America, Caribbean and Central Africa[1, 2.] It is spread from mother to child perinatally or by breast feeding. Transfer from one individual to another can also occur by sexual contact and infected blood. Although it is asymptomatic in the vast majority of the population, a relatively small (< 4%) but still significant number of individuals develops after several years from the onset of the infection, a severe adult T cell leukemia (ATL)[3] or the so-called tropical spastic paraparesis (TSP)[4], also known as a HTLV-I associated myelopathy (HAM), a neurological disorder characterized by a slow and progressive demyelination of the peripheral nerves and causing paraparesis and spasticity of the lower extremities. Moreover, HTLV-I can also cause a severe granulocytosis and eosinophilia[5] and in some cases an autoimmune chronic athritis[6].

HTLV-I shows a specific tropism for the lymphoid CD4+ T-cells[7] but it is also found in other cell types such as microglia and fetal astrocytes[4]. How HTLV-I can induce such different severe diseases is still unknown. The fact that HTLV-I, as in the case with other retroviruses, must integrate into the host genome in order to propagate, raised the question of whether HTLV-I induces host cell chromosomal rearrangements. A detailed analysis has been conducted in several patients with ATL. Trysomys of chromosomes 3 and 7 and rearrangements of the long arm of chromosome 6 have been found in HTLV-I infected lymphocytes[8]. However, due to the small number of patients that present chromosomal alterations, it is unlikely that chromosomal rearrangements are directly involved in HTLV-I associated diseases and instead suggests that the HTLV-I gene products must be responsible for the deregulation of cellular function.

In the past years, several studies have convincingly shown that a HTLV-I encoded regulator, called Tax, could play an important role in the genesis of these pathological disorders. As with many other oncogenic viral regulators such as the Adenovirus E1a[9, 10], Hepatitis B virus pX[11] and Herpes Simplex Virus VP16[12] proteins, Tax regulates the transcription of both viral and cellular genes and can transform cells in vitro or induce tumors when overexpressed in transgenic mice. Tax, therefore, represents an interesting candidate to understand HTLV-I pathogenesis.

Here we present an overview of the molecular biology of HTLV-I Tax protein and of the molecular mechanisms through which Tax deregulates cellular function and metabolism.

2. TAX: A TRANSACTIVATOR WITH MULTIPLE INDISPENSABLE DOMAINS

The HTLV-I genome has been completely cloned and sequenced[13,14]. Like other retroviruses, HTLV-I genome encodes several proteins required for the propagation and assembly of the viral progeny. These include a capsid protein (Gag 48 kD), an envelope protein (Env, 54 kD) and the reverse transcriptase (Pol, 99 kD). In addition HTLV-I 3' LTR contains several overlapping open reading frames that encode factors responsible for the regulation and the metabolism of the viral transcripts. One of these open reading frames, pX-IV and later called Tax, codes for a 40 kD transcriptional regulator that is essential for transcriptional activation of the HTLV-I LTR[15–18]. Tax is a phosphoprotein that is mainly localized in the nucleus[19–22] Apparently Tax is phosphorylated through the activation of the PKC pathway[23]. Phosphorylation occurs only on serines that are localized at the amino terminal domain of Tax. It is still unclear what is the effect of phosphorylation on Tax function, in that a recombinant non-phosphorylated Tax is still capable of inducing transactivation of its own LTR in vitro[24] However, mutants in the serine residues cannot activate the HIV-LTR[25]. Tax does not contain a typical nuclear localization signal, though several Tax regions contribute an essential function for its import into the nucleus. The most important one has been mapped at the amino terminal domain of Tax and encompasses amino acids 17–59[21, 26]. Interestingly this region contains several cysteines and histidines suggesting that it could form a zinc-binding structure. Accordingly Tax has been found to specifically bind zinc[21, 27–28] and other divalent cations such as Cu^{2+} and Ni^{2+} (ref.20). Moreover specific mutations of cys23, cys29 and cys36 show that these residues are essential for Tax nuclear import and suggest that the entire zinc-binding domain could serve as a nuclear localization signal[21]. Furthermore, other amino acids have been also found to affect the efficiency of nuclear import. In particular double substitutions in the region downstream the nuclear localization domain (amino acids 62–63, 73–74, 82–83, 102–103, 123–124, 130–131, 189–190, 194–195, 206–207) were shown to significantly reduce nuclear translocation of Tax[21].

Tax is a transcriptional regulator and is essential for the activation of several viral and cellular promoters. However, like several other viral activators, Tax does not bind DNA and requires cellular auxiliary factors to activate gene promoters. Several studies have shown that Tax functions through different unrelated cellular factors such as NF-κB CREB/ATF and SRF. Tax possesses domains that can specifically respond to these different factors. For example substitutions of amino acids 137 and 138 prevent Tax from transactivating NF-κB responsive promoters while they have no effect on the CREB/ATF responsive ones[21, 29]. Conversely, the substitution of amino acid 3 or 319 abolishes Tax response on promoters containing CREB/ATF binding sites but not on promoters that work through NF-κB factors. Mutations in the amino terminal region of Tax between amino acid 17 and 60 have been also described to affect Tax mediated HTLV-I LTR. However most of this mutations also affected the efficiency of Tax nuclear import suggesting that their inability to transactivate was caused by a reduced capability to localize to the nucleus[21,26].

Tax also possesses a specific transactivating domain that was mapped by deletion analysis at its carboxyl terminus[30]. In fact, in transfection assays, a chimeric protein containing the GAL4 DNA binding domain fused to the Tax region between amino acids 296 and 320 was sufficient to transactivate a promoter carrying multiple GAL4 DNA binding sites. Accordingly, single amino acid substitutions of the 296 and 320 residues drastically reduced Tax transactivating function. Moreover, the ability of Tax mutants to squelch activation by GAL4-Tax from a GAL4 sites-containing reporter plasmid, suggests that Tax could interact with a protein(s) of the general transcription machinery. Indeed, Tax has been found to contact TBP in vitro[31]. TBP is the fundamental component of the TFIID factor required to bind the TATA box and around which the general transcription machinery is assembled. However, in vivo experiments show that the mechanism through which Tax contacts the general transcription machinery is more complex than a simple Tax-TBP contact and that it must interact with an additional unidentified factor(s).

3. CELLULAR AND ANIMAL MODELS FOR IN VIVO STUDIES OF TAX FUNCTIONS

Tax is a viral oncoprotein that can immortalize and transform several mammalian cell lines such as NIH-3T3[32], Rat-1[29,32] and human CD4+ T lymphocytes[33]. In addition, transgenic mice overexpressing Tax under the control of the HTLV-I LTR develop tumors between 13 to 17 weeks[34]. However, other phenotypes have been observed in mice expressing Tax constitutively. For example in some cases, the accumulation of Tax in the thymus induces an involution of this organ[34]. As a consequence, mice grow very slowly and die from a severe immunodeficiency. In some other cases co-expression of Tax together with Env induces an erosion of the cartilage and bones resembling a form of rheumatoid arthritis typically found in patients with TPS/HAM[35]. Moreover, transgenic mice with high level of Tax develop an exocrinopathy resembling the Sjogren' s syndrome[36]. Despite the relevant number of pathological disorders that Tax generates in the mouse, none of the mice develop a T-cell leukemia and the Tax-induced tumors have instead the characteristics of mesenchymal tumors and neurofibromas[34]. To produce a HTLV-I associated ATL in an animal model may require the activation of a second oncogene. This hypothesis is strongly supported by the fact that co-transfection of Tax and the ras oncogene in rat embryo cells greatly increases the number of transformed cells thus suggesting that Tax can cooperate with other oncogenes to induce tumorigenesis[37].

4. PROMISCUOUS ACTIVATION OF VIRAL AND CELLULAR GENES

Like many other viral transactivators such as adenovirus E1a protein, HSV VP16 protein, HBV pX protein, Tax can target several viral and cellular promoters. These results are here briefly reviewed.

4.1 Activation of Viral Promoters

Tax is essential for the transactivation of the HTLV-I LTR. The LTR contains three 21 bp repeats that confer Tax responsiveness[38–40]. Each of these repeats contains a DNA sequence resembling the cAMP responsive element and ATF binding site (CRE)[41,42]. Several groups have found that a relatively large number of cellular factors can bind the LTR in vitro[42–45] These include CREB, TREB-1, TREB-2 TREB-3 TREB-4 TREB-5, TREB-7/ATF-2, TREB-36/ATF-1, TAXREB-67/ATF-4, HEF-1, HEF-1B, HEB1 and HEB2 (refs. 24, 46–50). These factors belong to the family of the bZIP proteins and all share a highly conserved DNA binding domain consisting of a basic amino acid enriched region (basic region) flanked by a leucine repeat (leucine zipper). Although Tax does not bind DNA it was suggested that it could be recruited to the LTR through the interaction with cellular factors. Several groups have isolated in vitro a ternary complex that contains Tax, CREB and the 21 base pair element of the LTR[24, 51–53]. Yet, it is unclear whether all the bZIP factors that bind to the LTR can recruit Tax to the promoter. So far only CREB and ATF-2[53] have been observed to form a stable ternary complex with Tax and DNA. Therefore, despite the wide number of bZIP factors that are able to recognize the LTR, only a subset of them are likely to mediate Tax responsiveness in vivo.

Tax can transactivate other viral promoters such as the HIV-I LTR[21,54] and the HBV enhancer[55]. To activate the HBV enhancer, Tax presumably requires proteins of the CREB/ATF family. In fact, the enhancer contains a sequence that resemble the CRE palindrome and that mediates the transcription of HBV genes. In contrast, Tax stimulates the HIV-LTR through a different set of proteins that belong to the NF-κB family.

4.2 Activation of Cellular Genes

Many of the genes regulated by Tax have been previously associated with cellular transformation. For example, Tax can stimulate the expression of several leucine zipper transcriptional factors such as c-Fos[56–58], Fra-1[58,59], JunD[58], and two zinc finger proteins Krox20 (Egr-1) and Krox24 (Egr-2)[60,61]. All of these are induced by serum stimulation and their activity has been correlated with the induction of cell proliferation. Tax activates these genes through different cis elements. For example several SRE (Serum Responsive Element) and CRE elements are required for Tax mediated activation of Krox-20 and Krox-24[60,61]. Stimulation of the c-fos promoter seems to be more complicated. In fact, four different types of DNA binding sites including SRE, CRE/AP1, SIE (v-sis conditioned medium inducible element) and DR (octanucleotide direct repeat element) sites are essential for Tax-mediated responsiveness[62]. Tax promotes the transcription of the vimentin gene through a NF-κB site[63,64]. Vimentin is an essential gene belonging to the family of the intermediate filaments and its deregulation has been proved to induce a high rate of cell proliferation. Altered expression of the vimentin gene could contribute to establish the transformed phenotype. Deregulated expression of the TGF-β1 gene is another way by which Tax could induce tumorigenesis. Tax increases TGF-β1 transcription through AP-1 cis-acting elements common to the two alternative promoters that control TGF-β1 expression[65]. In vivo and in vitro experiments suggest that Tax may require Jun/Fos heterodimers to transactivate.

Tax can also stimulate the transcription of several cytokines such as interleukin-2 (IL-2)[66, 67] and interleukin-3 (IL-3)[68]. In addition to IL-2, Tax can also activate the IL-2 receptor (IL-2Rα) in the T-cells, thus establishing an autocrine loop that can alter the growth rate of these cells[66, 67, 69–71]. Surprisingly, the up-regulation of IL-2 and IL-2Rα seems to induce inflammatory damage of the nervous system which could represent a first step for the development of the TSP/HAM. Co-expression of IL-2 and IL-2Rα has been found in the CD4+ T-cells of those patients with TSP/HAM but not in those with ATL[67]. As with the vimentin gene, NF-κB sites are essential to mediate Tax response in both IL-2 and IL-2Rα promoters[69,70] In contrast Tax enhances IL-3 transcription level through two lymphokine consensus sequences, CK-1 and CK-2 that bind unknown transcription factors[68]. Act-2, a general mediator of inflammation is also stimulated by Tax. The Act-2 Tax-mediated stimulation is dependent on the presence of an AP-1/CRE element in the Act-2 promoter[72]. Tax increases the expression of TFN-β and IgK light chain genes in lymphoid cells. Both genes respond to Tax through NF-κB elements[73,74]. However, the two genes show temporal differences in their expression in response to Tax suggesting that different NF-κB complexes could be involved[74]. TFN-β is an osteoclast-activating factor, which is involved in bone resorption. The deregulation of TNF-β could be correlated with the hypercalcemia that is frequently associated with ATL. Two other cytokines required for bone resorption are the granulocyte-macrophage colony stimulating factor (GM-CSF) and the granulocyte colony stimulation factor (G-CSF)[75,76]. Tax-mediated increase of GM-CSF and G-CSF expression occurs through NF-κB factors. However, an additional CREB/ATF factor is essential for transactivation of the GM-CSF promoter by Tax, while a maximal stimulation of G-CSF promoter occurs in the presence of the NF-IL6 factor. Surprisingly, the NF-kB site partially overlaps the CRE element in the GM-CSF promoter and is adjacent to the NF-IL6 site in the G-CSF promoter. Disruption of the relative position of these sites abolish Tax responsiveness[76]. It is possible that Tax reinforces a cooperative interaction between NF-kB and other DNA binding transcription factors. The Tax-mediated increase of GM-CSF and G-CSF expression levels can contribute to the appearance of the ATL-associated hypercalcemia, granulocytosis and eosinophilia.

Tax also affects transcription of the nerve growth factor (NGF)[77] and proenkephalin[78] genes. Promoters from both genes contain CRE/AP-1 sites that are Tax responsive. The CRE element in the NGF promoter is homologous to the CRE site of the 21 bp- repeats of the HTLV-I LTR. Interestingly the Tax-mediated regulation of the proenkephalin gene depends on the type of bZIP transcription factors present in the cells. For example, Tax stimulates the proenkephalin gene expression through the ATF-3 protein while it exerts a repressive function through JunB[78].

Tax also represses the transcription of the DNA polymerase β gene[79] However, no specific cis acting element in the DNA polymerase β promoter has been found to be Tax responsive. A possible explanation is that Tax represses this gene in an indirect way. In other words, Tax could sequesters some cellular factors that are essential for the activation of the DNA polymerase β gene.

5. MOLECULAR MODELS FOR A TAX-MEDIATED TRANSCRIPTIONAL ACTIVATION

How is possible that a single protein can function through so many different factors? Apparently Tax is composed of several domains that have evolved to interact specifically with a variety of cellular transcription factors. The biochemical mechanisms through which Tax stimulates gene transcription are briefly summarized below.

5.1 Transcriptional Activation Through NF-kB Factors

Several pieces of evidence indicate that Tax can interact specifically with p100 and p105 precursors of the p50 subunits of NF-kB and NF-κB2 factors respectively[80-83]. In both precursors the interaction with Tax is mediated through ankyrin-like regulatory domain. Under normal conditions, NF-κB dimers are in part retained in the cytoplasm through their association with the ankyrin domain of the p100 and p105 proteins and are translocated into the nucleus following a specific transmembrane signal. Tax, therefore, has an antagonistic effect on the association between NF-κB and p100/p105 precursors. The interaction of Tax with NF-KB precursors could result in a steric hindrance that prevents the association of the p100/p105 ankyrin-like domain with the NF-kB dimers (p50/p65). However, this is not the only mechanism that has been described for Tax-mediated stimulation of NF-κB activity. Figure 1 summarizes the different mechanisms through which Tax can activate NF-kB activity. For example Tax seems to induce the

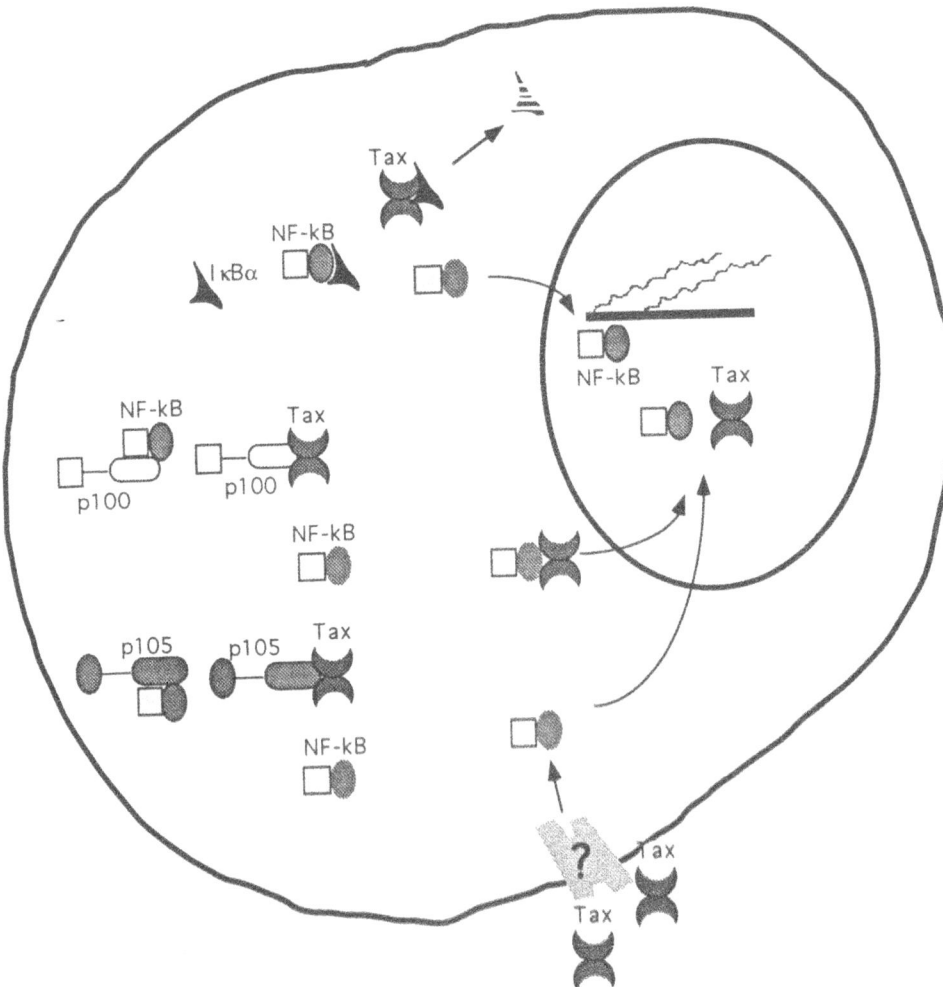

Figure 1. Model illustrating the different mechanisms through which Tax can regulate NF-kB activity.

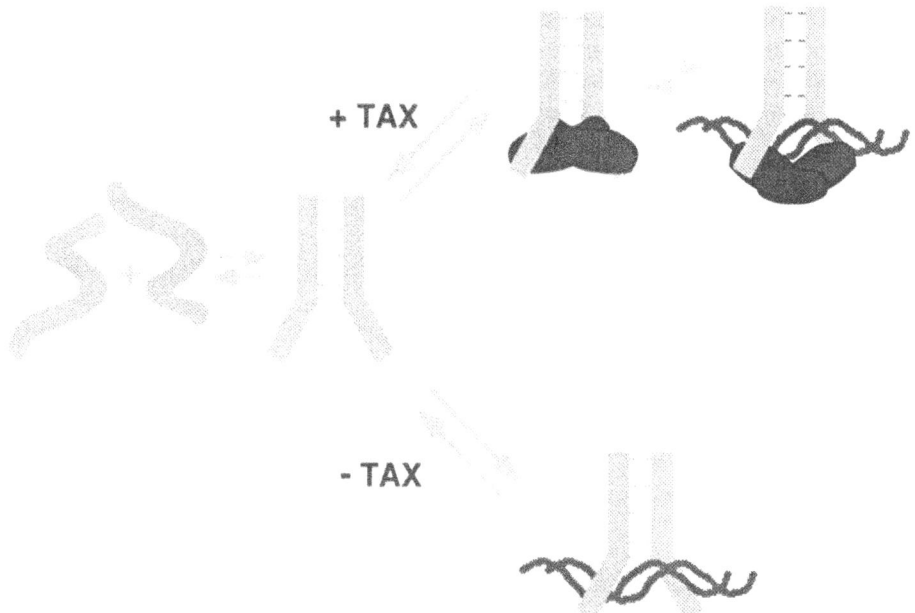

Figure 2. Model describing how Tax stimulates bZIP DNA binding. By interacting with the bZIP basic region Tax stabilizes a relatively unstable bZIP dimer, thus shifting the monomer-dimer equilibrium towards dimer formation. In addition, through its association with the bZIP-DNA complex, Tax affects bZIP DNA binding recognition.

phosphorylation of IκBα[84], an inhibitor of the p50/p65 heterodimer. IκBα interacts with NF-κB dimers and inhibits their translocation into the nucleus. Phosphorylation of IκBα prevents the association with NF-κB and promotes its degradation by specific proteases. Therefore, by promoting IkBα phosphorylation and its subsequent degradation, Tax facili tates the release of NF-κB dimers from the IκBα inhibitor and their fast transport to the nucleus. It was also found that Tax may function like an oxidative agent[85.] Oxidative stress is known to stimulate NF-κB activity[86]. It is possible that Tax increases the production of oxygen radicals that are required for NF-κB activation. In fact Tax-mediated effect on NF-κB activity is abolished when cells are treated with pyrrolidine dithiocarbamate (PDTC), a potent antioxidant reagent. It has been also found that Tax can enhance DNA binding of NF-κB dimers to their cognate DNA sites in vitro[87] suggesting that Tax could directly interact with the NF-κB factor and influence NF-kB DNA binding activity. These results are supported by recent studies showing that Tax can bind the p50 and p65 subunits of the NF-kB dimer[88,89]. Finally, additional results indicate that Tax could work like an extracellular cytokine. In fact, recombinant Tax can activate a signal transduction cascade that induces NF-κB nuclear translocation in lymphoid cells when directly supplied to the culture medium[71,73,90,91].

5.2 Transcriptional Activation through Basic Region-Leucine Zipper Factors

Most of viral and cellular promoters that are stimulated by Tax contain DNA binding sites for bZIP transcription factors. In several cases these cis-elements were shown to be necessary for Tax responsiveness suggesting that Tax stimulates gene transcription through a pathway alternative to the NF-κB pathway. bZIP proteins share a common DNA binding domain characterized by the presence of a basic region that contacts DNA and a flanking leucine repeats (leucine zipper) that mediates bZIP dimerization (see ref. 92 for review). Tax interacts specifically with this class of factors through their conserved DNA binding domain[51,93]. Several groups have found that Tax can increase the DNA binding activity of several bZIP factors such as, CREB, different ATF proteins (ATF-1, ATF-2, ATF-3), c-Jun, C/EBP and GCN4 the yeast homologue of c-Jun[24,51,87,93].

One possible mechanism for the Tax-mediated DNA binding increase is that Tax could modify the bZIP protein. Several efforts to identify such modifications have failed suggesting that a different mechanism is involved[51,87]. Indeed, Tax has been found present in a ternary complex with the bZIP and DNA, indicating that the enhancement of DNA binding may require the stable association of Tax to the bZIP-DNA complex. How does Tax increase bZIP DNA binding?

Recent findings indicate that Tax promotes bZIP dimerization[51]. bZIP proteins form homo- or heterodimers and bind DNA in a two-step reaction. In the first step the bZIP dimerizes followed by a second step in which the dimer binds DNA. However the two steps have different equilibrium constants and bZIP dimerization rate is the limiting step[94,95]. Therefore, by binding to a bZIP dimer, Tax increases the dimer lifetime and shifts the monomer-dimer equilibrium toward dimer formation. Recent results show that Tax recognizes the bZIP protein by interacting with the conserved basic region[96]. Specific mutations in the basic region completely abolish Tax responsiveness. Moreover, Tax is a stable dimer in solution. It is therefore possible that a Tax dimer, by interacting with the basic regions of an unstable bZIP dimer drives dimerization and thus promotes bZIP DNA binding. However quantitative analysis of the effect of Tax on bZIP-DNA binding reveals that, in addition to increasing the rate, of dimerization Tax must also influence bZIP recognition of DNA[97]. Accordingly it has been found that it alters the DNA site selection of the bZIP proteins[96]. Furthermore, increasing evidence suggests that the extent of Tax effect on bZIP DNA binding is strictly dependent on the DNA sequences that flanks the CRE/AP-1 core site [53, 96, 97, 98]

5.3 Activation through the p67 Serum Resposive Factor (SRF)

Tax interacts with the cellular factor p67[SRF], thereby activating the transcription of the cellular immediate early genes through CArG boxes[99]. In doing so, Tax relieves the requirement for a serum induced stimulation of the signal transduction pathway. Tax functions as a bridge between the p67[SRF] protein and the general transcription machinery. Tax carboxyl terminal region is necessary for the interaction with p67[SRF] (ref. 100). Apparently the stable interaction with factors that are specifically associated with the promoters allows Tax to contact the general transcription machinery and stimulate transcription. This model is consistent with studies of other viral transactivators, in particular the adenovirus E1a and the HSV VP16 protein.

6. DISCUSSION AND CONCLUSIONS

Although much has been learned about the molecular biology of Tax still many questions remain unanswered. For example, Tax can induce different pathological conditions in transgenic animals that in some cases resemble those found in humans. However every time new generations of transgenic animals were produced the results were completely different. A plausible explanation is that the sites of integration of the Tax vector in the host genome could affect the tissue specificity and the transcriptional level of the Tax gene. Moreover, small differences in the expression constructs such as the presence of part of other HTLV-I genes (for example env), produce results completely unexpected indicating that other regions of the HTLV-I genome could significantly contribute to the development of the HTLV-I associated diseases. Tax can induce different types of tumors in particular mesenchymal tumors and neurofibrosarcomas. However, there are no examples of Tax-induced T-cell leukemias. One possibility is that the mouse background is inadequate to develop this kind of tumor. A second one is that the activation of other oncogenes could be required. Generally, this event is very rare and could not occur during the short lifetime of the transgenic animal. Third, since Tax expression starts at the very beginning of embryonic development, it is possible that the thymus selectively removes those subpopulations of lymphocytes that could induce leukemia during adult life.

A fascinating aspect of Tax biology is its ability to transcriptionally activate large number of cellular genes. Interestingly the majority of the genes code for cytokines or growth factors. On one hand it is clear the role that these gene may play in the deregulation of the biology of T-cells, on the other hand it is not obvious what is the cause-effect relationship between the deregulation of these factors and neurological disorders. Nevertheless, an increasing number of reports shows that cytokines and their receptors are expressed in tissue of the nervous system (see ref. 101 for review). Growth factors such as TGF-β, TNF and NGF are expresses in the peripheral nervous system following nerve and tissue injury and can induce the expression of other cytokines such as IL-1 IL-6 and neurothophins. The expression of these growth factors is not restricted to immune cells. For example, Schwann cells express TGF-β, while microglia and astrocytes can express almost the entire array of known cytokines and growth factors. These cytokines and growth factors are released from the nerve tissues concomitant with a nerve tissue damage and they are supposed to promote survival and repair of the tissue. It is therefore possible that Tax by altering the balanced homeostatis of these factors establishes a condition resembling that of an injury in the nerve tissue which will eventually result in a permanent damage of the nerve.

Another amazing aspect is Tax ability to interact with an almost unlimited number of cellular factors. Most of these results have been obtained in vitro and so far there is little evidence for a Tax function in vivo. For example many groups have shown that Tax can induce NF-κB activity by interacting with NF-κB precursors or with the IκBα inhibitor. Not only this interaction is weak, but these results are difficult to understand because Tax is almost entirely localized in the nucleus, while NF-κB precursors and IκBα are restricted to the cytoplasm.

It is also important to verify whether Tax-mediated DNA binding increase of bZIP factors occurs in vivo. Moreover it is not clear how Tax modifies DNA site selection. One possibility is that Tax reorients the bZIP so that it contacts DNA differently. For example amino acids in the basic region that normally do not contact DNA might be reoriented by Tax to contact the phosphodiester backbone or the bases. Another possibility is that Tax can bind DNA following a conformational change induced by the interaction with the basic region. In any case, it is now clear that the Tax responsive elements are more complex than the simple CRE/AP-1 core site and that the flanking sequences contribute an important function for Tax-mediated stimulation of DNA binding.

Appropriate development of in vivo models as well as biophysical studies and crystallographic analysis will be extremely useful to refine the mechanism through which Tax can interact with various cellular factors, regulate transcription and promote pathogenesis.

ACKNOWLEDGMENTS

We would like to thank all the members of Green' s lab and especially S. Roberts, J. Valcarcel and S. Wagner for their suggestions and support. G. P. and M. R. G. are respectively postdoctoral associate and Investigator of the Howard Hughes Medical Institute.

REFERENCES

1. Woong-Staal, F., and Gallo, R. C. (1985). Human lymphotrophic retroviruses. *Nature*. 317, 395.
2. Manns, A., and Blatter, W. A. (1991). The hepidemiology of the human T-cell lymphotrophic virus type I and type II: etiologic roles in human disease. *Transfusion*. 31, 67.
3. Yip, M. T., and Chen, I. S. Y. (1990). Modes of transformations by the Human T-cell leukemia viruses. *Mol. Biol. Med*. 7, 33.
4. Bangham, C. R. M. (1993). Human T-cell leukemia virus type I and neurological disease. *Current Opinion in Neurobiology*. 3, 773.
5. Wachsman, W., Golde, D. W., and Chen, I. S. Y. (1986). HTLV and human leukemia: perspectives 1986. *Semin. Hemat*. 23, 246.
6. Kitajima, I., Maruyama, I., Maruyama, Y., Ijichi, S., Riraku, N., Mimura, Y., and Osame, M. (1989). Polyarthritis in human T lymphotrophic virus type I-associated myelopathy. *Arthritis Rheum*. 32, 1344.
7. Gazzolo, L., and Duc Dodon, M. (1987). Direct activation of resting lymphocytes by human T-lymphotropic virus type I. *Nature*. 326, 714.
8. Fujita, K., Yamasaki, Y., Sawada, H., Izumi, Y., Fukuhara, S., and Uchino, H. (1989). Cytogenetic studies on the adult T-cell leukemia in Japan. *Leuk. Res*. 13, 535.
9. Liu, F., and Green, M. R. (1990). A specific member of the ATF transcription factor family can mediate transcription activation by Adenovirus E1a protein. *Cell*. 61, 1217.
10. Liu, F., and Green, M. R. (1994). Promoter targeting by Adenovirus E1a through interaction with different cellular DNA-binding domains. *Nature*. 368, 520.
11. Maguire, H. F., Hoeffler, J. P., and Siddiqui, A. (1991). HBV X protein alters the DNA binding specificity of CREB and ATF-2 by protein-protein interaction. *Science*. 252, 842.
12. Stern, S., Tanaka, M., and Herr, W. (1989). The Oct-1 homeodomain directs formation of a multiprotein-DNA complex with the HSV transactivator VP16. *Nature*. 341, 624.
13. Seiki, M., Hattori, S., Hirayama, Y., Yoshida, M. (1983). Human adult T-cell leukemia virus; complete nucleotide sequence of the provirus genome integrated in leukemia cell DNA. *Proc. Natl. Acad. Sci. USA*. 80, 3618.
14. Josephs, S. F., Wong-Staal, F., Manzari, V., Gallo, R. C., Sodroski, J. G., Trus, M. D., Perkins, D., Patarca, R., and Haseltine, W. A. (1984). Long terminal repeat structure of an american isolate of type I human T-cell leukemia virus. *Virology*. 139, 340.
15. Cann, A. J., Rosenblatt, J. D., Wachsman, W., Shah, N. P., and Chen, I. S. Y. (1985). Identification of the gene responsible for T-cell leukemia virus transcriptional regulation. *Nature*. 318, 571.
16. Slamon, D., Press, M. F., Souza, L. M., Murdock, D. C., Cline, M. J., Golde, D. W., Gasson, J. C., Chen, I. S. Y. (1985). Studies of the putative transforming protein of the type I human T-cell leukemia virus. *Science*. 228,1427.
17. Sodroski, J., Rosen, C., Goh, W. C., and Haseltine, W. (1985). A transcriptional activator protein encoded by the x-lor region of the human T-cell leukemia virus. *Science*. 228, 1430..
18. Seiki, M., Inoue, J., Takeda, T., and Yoshida, M. (1986). Direct evidence that p40x of human T-cell leukemia virus type is a trans-acting transcriptional activator. *EMBO J*. 5, 561.
19. Goh, W, S., Sodroski, J., Rosen, C., Essex, M., and Haseltine, W. A.(1985). Subcellular localization of the product of the long open reading frame of the human T-cell leukemia virus type I. *Science*. 227, 1227.
20. Slamon, D. J. , Boyle, W. J. Keith, D. E., Press, M. F. Golde, D. W. and Souza, L. M. (1988). Subnuclear localization of the Trans-activating protein of human T-cell leukemia virus type I. *J. Virol*. 62, 680.
21. Smith, M. R., and Greene, W. C. (1990). Identification of the HTLV-I Tax trans-activator mutants exhibiting novel transcriptional phenotypes. *Genes Dev*. 4, 1875.
22. Gitlin, S. D., Lindholm, P. F., Marriot, S. J., and Brady, J. N. (1991). Transdominant human T-cell lymphotrophic virus type I Tax1 mutant fails to localize to the nucleus. *J. Virol*. 65, 2612.
23. Fontes, J. D., Strawhecker, J. M., Bills, D. N., Lewis, R. E., and Hinrichs, S. H. (1993). Phorbol esters modulate the phosphorylation of human T-cell leukemia virus type I Tax. *J. Virol*. 67, 4436.

24. Zhao, L.-J. and Giam, C.-Z. (1992). Human T-cell lymphotrophic virus type I (HTLV-I) transcriptional activator, Tax, enhances CREB binding to HTLV-I 21-base-pair repeats by protein-protein interaction. *Proc. Natl. Acad. Sci. USA*. **89**: 7070.

25. Semmens, O., and Jeang, K.-T. (1992). Mutational analysis of human T-cell leukemia virus type I Tax: regions necessary for function determined with 47 mutant proteins. *J. Virol.* **66**, 7183.

26. Smith, M. R., and Greene, W. C. (1992). Characterization of a novel nuclear localization signal in the HTLV-I Tax transactivator protein. *Virology*, **187**, 316.

27. Semmens, O., and Jeang, K.-T. (1992). HTLV-I Tax is azinc binding protein: role for zinc in Tax structure and function. *Virology*. **188**, 754.

28. Lindholm, P. F., Marriott, S. J., Gitlin, S. D., and Brady, J. N. (1991). Differential precipitation and zinc chelate chromatography purification of biologically active HTLV-I Tax1 expressed in E. coli. *J. Biochem. Biophys. Methods*. **22**, 233.

29. Smith, M. R., and Greene, W. C. (1991). Type I human T-cell leukemia virus Tax protein transforms Rat fibroblasts through the cyclic adenosine monophosphate response element binding protein/activating transcription factor pathway. *J. Clin. Invest.* **88**, 1038.

30. Semmens, O:J., and Jeang, K.-T. (1995). Definition of a minimal activation domain in human T-cell leukemia virus type I Tax. *J. Virol.* **69**, 1827.

31. Caron, C., Rousset, R., Beroud, C., Moncollin, V., Egly, J.-M., and Jalinot, P. (1993). Functional and biochemical interaction of the HTLV-I Tax1 transactivator with TBP. *EMBO J.* **12**, 4269.

32. Tanaka, A., Takahashi, C., Yamaoka, S., Nosaka, T., Maki, M., and Hatanaka, M. (1990). Oncogenic transformation by the Tax gene of the human T-cell leukemia virus type I in vitro. *Proc. Natl. Acad. Sci. USA*. **87**, 1071.

33. Grassmann, R., Berchtold, S., Radant, I., Alt, M., Fleckeenstein, B., Sodroski, J. G., Haseltine, W.A., and Ramsted, U. (1992). Role of the human T-cell leukemia virus type I X region proteins in immortalization of primary human lymphocytes in culture. *J. Virol.* **66**, 4570.

34. Nerenberg, M., Hinrichs, S. H., Reynolds, R. K., Khoury, G., and Jay, G. (1987). The tat gene of human T-lymphotrophic virus type I induces mesenchymal tumors in transgenic mice. *Science*. **237**, 1324.

35. Iwakura, Y., Tosu, M., Yoshida, E., Takiguchi, M., Sato, K., Kitajima, I., Nishioka, K., Yamamoto, K., Takeda, T., Hatanaka, M., Yamamoto, H., and Sekiguchi, T. (1991). Induction of inflammatory arthropathy resembling rheumatoid arthritis in mice transgenic for HTLV-I. *Science*. **253**, 1026.

36. Green, S. J., Hinrichs, S. H., Vogel, J., and Jay, G. (1989). Exocrinopathy resembling Sjogren-s syndrome in HTLV-I Tax transgenic mice. *Nature*. **341**, 72.

37. Pozzati, R., Vogel, J., Jay, G. (1990). The human T-lymphotrophic virus type I Tax gene can cooperate with the ras oncogene to induce neoplastic transformation of cells. *Mol. Cell. Biol.* **10**, 413.

38. Paskalis, H. Felber, B. K., and Pavlakis, G. N. (1986). Cis-acting sequences responsible for the transcriptional activation of the human T-cell leukemia virus type I constitute a conditional enhancer. *Proc. Natl. Acad. Sci. USA*. **83**, 6558.

39. Shimonotohno, K., Takano, M., Teruuchi, T., and Miwa, M. (1986). Requirement of multiple copies of a 21-nucleotide sequence in the U3 regions of human T-cell leukemia virus type I and type II long terminal repeats for trans-acting activation of trancription. *Proc. Natl. Acad. Sci. USA*. **83**, 8112.

40. Brady, J., Jeang, K.-T., Duvall, J., and Khoury, G. (1987). Identification of p40x-responsive regulatory sequences within the human T-cell leukemia virus type i long terminal repeat. *J. Virol.* **61**, 2175.

41. Rosen, C. A., Park, R., Sodroski, G. J., and Haseltine, W. A. (1987). Multiple sequence elements are required for regulation of human T-cell leukemia virus gene expression. *Proc. Natl. Acad. Sci. USA*. **84**, 4919.

42. Giam, C.-Z., and Xu, Y-L. (1989). HTLV-I Tax gene product activates transcription via pre-existing cellular factors and c-AMP responsive elements. *J. Biol. Chem.* **264**, 15236.

43. Xu, Y.-L., Adya, N., Siores, E., Gao, Q., and Giam, C.-Z. (1990). Cellular factors involved in the transcription and Tax-mediated trans-activation directed by the TGACGT motifs in the human T-cell leukemia virus type I promoter. *J. Biol. Chem.* **265**, 20285.

44. Poteat, H. T., Chen, F. Y., Kadison, P., Sodroski, J. G., and Haseltine, W. A. (1990). Protein kinase A-dependent binding of a nuclear factor to the 21-base-pair repeat of the human T-cell leukemia virus type I long terminal repeat. *J. Virol.* **64**, 1264.

45. Zhao, L-J., and Giam, C-Z. (1991). Interaction of human T-cell lymphotrophic virus type I (HTLV-I) transcriptiona activator Tax with cellular factors that bind specifically to the 21-base-pair repeats in HTLV-I enhancer. *Proc Natl. Acad. Sci. USA*. **88**, 11445.

46. Tan, T.-H., Horikoshi, M., and Roeder, R. (1989). Purification and characterization of multiple nuclear factors that bind to the Tax-inducible enhancer within the human T-cell leukemia virus type I long terminal repeat. *Mol. Cell. Biol.* **9**, 1733.

47. Yoshimura, T., Fujisawa, J., and Yoshida, M. (1990). Multiple cDNA clones encoding nuclear proteins that bind to the Tax-dependent enhancer of HTLV-I: all contain a leucine zipper structure and basic amino acid domain. *EMBO J.* **9**, 2537.

48. Tsujimoto, A., Nyunoya, H., Morita, T., Sato, T., and Shimitohono, K. (1991). Isolation of cDNAs for DNA-binding proteins which specifically bind to a Tax-responsive enhancer element in the long terminal repeat of the human T-cell leukemia virus type I. *J. Virol.* **65**, 1420.

49. Beraud, C., Lombard-Platet, G., Michal, Y., and Jalinot, P. (1991). Binding of the HTLV-I Tax1 trabsctivator to the inducible 21 bp enhancer is mediated by the cellular factor HEB1. *EMBO J.* **10**, 3795.

50. Lombard-Platet, G., and Jalinot, P. (1993). Purification by DNA affinity precipitation of the cellular factors HEB1-p67 and HEB1-p94 whcich bind specifically to the human T-cell leukemia virus type-I 21 bp enhancer. *Nucleic Acids Res.* **21**, 3935.

51. Wagner, S., and Green, M. R. (1993). HTLV-I Tax protein stimulation of DNA binding of bZIP proteins by enhancing dimerization. *Science.* **252**, 395.

52. Adya, N., Zhao, L.-J., Huang, W, Boros, I., Giam, C.-Z. (1994). Expansion of CREB' s DNA recognition specificity by Tax results from interaction with Ala-Ala-Arg at position 282–284 near the conserved DNA-binding domain of CREB. *Proc. Natl. Acad. Sci. USA.* **91**, 5642.

53. Brauweiler, A., Garl, P., Franklin, A.A., Giebler, H.A., and Nyborg, J.K. (1995). A molecular mechanism for human T-cell leukemia virus latency and Tax transactivation. *J. Biol Chem.* **270**, 12814.

54. Zimmermann, K., Dobrovnik, M., Ballaun, C., Bevec, D., Hauber, J., and Bohnlein, E. (1991). Trans-activation of the HIV-LTR by the HIV-1 Tat and HTLV-I Tax proteins is mediated by different cis-acting sequences. *Virology.* **182**, 874.

55. Faktor, O., and Shaul, Y. (1990). The identification of hepatitis B virus X gene responsive elements reveals functional similiraty of X and HTLV-I Tax. *Oncogene.* **5**, 867.

56. Fujii, M., Sassone-Corsi, P., and Verma, I. M. (1988). c-fos promoter trans-activation by the Tax1 protein of the human T-cell leukemia virus. *Proc. Natl. Acad. Sci. USA.* **85**, 8526.

57. Nagata, K., Ohtani, k., Nakamura, M., and Sugamura, K. (1989). Activation of endogenous c-fos proto-oncogene expression by the human T-cell leukemia virus type I encoded p40[tax] protein in the human T-cell line, Jurkat. *J. Virol.* **63**, 3220.

58. Fujii, M., Niki, T., Mori, T., Matsuda, T., Matsui, M., Nomura, N., and Seiki, M. (1991). HTLV-I Tax induces expression of various immediate early serum responsive genes. *Oncogene.* **6**, 1023.

59. Tsuchiya, H., Fujii, M., Niki, T., Tokuhara, M., Matsui, M., and Seiki, M. (1993). Human T-cell leukemia virus type I Tax activates transcription of the human fra-1 gene through multiple cis elements responsive to transmembrane signals. *J. Virol.* **67**, 7001.

60. Alexandre, C., Charnay, P., and Verrier, B. (1991). Transactivation of Krox-20 and Krox-24 promoters by the HTLV-I Tax protein through common regulatory elements. *Oncogene.* **6**, 1851.

61. Sakamoto, K. M., Nimer, S. D., Rosenblatt, J. D., and Gasson, J. C. (1992). HTLV-I and HTLV-II Tax trans-activate the human EGR-1 ptomoter through different cis-acting sequences. *Oncogene.* **7**, 2125.

62. Alexandrem C., and Verrier, B. (1991). Four regulatory elements in the human c-fos promoter mediate transactivation by the HTLV-I Tax protein. *Oncogene.* **6**, 543.

63. Lilienbaum, A., Duc Dodon, M., Alexandre, C., Gazzolo, L., and Paulin, D. (1990). Effect of human T-cell leukemia virus type I Tax protein on the activation of human vimentin gene. *J. Virol.* **64**, 256.

64. Lilienbaum, A., and Paulin, D. 1993. Activation of the human vimentin gene by the Tax human T-cell leukemia virus I. *J. Biol. Chem.* **268**, 2180.

65. Kim, S.-J., Winokur, T. S., Lee, H.-D., Danielpour, D., Kim, K. Y., Geiser, A. G., Chen, L.-S., Sporn, M. B., Roberts, A. B., and Jay, G. (1991). Overexpression of the Transforming Growth Factor-β in transgenic mice carrying the human T-cell leukemia virus type I Tax gene. *Mol. Cell. Biol.* **11**, 5222.

66. Wano, Y., Feinberg, M., Hoskin, J. B., Bogerd, H., and Greene, W. C. (1988). Stable expression of Tax gene of type I human T-cell leikemia virus in human T cells activates specific cellular genes involved in growth. *Proc. Natl. Acad. Sci USA.* **85**, 9733.

67. Tendler, C. L., Greenberg, S. J., Blattner, W. A., Manns, A., Murphy, E., Fleisher, T., Hanchard, B., Morgan, O., Burton, J. D., Nelson, D. L., and Waldmann, T. A. (1990). Transactivation of interleukin 2 and its receptor induces immune activation in human T-cell lymphotropic virus type I-associated myelopathy: pathogenic implications and a rationale for immunotherapy. *Proc. Natl. Acad. Sci. USA.* **87**, 5218.

68. Wolin, M., Kornuc, M., Hong, C., Shin, S.-K., Lee, F., Lau, R., and Nimer, S. (1993). Differential effect of the HTLV infection and HTLV Tax on interleukin 3 expression. *Oncogene.* **8**, 1905.

69. Leung, K., and Nabel, G. J. (1988). HTLV-I transactivator induces interleukin-2 receptor expression through an NF-κB-like factor, *Nature.* **333**, 776.

70. Ballard, D. W., Bohnlein, E., Lowenthal, J., W., Wano, Y., Franza, B. R., and Greene, W. C. (1988). HTLV-I Tax induces cellular proteins that activate the κB element in the IL-2 receptor α gene. *Science.* **241**, 1652.

71. Marriot, S. J., Trinh, D., and Brady, J. N. (1992). Activation of interleukin-2 receptor alpha expression by extracellular HTLV-I Tax protein1: a potential role in HTLV-I pathogenesis. *Oncogene.* **7**, 1749.

72. Napolitano, M., Modi, W. S., Cevario, S. J., Gnarra, J. R., Seuanez, H. N., Leonard, W. J. (1991). The gene encoding the the Act-2 cytokine. *J. Biol. Chem.* **266**, 17531.

73. Lindholm, P. F., Reid, R. L., and Brady, J. (1992). Extracellular Tax1 protein stimulates Tumor Necrosis Factor-β and Immunoglobulin kappa light chain expression in lymphoid cells. *J. Virol.* **66**, 1294.

74. Paul, N. L., Lenardo, M. J., Novak, K. D., Sarr, T., Tang, W.-L., and Ruddle, N. H. (1990). Lymphotoxin activation by human T-cell leukemia virus type I-infected cell lines: role for NF-kB. *J. Virol.* **64**, 5412.

75. Nimer, S. D., Gasson, J. C., Hu, K., Smalberg, I., Williams, J. L., Chen, I. S. Y. and Rosenblatt, J. D. (1989) Activation of the GM-CSF promoter by HTLV-I and -II Tax proteins. *Oncogene* . **4**, 671.

76. Himes, S. R., Coles, L. S., Katsikeros, R., Lang, R. K., and Shannon, M. F. (1993). HTLV-I Tax activation of the GM-CSF and G-CSF promoters requires the interaction of NF-κB with other transcription factors families. *Oncogene.* **8**, 3189.

77. Green, J. E. (1991). Transactivation of the Nerve Growth Factor in transgenic mice containing the human T-cell leukemia lympothrophic virus type I Tax gene. *Mol. Cell. Biol.* **11**, 4635.

78. Low, G. K., Chu, H-M., Tan, Y., Schwartz, P.M., Daniels, G. M., Melner, M.H., and Comb, M. J. (1994). Novel interaction between human T-cell leukemia virus type I Tax and Activating Transcription Factor 3 at the cyclic AMP-responsive element. *Mol. Cell. Biol.* **14**, 4958.

79. Jeang, K.-T., Widen, S. G., Semmes, O. J. IV, and Wilson, S. H. (1990). HTLV-I trans-activator protein, Tax, is a trans-repressor of the human β-polymerase gene. *Science.* **247**, 1082.

80. Beraud, C., Sun, S.-C., Ganchi, P., Ballard, D. W., and Greene, W. C. (1994). Human T-cell leukemia virus type I tax associates with and is negatively regulated by the NF-kB2 p100 gene product: implication for viral latency. *Mol. Cell. Biol.* **14**, 1374.

81. Kanno, T., Franzoso, G., and Siebenlist, U. (1994). Human T-cell leukemia virus type I Tax-protein-mediated activation of the NF-κB from p100 (NF-κB2)-inhibited cytoplasmic reservoirs. *Proc. Natl. Acad. Sci. USA.* **91**, 12634.

82. Hirai, H., Fujisawa, J., Suzuki, T., Ueda, K., Muramatsu, M., Tsuboi, A., Arai, N., and Yoshida, M. (1992). Transcriptional activator Tax of HTLV-I binds to the NF-κB precursor p105. *Oncogene.* **7**, 1737.

83. Watanabe, M., Muramatsu, M., Hirai, H., Suzuki, T., Fujisawa, J., Yoshida, M., Arai, K., and Arai, N. (1993). HTLV-I encoded Tax in association with NF-κB precursor p105 enhances nuclear localization of NF-κB p50 and p65 in transfected cells. *Oncogene.* **8**, 2949.

84. Sun, S.-C., Elwood, J., Beraud, C., and Greene, W. (1994). Human T-cell leukemia virus type I Tax activation of the NF-κB/Rel involves phosphorylation and degradation of the IκBα and RelA (p65)-mediated induction of the c-rel gene. *Mol. Cell. Biol.* **14**, 7377.

85. Schreck, R., Grassmann, R., Fleckenstein, B., and Baeuerle, P. A. (1992). Antioxidants selectively suppress activation of NF-κB by Human T-cell leukemia virus type I Tax protein. *J. Virol.,* **66**, 6288.

86. Schreck, R., Rieber, P., and Baeuerle, P. A. (1991) Reactive oxygen intermediates as apparently widely used messenger in the activation of the NF-κB transcription factor and HIV-1. *EMBO J.* **10**, 2247.

87. Armstrong, A. P. Franklin, A. A., Uittenbogaard, M. N., Giebler, H. A., and Nyborg, J. K. (1993). Pleiotropic effect of the human T-cell leukemia virus Tax protein on the DNA binding activity of eukaryotic transcription factors. *Proc. Natl. Acad. Sci. USA.* **90**, 7303.

88. Suzuki, T., Hirai, H., Fujisawa, J., Fujita, T., and Yoshida, M. (1993). A trans-activator Tax of the human T-cell leukemia virus type I binds to NF-kB p50 subunits and serum response factor (SRF) and associates with enhancer DNAs of the NF-κB site and CArG box. *Oncogene.* **8**, 2391.

89. Suzuki, T., Hirai, H., and Yoshida, M. (1994). Tax protein of HTLV-I interacts with the rel homology domain of NF-κB p65 and c-Rel proteins bound to to the NF-κB binding site and activates transcription. *Oncogene.* **9**, 3099.

90. Lindholm, P. F., Marriot ,S. J., Gitlin, S. D., Bohan, C. A., and Brady, J. N. (1990). Induction of nuclear NF-kB DNA binding activity after exposure of lymphoid cells to soluble Tax1 protein. *New Biol.* **2**, 1034.

91. Marriot, S. J., Trinh, D., Reid, R. L., and Brady, J. N. (1991). Soluble HTLV-I Tax1 protein stimulates proliferation of human peripheral blood lymphocytes. *New Biol.* **3**, 678.

92. Hurst, H. C.(1994). Transcription factors 1: bZIP proteins. *Protein Profile.* Vol. **1**, issue **2**, 122.

93. Franklin, A. A., Kubik, M. F., Uittenbogaard, M. N., Brauweiler, A A., Utaisincharoen, P., Matthews, M.-A. H., Dynan, W. S., Hoeffler, J. P., and Nyborg, J. K. (1993). Transactivation by the human T-cell leukemia virus Tax protein is mediated through enhanced binding of Activating transcription factor-2 (ATF-2) response and cAMP element-binding protein (CREB). *J. Biol. Chem.* **268**, 21225.

94. O'Shea, E. K., Rutkowski, R., and Kim, P. S. (1989). Evidence that the leucine zipper is a coiled coil. *Science.* **243**, 538.

95. Weiss,. M. A., Ellenberger, T., Wobbe, C. R., Lee, J. P., Harrison, S. C., and Struhl, K. (1990). Folding transition in the DNA-binding domain of GCN4 on specific binding to DNA. *Nature*. **347**, 575.

96. Perini, G., Wagner, S., and Green, M. R. (1995). Recognition of bZIP proteins by the human T-cell leukemia virus transactivator Tax. *Nature*, in press.

97. Anderson, M. G., and Dynan, W. S. (1994). Quantitative studies of the effect of HTLV-I Tax protein on CREB-protein - DNA binding. *Nucleic Acids Res.* **22**, 3194.

98. Paca-Uccaralertkun, S., Zhao, L.-J., Adya, N., Cross, J. V., Cullen, B. R., Boros, I. M., and Giam, C.-Z. (1994). In vitro selection of DNA elements highly responsive to the human T-cell lymphotrophic virus type I transcriptional activator Tax. *Mol. Cell. Biol.* **14**, 456.

99. Fujii, M., Tsuchiya, H., Chuhjo, T., Akizawa, T., and Seiky, M. (1992). Interaction of the HTLV-I Tax I with the $p67^{SRF}$ causes the aberrant induction of cellular immediate early genes through CArG boxes. *Genes Dev.* **6**, 2066.

100. Fujii, M., Tsuchya, H., Chuhjo, T., Minamino, T., Miyamoto, K.-I., and Seiki, M. (1994). Serum Response Factor has functional roles both in the indirect binding to the CArG box and in the transcriptional activation function of the Human T-cell leukemia virus type I. *J. Virol.* **68**, 7275.

101. Hopkins, S. J., and Rothwell, N. J. (1995). Cytokines and the nervous system I: expression and recognition. *Trends in Neurosciences.* **18**, 83.

DISCUSSION

M. Oren: Is there any evidence that other monomeric or tetrameric proteins also take advantage of cellular "glues" to assemble, and what do you think of the report that HBV-X binds to p53?

M. Green: Right, so those are two very different questions. I will take the first one. The first one has to do, I think, with whether there are other examples of chaperones forming complexes with transcription factors. So the best example, in fact, is in the case of steroid hormone receptors in which HSP-90 very clearly plays an important role in at least certain steroid hormones receptors. There is also some work in prokaryotic cases in which proteins chaperones have been known to play roles, in bacterial and I think in yeast transcription. The second question you asked has to do with p53 and pX; I have been asked this before. I am uncomfortable with the fact that p53 binds so many things. I am not a p53 expert and I do not really feel qualified to comment on how meaningful that is in terms of pX function. You would probably be in a better position to do it than I would, but I would be interested in hearing what you had to say about that.

F. Rauscher: You showed a really convincing GRO-EL co-transfection assay for b-Zip activation; can the same be said of GRO-EL when co-transfection is in the same situation?

M. Green: So the question is can we, something like GRO-EL, express it in the nucleus of a HeLa cell and increase b-Zip? That is something very much we want to do. We would actually prefer to do it with a cellular protein BEF and we have been holding off to do that experiment. I am becoming increasingly impatient at our difficulty in cloning this, so we may do the GRO-EL experiment.

F. Rauscher: So you also argue that Tax-like molecules are ordering the basic region whereas GRO-EL-like molecules are ordering the zipper region?

M. Green: I presume they probably do order the basic region, but I have no direct evidence for that. What I think is that Tax itself is a stable dimer and I think each subunit of the dimer binds to a basic region in the unstable dimer form of the b-Zip, and therefore, stabilizes the b-Zip.

F. Rauscher: Why do you think that virus has only targeted this type of DNA binding domain as proposed to all the other types of cellular binding domains for this kind of promiscuous activator as opposed to a zinc finger-like protein or a homeo-domain protein which can be just as well ordered?

M. Green: I think that is a good question. You have at least three different viruses, which are not related adenovirus, hepatitis-B and HTLV-1 and all three of them have ATF sites as playing a crucial role in the readout of some of their genes. Now, that is not the only case. There are other types of transcription factors that viruses play upon; I mean E2F is a very good example. Viruses play upon in the SV-40 early promoter. SP-1 is another good example of important transcription factor that plays also an important role. But, b-Zips do come up more often than not, and I think maybe one of the reasons is because they provide a large reservoir of proteins. I think the virus wants to activate both viral and cellular genes. There is a large reservoir that can be tapped upon to form both homo- and heterodimers which play an important role in a lot of cellular genes.

D. Livingston: Now, do you think cells make Tax-equivalents or only BEF equivalents? Because you would think once Tax-equivalents were synthesized, the game was over.

M. Green: Yes, you might, but no.

D. Livingston: That is a novitiate thought but, nonetheless, if you assay the other way, if you assay for synergy with BEF, can you detect the cellular Tax?

M. Green: We have not done that. Historically, of course, we were looking for equivalents in our experiment. This is exactly what we were looking for when we started out and did not find them, that is to say, that when we took a nuclear extract and tried to stimulate b-Zip binding under the same conditions, namely minus ATP, that we were doing for BEF for a lot of reasons, negative result and both came out when we added ATP. Now that we have both we have not looked for synergizers, like you say, and it might be something that we would see in that assay and miss in our original assay.

D. Livingston: In some sense, there is a cellular Tax. Might it be an oncogene?

M. Green: Exactly, that is something that I was running out of time so I speculated on last. But, yes, we think Tax is an oncoprotein, and we are not the only ones who think that. It is by increasing the activity of cellular transcription factors such as AP-1 and c-Jun; the prediction is that if we over express BEF that we might also be able to see it as an oncoprotein. So again, we have held off that experiment till we get a molecular clone for BEF, but once we have it in hand that is something that we would really like to do.

T. Graf: Besides the difference in ATP dependence between BEF and typical chaperones, is there also a difference in specificity for recognition of sequences? And, for example, would Tax be negative in any kind of chaperone assay?

M. Green: I am not sure I understand your question. But, if you are asking aboutTax and pX and E1A, none of those proteins have any chaperone activity - I should say they do not have any signature sequences of a chaperone. So they are promoting binding but simply through protein-protein interactions and binding to the dimerized form of the b-Zip.

T. Graf: I see, so you think they are more like a glue?

M. Green: They are, if you want to think of them like a glue, but a weak glue. They are very simple, they just bind to the dimerized form and not the undimerized form, and just by doing that, they pull the equilibrium.

P. Sassone-Corsi: Is the on-rate binding or off-rate binding affected by BEF?

M. Green: It would be the on-rate. We have done it and published it for Tax and it is the on-rate and not the off-rate that is affected.

P. Sassone-Corsi: I am wondering about the specificity of the site. There are sites, like CRE sites, that as you know, are not perfectly canonical but that will still bind proteins. My question is: Is BEF or Tax going to specify in a differential fashion binding to different sites?

M. Green: Certainly, Tax can do that, but it may have also a negative effect on that site. What I hope I stressed is that it is, at the moment, completely empirical with a particular b-Zip Tax combination what that specificity will be. We have taken 5 different b-Zip's, on four sites, we felt completely unpredictable and different ways in which the binding specificity is changed. So Tax can very well promote CREB binding to a non-consensus site. On the other hand, it could have a negative effect - it may make the binding less well to that relative to another site.

P. Sassone-Corsi: So what do you think this has to do with, in general, transcriptional activation? Can association with other proteins, such as CBP be involved, and whether maybe phosphorylation of the transcription factors might be affected by Tax or BEF binding?

M. Green: CBP is working on a completely different part, as I understand it, from CREB, so it has nothing to do with the DNA binding domain in getting CREB to DNA. So I would say it is not relevant except for the fact that for CBP to work it is a prerequisite that CREB sits on DNA.

C. Goding: How much specificity do you see in the BEF regulation of the zipper? Can you see BEF effects on the zippers of bHLH proteins?

M. Green: With every b-Zip that we have offered to BEF that has a haptad repeat it has worked - we have seen no effect on the members of the HLH proteins that we have acted upon, but I think the reason is that, if you measure the dimerization constants for HLH proteins they are about 100 fold higher than they are for b-Zip proteins.

C. Goding: This is bHLH-related proteins with zippers on?

M. Green: No. I think you asked me that yesterday. No, the only ones we have looked at are myogenin and MyoD. But I think for myc as well, I do not know for sure, but I think the dimerization constants is pretty robust. That would be an experiment worth doing. We have only done it for the myogenin and MyoD and saw no effect under those circumstances.

G. Evan: To tie that together with the question that Frank asked; why do you think it is then that these viruses do not target myc? Or indeed, if you have not done that experiment, do you think they might be targeting myc as well? It is an obvious candidate, but E1A, for example, all the data argue that it replaces myc rather than induces myc or activates myc.

M. Green: Well, E1A replaces myc in certain types of transformation assays, in a lot of transcription assays, it does not. So I do not know. I myself know of no virus that has a myc. You undoubtedly know, probably better than I do, which has myc binding sites. So why the viruses have not figured out to target myc, I really have no intelligent thing to offer.

F. Rauscher: Is BEF in the complex, in the gel shifted complex as opposed to Tax; are they both not in the complex?

M. Green: No, Tax is in the complex. You have to work hard to see it. But BEF is not, BEF releases, remember, BEF as a good chaperone would release the balance substrate. And comparable experiments I did not show you BEF has no change - does not change the DNA binding specificity of b-Zips whereas Tax does.

T. Taniguchi: Do you know, in addition to Tax functioning as ATF family members, which also have to have other transcription factors in like NFκB, in this case perhaps there is a mechanism by which Tax activates NFκB.

M. Green: That is a very good point, and one that I should have touched upon but did not. Tada brings out the fact that I have talked only about a small part of the Tax protein - Tax is 350 amino acids and like other viral proteins, such as E1A there are other domains that do other things, one of the domains that Tada is referring to is a domain that acts through NFκB and, by what I still think are mysterious mechanisms, activates NFκB. That part of Tax is completely dissociable from the part of Tax that I talked about in acting through b-Zip studies. A number of genetic experiments have shown that. It is another way in which Tax is promiscuous - I do not want for people to think that the promiscuity mechanism I described is the only way. Similarly, for E1A I talked only about E1A region-3 and you will hear, I presume, that there are other regions of E1A that work on transcription through other mechanisms.

P. Sassone-Corsi: Several of these proteins are, like fos and jun, early response genes responding very quickly to mytogenic stimuli. Did you try to see whether the BEF endogenous activity changes upon mytogenic stimuli or during the cell cycle?

M. Green: So that relates to the question that Erich Nigg asked and that is: Is there any regulation of BEF activity and the only way we would do that experiment now is to make extracts of various synchronized cells. That experiment does not appeal to me. So what we are waiting for is to get a clone for BEF which we could have an anti-body and then follow it through antibody activity because one of the problems that we have had with purifying BEF, which is characteristic of chaperones, is that they do not purify very well - that is because they bind to a lot of endogenous protein substrates along the way to fractionate them.

F. Blasi: Does Tax preferentially increases dimerization of homodimers versus heterodimers?

M. Green: No, it does not. It will work on homo- or heterodimers; in the experiments we have done, we have not seen particular preferences. Again, if there are mutations in the basic region which render it not responsive then, of course, it would be preferential, but if basis regions are good, it will do both homo and hetero dimers.

T. Beerman: The presentation describes a dimerization event and then a reaction with Tax.. Since dimerization could be a limiting event, is it possible that a monomer form can interact with Tax and then generate a dimer with Tax?

M. Green: The question is, is there any evidence that Tax combines to monomer forms and recruit them? I guess, one does not formally have any way of knowing the order in which those events occur. We are only measuring the equilibrium and that there is a shift of equilibrium to the dimer form. So I guess we thought about it, that when the dimer forms, it sees that and binds to it most stabley - but we have no evidence against the possibility that there is a Tax-monomer complex which then goes and dimerizers.

P. Amati: Have you any evidence about which part of Tax makes contact with the dimers?

M. Green: Yes, it is the amino terminal region of Tax which has a zinc finger.

P. Amati: Is there any similarity between the contacting region of Tax U and A and X proteins?

M. Green: Yes, there is homology. In fact, I pulled the slide because of lack of time. All three of these viral proteins have zinc binding sites. So, there are a number of examples, in which you find metal binding sites interacting with losing zippers. This was first shown in the case of steroid hormone receptors where jun and fos members were shown through their loosing zippers to interact with the DNA binding domain which is a metal binding site steroid hormone receptor.

D. Oren: A comment and two questions. The comment is that a number of years ago, several labs, including ours, showed that p53 can interact with HSP-70 and Joan Miller has recently presented formal evidence that HSP can facilitate the folding of p53 into DNA competent binding form. So that may be another example of the chaperone doing the same thing. Now the question is, is there any evidence that E1A also forms stable homodimers either before or after interaction with ATF's which would account for a similar activity as Tax? And the other question is; if BEF facilitates folding of the looser zipper into a proper confirmation would you expect that using conformation-specific monoclonal antibodies, you could show generation of specific apoptosis in the presence of BEF which would not be there in the absence of it? That could be a very useful assay for the proper folding if you try to do something of this kind.

M. Green: I know certainly that we have not done that. So the question is have we looked for confirmational specific antibodies? No, we have not done that. We have really used up to this point, gluteraldehyde cross-linking as a read out of dimerization. The first question was about E1A? Yes, there is no evidence as far as I know, we have not looked for it ourselves, but I know that Ed Harlow has looked hard to see if E1A is ever anything but a monomer, and all his experiments were negatives, so he also thinks E1A is a monomer.

D. Oren: So how does it work here? How does it bring together two monomers of ATF?

M. Green: We have never done these experiments with E1A. Our experiments with E1A were completely different and had to do with protein fusion and *in vivo* recruiting and showing that it could recruit to a minimal b-Zip domain. But we do not formally know that E1A promotes b-Zip binding, in contrast to the case with Tax and pX.

T. Graf: I have another question which reflects my ignorance about chaperones. I guess they do not have any specificity for recognizing proteins, right? Would you not expect then, that BEF would be helping other transcription factors which act as homodimers or heterodimers such as homeodomain proteins as well as b-Zip proteins? Do you see a specificity or did you not look for that?

M. Green: No, we looked for it. It is not that they have no specificity, they just have broad specificity. So, for example, they have families of chaperones and different ones like the HSP-60's and the HLH-70's and each one of those can act on a variety of substrates but in different set of substrates than the other one can. Often, as I alluded to briefly, they are looking for signature sequences that are characteristic of unfolded protein, for example, surface exposed hydrophobic residues. With regard to your second question; why does not it act on a wide variety of transcription factors; I think one of the reasons is that b-Zips are unusual in primarily existing in the unfolded form, HLH proteins and zinc finger proteins are primarily folded, they have much more robust dimerization constants. And so, these may not be the best targets for chaperones. Just because they are already pre-folded for the most part in the nucleus.

A. Matter: Is there any sort of Tax-like function that is affecting steroid hormone receptors? Is there a Tax-like function of any protein that is regulating steroid hormone complexes?

M. Green: A Tax-like function? Well, I would say, not to my knowledge. There is a chaperone-like function that affects steroid hormone HFP-90.

A: Matter: But DNA binding?

M. Green: To my knowledge, no.

P. Sassone-Corsi: Is there any BEF in the cytoplasm?

M. Green: That is a good question. When we refractionate, we get a nuclear endocytoplasmic fraction and most of it is nuclear. But we do see some in the cytoplasm. We see the same thing for any transcription of splicing factor we have ever looked at, so the only way to really know that, is to get an antibody and do indirect amino florescence.

8

CREM

Transcriptional Pacemaker of the cAMP Response

Janet S. Lee, Monica Lamas, Katherine Tamai, Emmanuel Zazopoulos, Lucia Penna, Nicholas S. Foulkes, François Nantel, Enzo Lalli and Paolo Sassone-Corsi

Institut de Génétique et de Biologie Moléculaire et Cellulaire
B. P. 163, 67404 Illkirch-Cédex
C. U. de Strasbourg, France

INTRODUCTION

Transcription factors are elements able to integrate information from promoter sequences and signal transduction pathways to control the rate of gene expression. Several transcription factors have been characterised at both the structural and functional level. Their organization is intrinsically modular, in most cases including a DNA binding domain and an activation domain. It has been shown that these domains can be interchanged between different factors and still retain their functional properties. This modularity suggests that, during evolution, increasing complexity of gene expression may have resulted not only by duplication and divergence of existing genes, but also by a domain shuffling process to generate factors with novel properties[1].

An important step forward in the study of transcription factors has been the discovery that many constitute final targets of specific signal transduction pathways. The two major signal transduction systems are those including cAMP and diacylglycerol (DAG) as secondary messengers[2]. Each pathway is also characterized by specific protein kinases (Protein Kinase A and Protein Kinase C, respectively) and its ultimate target DNA control element (cAMP-responsive element (CRE) and TPA-responsive element (TRE), respectively). Although initially characterized as distinct systems, accumulating evidence points towards extensive cross-talk between these two pathways[3–5].

Intracellular levels of cAMP are regulated primarily by adenylate cyclase. This enzyme is in turn modulated by various extracellular stimuli mediated by receptors and their interaction with G proteins[6]. The binding of a specific ligand to a receptor results in the activation or inhibition of the cAMP-dependent pathway. cAMP, in turn, binds cooperatively to two sites on the regulatory subunit of protein kinase-A (PKA), releasing the active catalytic subunit[7, 8]. These are translocated from cytoplasmic and Golgi complex anchoring sites and phosphorylate a number of cytoplasmic and nuclear proteins on serines in the context X-Arg-Arg-X-<u>Ser</u>-X[6,8]. In the nucleus, PKA-mediated phosphorylation ultimately influences the transcriptional regulation of various genes through distinct, cAMP-inducible promoter responsive sites[9,10].

GENES RESPONSIVE TO cAMP

The analysis of promoter sequences of several genes allowed the identification of promoter elements which mediate the transcriptional response to changes in the levels of intracellular cAMP. A number of sequences have been identified of which the best characterised is the CRE[7,9,10]. A consensus CRE site is constituted by an 8 bp palindromic sequence (TGACGTCA) with a higher conservation in the 5' half of the palindrome with respect to the 3' sequence. Several genes which are regulated by a variety of endocrinological stimuli contain similar sequences in their promoter regions although at different positions[10]. However, the CRE consensus sequence has also been found in the context of other distinct promoter elements where they apparently confer different transcriptional properties[11,12]. Another extensively studied example is the ATF (activating transcription factor) element which is present in the early promoters of adenovirus and mediates transcriptional activation by the viral oncogenic protein E1A[13,14].

A MULTIGENE FAMILY OF TRANSCRIPTION FACTORS

The first CRE-binding factor to be characterised was CREB (CRE-binding protein; ref. 15) but subsequently at least ten additional CRE-binding factor cDNAs have been cloned (Figure 1). They were obtained by screening a variety of cDNA expression libraries, with CRE and ATF sites[16,17]. Some key features of these transcription factors:

   a. They all belong to the bZip transcription factor class (Figure 1). The number of leucines in the zipper heptad repeat varies from 4 to 6.
   b. Outside of the bZip region, homology between these factors is relatively poor. Based upon regions of sequence similarity however, they can be divided into subfamilies.
   c. The different factors are able to heterodimerize with each other but only in certain combinations. A "dimerization code" exists which seems to be a property of the leucine zipper structure of each factor. Some ATF/CREB factors are able to heterodimerize with Fos and Jun, and this may change the specific affinity of binding to a CRE with respect to a Fos-Jun binding site[18]. This property is likely to reside in the similarity between the CRE (TGACGTCA) and TRE (TGAC-TCA) sequences[4,19] and demonstrates the versatility of the transcriptional response to signal transduction.
   d. Alternative splicing of CRE-binding bZip factors seems common. The CREM gene generates a large family of alternatively spliced transcripts although unlike CREB, the function and physiological role of many of these isoforms has been determined[20–22]. Alternative polyadenylation and translation initiation have also been observed in the CREM gene[23,24].
   e. CRE-binding proteins act as both activators and repressors of transcription. Some alternatively spliced CREM isoforms act as antagonists of cAMP-induced

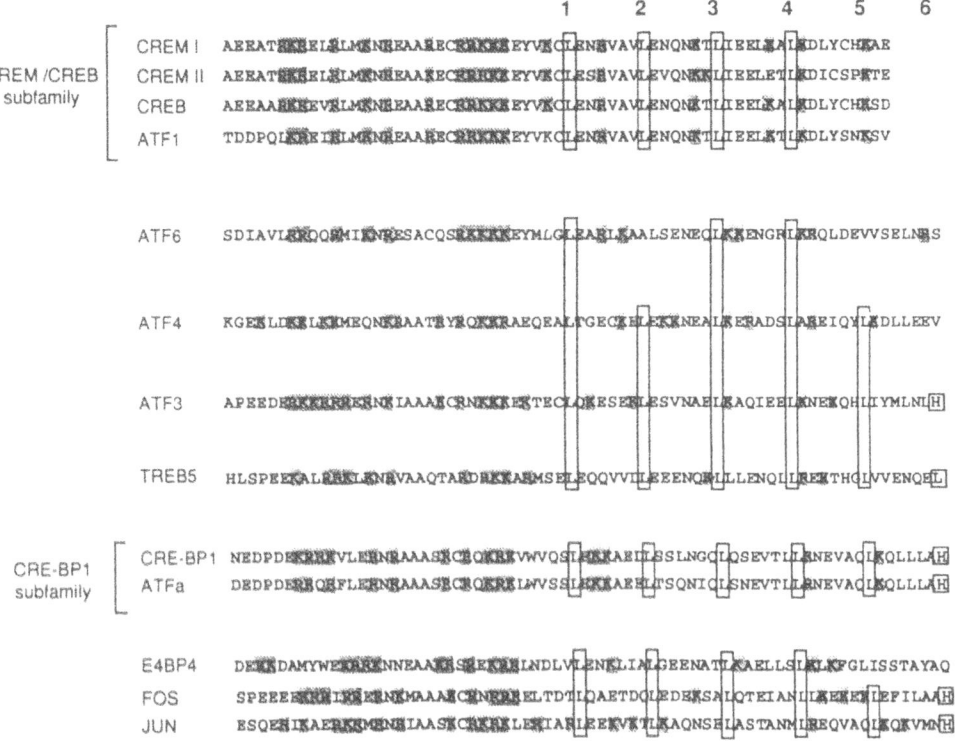

Figure 1. Sequence comparison of the bZip domains of all CRE-binding proteins described to date. The sequences of c-Fos and c-Jun are included for comparison. The boxed histidine residues at the C-terminus of some of the sequences may substitute for leucine to extend the zipper structure At position 2 in the leucine zipper of ATF6, an alanine substitutes for a leucine. Related sequences constituting the CREM/CREB and CREBP1 subfamilies are indicated.

transcription. The cAMP-inducible ICER product deserves special mention since it is generated from an alternative promoter of the CREM gene[25,26], and which is responsible for its early response inducibility which is unique amongst CRE-binding factors.

PHOSPHORYLATION-DIRECTED TRANSCRIPTIONAL ACTIVATION

Important steps in the understanding of the control of transcription factor function by phosphorylation have been made with the characterisation of the transcriptional activators CREB and CREM[20,27]. Figure 2 shows the general structure of the activator proteins. Interestingly, the relative position of the different functional domains is well conserved among various other CRE-binding proteins such as ATF1 and ATF2[16]. The transcriptional activation domain contains two independent regions[7]. The first, known as the phosphorylation box (P-box) or kinase inducible domain (KID), contains several consensus phosphorylation sites for various kinases, such as PKA, PKC, p34[cdc2], glycogen synthase kinase-3

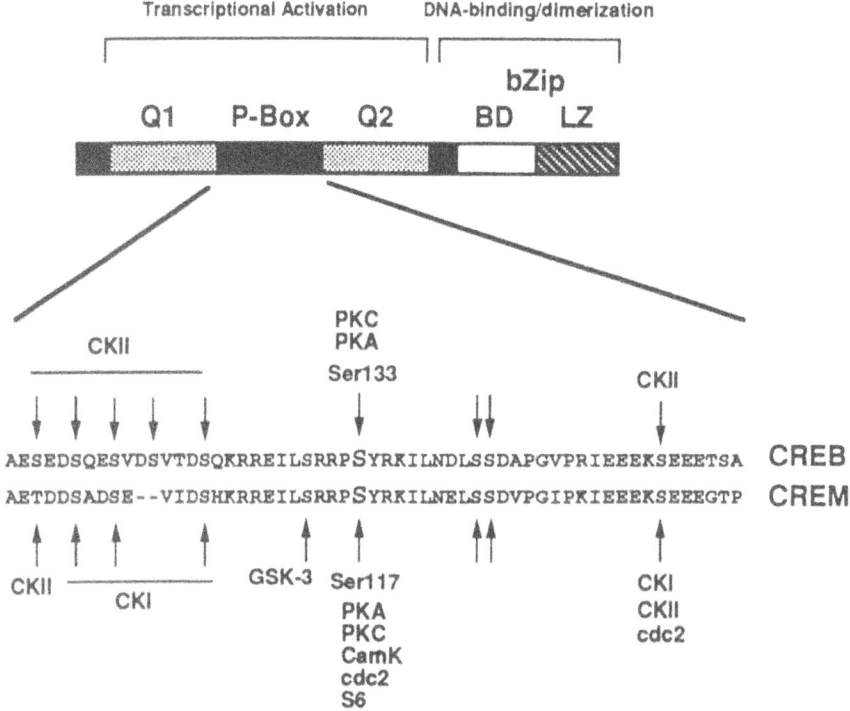

Figure 2. Structure of a CRE-binding protein activator. The two glutamine-rich domains (Q1 and Q2) and the bZip region (BD and LZ) are indicated in addition to the P-Box. This schematic representation is valid for the transcriptional activators CREB and CREM. The detailed amino acid sequence of the CREM and CREB P-box domains. Arrows indicate the serine and threonine residues in CREB and CREM which have been demonstrated in vivo or in vitro to be phosphorylated by the indicated kinases.

and casein kinases (CK) I and II[27–30]. The second region, divided in two parts, flanks the P-box, and is constituted by domains rich in glutamine residues[7].

Upon activation of the adenylyl cyclase pathway, a serine residue at position 133 of CREB and at position 117 of CREM is phosphorylated by PKA[27,29]. The major effect of phosphorylation is to convert CREB and CREM into powerful transcriptional activators. Within the P-box, serine 133/117 is located in a region of about 50 amino acids containing an abundance of phosphorylatable serines and acidic residues which was shown to be essential for transactivation by CREB and CREM[28,29]. It is apparent that this domain represents the convergence point for phosphorylation events stimulated by several signal transduction pathways. Indeed, it has been shown that the residue Ser 117 in CREM is the target for phosphorylation by PKC, CamK, p34[cdc2] as well as PKA in vitro (Figure 2)[29,30]. These phosphorylation events are relevant in vivo, since treatment with forskolin, TPA or the Ca^{2+} ionophore A23187 all lead to the enhanced phosphorylation of Ser 117. In PC12 cells, increases in the levels of intracellular Ca^{2+} by membrane depolarization have been shown to increase the phosphorylation of serine 133 in CREB and a concomitant induction of c-*fos* gene expression mediated by a CRE in the c-*fos* promoter[31,32]. Although Ca^{2+}-dependent CamK was shown to be able to phosphorylate serine 133 in vitro[33], the in vivo significance remains unclear, since PKA also seems to be necessary for c-*fos* induction mediated by Ca^{2+} influx in PC12 cells[34]. Although phosphorylation appears indispensable for activation by CREB, it is not sufficient for full activity. An acidic region just downstream of serine 133 (140-DLSSD) has been shown to be important for CREB function[28].

An interesting finding that reveals the complexity of the transcriptional response elicited by these factors concerns the mitogen-induced p70 S6 kinase, which phosphorylates and activates CREM[35]. This finding implicates p70[s6k], a kinase generally considered cytoplasmic, in the mitogenic response also at the nuclear level. Interestingly, since CREM and other factors of the CREB/ATF family represent the final targets of the cAMP-pathway, these results show that they may also act as effectors of converging signalling systems and possibly as mediators of pathway cross-talk[35].

THE GLUTAMINE-RICH ACTIVATION DOMAIN

The two domains flanking the P-box contain about three-times more glutamine residues than in the remainder of the protein in both CREB and CREM. Glutamine-rich domains have been characterized in other factors, such as AP-2 and Sp1[36,37] as transcriptional activation domains. The current notion is that they constitute surfaces of the protein which can interact with other components of the transcriptional machinery. The Q2 domain appears to make a more significant contribution to the transactivation function than Q1[22]. Furthermore, ATF1 lacks a counterpart of the Q1 domain, and still functions as an efficient transcription activator[38]. Thus, the P-box region and the Q2 domain are sufficient to mediate cAMP-induced transcription.

It is apparent that the activation domain is inherently a modular structure. Indeed, the Q2 domain when fused to a heterologous DNA binding domain, still retains a non-inducible activation function, while the P-box is able to confer PKA inducibility on a heterologous acidic activation domain (eg. GAL4)[22]. Furthermore, the P-box is able to confer this inducibility in *trans* as well as in *cis*. Thus, theoretically, the P-box could be involved in the regulation not only of the adjacent Q domains but also in controlling the activation function of other factors bound to separate promoter elements[7].

MECHANISMS OF REPRESSION

Dephosphorylation appears to represent a key mechanism in the negative regulation of CREB activation function. It has been proposed that a mechanism to explain the attenuation of CREB activity following induction by forskolin is dephosphorylation by specific phosphatases[39]. After the initial burst of phosphorylation in response to cAMP, CREB is dephosphorylated in vivo by protein phosphatase-1 (PP-1). However, the situation is more complex since it has been shown that both PP-1 and PP-2A can dephosphorylate CREB in vitro[40] resulting in an apparent decreased binding to low affinity CRE sites in vitro. Therefore, the precise role of PP-1 and PP-2A in the dephosphorylation of CREB remains to be determined.

The discovery of the CREM gene opened a new dimension in the study of the transcriptional response to cAMP[21]. The dynamic and versatile pattern of CREM expression combined with its tissue- and developmental-specific pattern, contrasts with that of the remaining members of the CRE-binding factor family which seem to be constant and ubiquitous[10, 16]. A striking feature of the CREM gene is the presence of two bZip domains used alternatively by differential splicing (DBDI and DBDII; Figure 3). These features offered the first clue that CREM occupied a priviliged position amongst this group of factors and pointed further to it fulfilling a pivotal role in the nuclear response to cAMP.

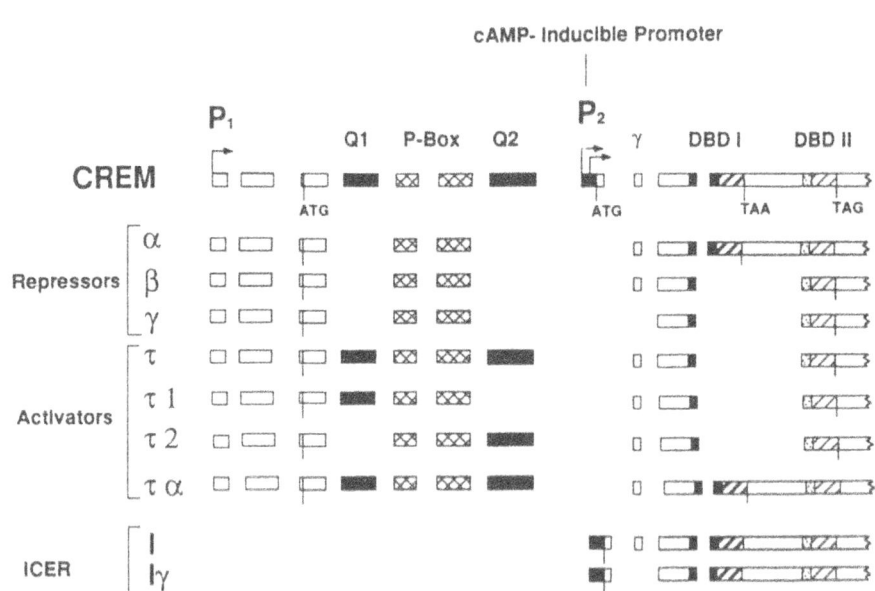

Figure 3. Activators and repressors from the same gene. Schematic representation of the CREM gene. The various activator and repressor CREM isoforms are indicated. The P1 promoter is GC-rich and directs a non-inducible pattern of expression, while the P2 promoter is strongly inducible by activation of the cAMP-dependent signaling pathway.

Various studies have established that differential transcript processing is central to the regulation of CREM expression. The importance of this mechanisms is reinforced by the fact that all the CREM isoforms which incorporate the P-box exons (Figure 3) are generated from a GC-rich promoter (P1) which has been shown to behave as a housekeeping promoter directing a non-inducible pattern of expression[25,26].

INDUCIBLE REPRESSOR ICER

An alternative promoter lying within an intron near the 3' end of the CREM gene, directs the transcription of a truncated product, termed ICER (Inducible cAMP Early Repressor)[25,26]. The ICER open reading frame is constituted by the C-terminal segment of CREM (Figure 3). The predicted open reading frame encodes a small protein of 120 amino acids with an expected molecular weight of 13.4kD. This protein, compared with the previously described CREM isoforms, essentially consists of only the DNA binding domain, which is constituted by the leucine zipper and basic region. The provocative structure of ICER is suggestive of its function and makes it one of the smallest transcription factors ever described[25].

The intact DNA binding domain directs specific ICER binding to a consensus CRE element. Importantly, ICER is able to heterodimerize with the other CREM proteins and with CREB. ICER functions as a powerful repressor of cAMP-induced transcription in transfection assays using an extensive range of reporter plasmids carrying individual CRE elements or cAMP-inducible promoter fragments[25]. Interestingly, ICER-mediated repression is obtained at substoichiometric concentrations, similarly to the previously described CREM antagonists[22]. ICER escapes from PKA-dependent phosphorylation and thus constitutes a new category of CRE binding factor, for which the principle determinant of their activity is their intracellular concentration and not their degree of phosphorylation.

The expression of ICER was first described in the pineal gland where it is the subject of a dramatic circadian pattern of expression[26]. However, recent data implicates dynamic ICER expression as a general feature of neuroendocrine systems (ref. 26; E. Lalli, N. S. Foulkes and L. Monaco, unpublished). An important feature about ICER is its inducibility. This makes ICER the only CRE-binding protein whose function is physiologically regulated by altering its cellular concentration.

CREM IS AN EARLY RESPONSE GENE

During studies of CREM expression within the neuroendocrine system, an unexpected new facet emerged: namely the transcription of the CREM gene is inducible by cAMP[25]. Furthermore, the kinetics of this induction is that of an early response gene[41]. This important finding further reinforces the notion that CREM products play a fulcral role in the nuclear response to cAMP since the expression of no other CRE-binding factor has been shown to be inducible to date. For example, the recently characterised CREB promoter is GC-rich and reminiscent of the promoters of constitutively expressed, housekeeping genes[42]. Similarly, the promoter which directs expression of the other CREM isoforms (P1) is not cAMP inducible[25].

Clues that the CREM gene was cAMP inducible first came from the demonstration that adrenergic signals direct CREM transcription in the pineal gland[26]. The inducibility phenomenon was then characterised in detail in the pituitary corticotroph cell line AtT20. In unstimulated cells the level of CREM transcript is below the threshold of detectability. However, upon treatment with forskolin (or other cAMP analogs), within 30 minutes there is a rapid increase in CREM transcript levels which peak after 2 hours and then progressively decline to basal levels by 5 hours. This characteristic kinetic classifies CREM as an "early response gene" and thus directly implicates the cAMP pathway in the cell's early response for the first time. CREM inducibility is specific for the cAMP pathway since it is not inducible by TPA or dexamethasone treatment[25].

The 5' end of the ICER clones correspond to an alternative transcription start site. The start of transcription, which identifies the so-called P2 promoter, is within the 10kb intron which is C-terminal to the Q2 glutamine-rich domain exon. In contrast to the promoter which generates all the previously characterised CREM isoforms (P1) which is GC-rich and not inducible by cAMP (N. S. Foulkes, unpublished), the P2 promoter has a normal A-T and G-C content and is strongly inducible by cAMP. It contains two pairs of closely-spaced CRE elements organized in tandem, where the separation between each pair is only three nucleotides. These features make P2 unique amongst cAMP-regulated promoters and are suggestive of cooperative interactions among the factors binding to these sites.

A NEGATIVE AUTOREGULATORY LOOP

Upon cotreatment with cycloheximide, the kinetics of CREM gene induction by forskolin are altered in that there is a significant delay in the post-induction decrease in

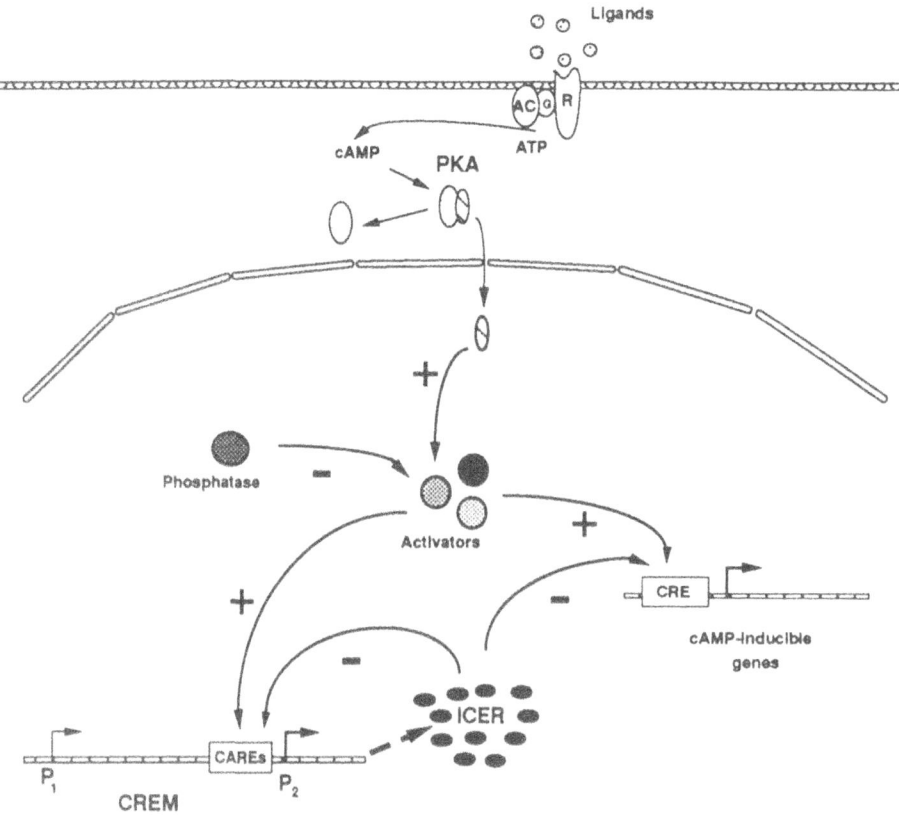

Figure 4. The cAMP signal transduction pathway. Schematic representation of the route whereby ligands at the cell surface interact with membrane receptors (R) and result in altered gene expression. Ligand binding activates coupled G-proteins (G) which in turn stimulates the activity of the membrane-associated adenylyl cyclase (AC). This converts ATP to cAMP which causes the dissociation of the inactive tetrameric protein kinase A (PKA) complex into the active catalytic subunits and the regulatory subunits. Catalytic subunits migrate into the nucleus where they phosphorylate and thereby activate transcriptional activators. Attenuation of the activators may occur via a nuclear phosphatase. Activators interact with the cAMP response enhancer element (CRE) found in the promoters of cAMP-responsive genes to activate transcription. Phosphorylated factors activate also transcription from the CREM P_2 promoter via the CARE elements and ultimately lead to a rapid increase in ICER protein levels. ICER represses cAMP-induced transcription, including that from its own promoter. The consequent fall in ICER protein levels eventually leads to a release of repression and permits a new cycle of transcriptional activation.

the transcript; elevated levels persist for as long as 12 hours. This implicates a *de novo* synthesised factor which might downregulate CREM transcription[25]. This observation combined with the presence of CRE elements in the P2 promoter, suggested that the transient nature of the inducibility could be due to ICER. Consistently, the CRE elements in the P2 promoter have been shown to bind to the ICER proteins. Detailed studies have demonstrated that the ICER promoter is indeed a target for ICER negative regulation[25]. Thus, there exists a negative autoregulatory mechanism controlling ICER expression (Figure 4). The CREM feedback loop predicts the presence of a refractory inducibility period in the gene's transcription[43]. Recent results are consistent with this hypothesis (M. Lamas, unpublished).

ROLE OF CREM IN SPERMATOGENESIS

CREM is a highly abundant transcript in adult testis while in prepubertal animals is expressed at very low levels. Thus, in testis CREM is the subject of a developmental switch in expression[20]. Further charaterisation revealed that the the abundant CREM transcript encodes exclusively the activator form, while in prepubertal testis only the repressor forms were detected at low levels. Thus, the developmental switch of CREM expression also constitiutes a reversal of function[21].

Spermatogenesis is a process occurring in a precise and coordinated manner within the seminiferous tubules[44]. During this entire developmental process the germ cells are maintained in intimate contact with the somatic Sertoli cells. As the spermatogonia mature, they move from the periphery towards the lumen of the tubule until the mature spermatozoa are conducted from the lumen to the collecting ducts.

CREM activator protein is detected in mature germ cells, such as round spermatids, which have undergone meiosis[45]. Thus, CREM transactivator function must be restricted to the late phase of transcription before the compaction of the DNA. Interestingly, several genes have been identified which are transcribed at the time of appearance of the CREM protein and which include CRE-like sequences in their promoter regions[45]. Several lines of evidence demonstrate that CREM constitutes the first step of a transcriptional cascade which is responsible for the activation of several germ specific genes. To date at least three genes, RT7[45], transition protein-1[46] and claspermin[47] have been shown to be targets of CREM-mediated transactivation in germ cells. Importantly, the dramatic increase in the levels of CREM protein correlates with its concomitant phosphorylation at serine 117 by a cAMP-stimulated PKA activity in round spermatid extracts[45]. Thus, CREM appears to participate in the testis-specific promoter activation of numerous haploid-expressed genes.

A remarkable aspect of the CREM developmental switch in germ cells is constituted by its exquisite hormonal regulation. The spermatogenic differentiation program is under the tight control of the hypothalamic-pituitary axis[44]. The regulation of CREM function in testis seems to be intricately linked to FSH both at the level of the control of transcript processing and at the level of protein activity. For example, surgical removal of the pituitary gland leads to the loss of CREM expression in the rat adult testis[23]. Furthermore hypophysectomisation in prepubertal animals, prevents the switch in CREM expression at the pachytene spermatocyte stage, thus implicating the pituitary directly in the maintenance of as well as the switch to high levels of CREM expression. Injections of FSH leads to a rapid and significant induction of the CREM transcript[23]. The hormonal induction of CREM by FSH is not transcriptional, as expected by the housekeeping nature of the P1 promoter. Instead, by a mechanism of alternative polyadenylation, AUUUA destabilizer elements present in the 3′ untranslated region of the gene are excluded, dramatically increasing the stability of the CREM message. CREM is the first example of a gene whose expression is modulated by a pituitary hormone during spermatogenesis[23]. The implication of these findings is that hormones can regulate gene expression at the level of RNA processing and stability. Importantly the effect of FSH can not be direct since germ cells do not have FSH receptors. Recent results show that another hormonal message originating from the Sertoli cells upon FSH stimulation is mediating CREM activation in germ cells (L. Monaco, unpublished).

ROLE OF CREM IN CIRCADIAN RHYTHMS

Crucial elements for the synchronization of biological rhythms in mammals are the pineal gland[48] and the suprachiasmatic nucleus (SCN)[49]. Environmental lighting conditions are transduced by the pineal gland from a neuronal to an endocrine message, the rhythmic secretion of melatonin[48]. This hormone synthesis is controlled by the SCN, being elevated at night and low during the day[49]. The cAMP-dependent signal transduction pathway serves as a relay to stimulate melatonin synthesis. Thus, from neuronal pathways which include the retina and the SCN, the pineal gland acts as a temporal regulator for the function of the hypothalamic-pituitary-gonadal axis[48].

The study of CREM expression in the rat brain indicated a specific pattern of expression[50]. Analysis of CREM expression in the pineal gland has revealed a dramatic day-night regulation, with peak during the night. The CREM isoform in the pineal gland corresponds to ICER, the early response repressor known to be cAMP-inducible in endocrine cells[26]. The transcript shows a very characteristic and reproducible kinetic of expression. It appears likely that the autoregulatory loop shown to control ICER transient inducibility[25] would also play a role in the day-night cyclic expression in the pineal gland (N. S. Foulkes, unpublished).

By a series of physiological experiments, the mechanism controlling this pattern of ICER expression was determined and found to require clock-distal elements. Indeed, it is known that at night, postganglionic fibers originating from the superior cervical ganglia (SCG) release norepinephrine which in turn regulates melatonin synthesis via adrenergic receptors. These analyses have shown that signals from the SCN direct the induction of CREM expression[26].

The question of possible targets for downregulation by ICER in the gland is of particular interest. It has been proposed that a reasonable target could be the enzyme which catalyses the rate-limiting step of melatonin synthesis, namely N-acetyl transferase or factors which regulate its activity (J. H. Stehle and N. S. Foulkes, unpublished).

Another important finding concerning the role of CRE-binding factors in circadian rhythms concerns the cyclic phosphorylation of CREB in the suprachiamatic nucleus[51]. During the night, upon light stimuli which pahse-shift the clock, CREB appears to be efficiently phosphorylated by an SCN-endogenous kinase at the serine 133 residue. Phosphorylation at this site turns CREB into an activator and may be obtained by a number of kinases[7]. While the nature of the SCN-endogenous kinase has not been established, it seems likely that it could be PKA[51]. This result would suggest a key role for this kinase or of a counteracting phosphatase in the regulation of the clock function. The target genes for the activated CREB in the SCN have yet to be established.

CONCLUSIONS AND PERSPECTIVES

To date much of the research in transcription factor biology has been devoted to understanding the structure and function relationship of these factors. Progress has been extremely rapid and now the basic principles of transcription factor function are close to being elucidated. As a result of this work, new questions have been raised and so it is clear we still have a long way to go before we understand completely how the promoters and enhancers of genes execute transcriptional control. However a much greater challenge lies ahead and that is to relate transcriptional control mechanisms to the physiology and biology of the organism. The use of homologous recombination to inactivate specific gene products offers a powerful tool to address such questions. Paradoxically however, in some cases it has complicated our understanding since it is clear that many important factors operate in the context of networks where there is considerable overlap of function. Thus, it is possible that the phenotype obtained by loss of a single factor could reflect more the compensatory adjustments made by other factors in its network rather than the function of the target factor itself. CRE-binding proteins appear to play a central role in the physiology of the neuroendocrine system. Further studies of their molecular and functional characteristics will therefore represent another major step forward in our understanding of hormonal regulation and metabolism.

REFERENCES

1. S.C. Harrison, A structural taxonomy of DNA-binding domains. *Nature* 353: 715–719 (1991)
2. Y. Nishizuka, Studies and perspectives of protein kinase C. *Science* 233: 305–312 (1986)
3. J.C. Cambier, N.K. Newell, L.B. Justement, J.C. McGuire, K.L. Leach and Z.Z.Chen, Iα binding ligands and cAMP stimulate nuclear translocation of PKC in β lymphocytes. *Nature* 327: 629–632 (1987)
4. D. Masquilier and P. Sassone-Corsi, Transcriptional cross-talk: nuclear factors CREM and CREB bind to AP-1 sites and inhibit activation by Jun. *J. Biol. Chem.* 267: 22460–22466 (1992)
5. T. Yoshimasa, D. R. Sibley, M. Bouvier, R.J. Lefkowitz and M.G. Caron, Cross-talk between cellular signalling pathways suggested by phorbol ester adenylate cyclase phosphorylation. *Nature* 327: 67–70 (1987)
6. S.G. McKnight, C.H. Clegg, M.D. Uhler, J.C. Chrivia, G.G. Cadd and L.L. Correll, Analysis of the cAMP-dependent protein kinase system using molecular genetic approaches. *Rec. Progr. Horm. Res.* 44: 307–335 (1988)
7. E. Lalli and P. Sassone-Corsi, Signal Transduction and Gene Regulation: The nuclear Response to cAMP. *J. Biol. Chem.* 269: 17359–62 (1994)
8. W.J. Roesler, G.R. Vanderbark and R.W. Hanson, Cyclic AMP and the induction of eukaryotic gene expression. *J. Biol. Chem.* 263: 9063–9066 (1988)
9. E.B. Ziff, Transcription factors: a new family gathers at the cAMP response site. *Trends Genet* 6: 69–72 (1990)
10. E. Borrelli, J.P. Montmayeur, N.S. Foulkes and P. Sassone-Corsi, Signal transduction and gene control: the cAMP pathway. *Critical Rev Oncogenesis* 3: 321–338 (1992)
11. H.C. Liou, M.R. Boothby and L.H. Glimcher, Distinct cloned class II MHC DNA-binding proteins recognize the X-box transcription element. *Science* 242: 69–71 (1988)
12. S. Wagner and M.R. Green, HTLV-I *tax* protein stimulation of DNA-binding of bZip proteins by enhancing dimerization. *Science* 262: 395–399 (1993)
13. P. Sassone-Corsi, Cyclic AMP induction of early adenovirus promoters involves sequences required for E1A-transactivation. *Proc. Natl. Acad. Sci. U.S.A.* 85: 7192–7196 (1988)
14. K.A.W. Lee, S.J. Fink, R.H. Goodman and M.R. Green, Distinguishable promoter elements are involved in transcriptional activation by E1A and cyclic AMP. *Mol. Cell. Biol.* 9: 4390–4397 (1989)
15. J.P. Hoeffler, T.E. Meyer, Y. Yun, J.L. Jameson and J.F. Habener, Cyclic AMP- responsive DNA-binding Protein: Structure Based on a Cloned Placental cDNA. *Science* 242: 1430–1433 (1988)
16. T.Y. Hai, F. Liu, W.J. Coukos and M.R. Green, Transcription factor ATF cDNA clones: An extensive family of leucine zipper proteins able to selectively form DNA binding heterodimers. *Genes & Dev.* 3: 2083–2090 (1989)
17. N.S. Foulkes, E. Borrelli and P. Sassone-Corsi, CREM gene: Use of alternative DNA binding domains generates multiple antagonists of cAMP-induced transcription. *Cell* 64: 739–749 (1991)
18. T.Y. Hai and T. Curran, Cross-family dimerization of transcription factors Fos:Jun and ATF/CREB alters DNA binding specificity. *Proc. Natl. Acad. Sci. U.S.A.* 88: 3720–3724 (1991)
19. P. Sassone-Corsi, L.J. Ransone and I.M. Verma, Cross-talk in signal transduction: TPA-inducible factor Jun/AP-1 activates cAMP responsive enhancer elements. *Oncogene,* 5: 427–431 (1990)
20. N.S. Foulkes, B. Mellström, E. Benusiglio and P. Sassone-Corsi, Developmental switch of CREM function during spermatogenesis: from antagonist to transcriptional activator. *Nature* 355: 80–84 (1992)
21. N.S. Foulkes and P. Sassone-Corsi, More is better: Activators and Repressors from the Same Gene. *Cell* 68: 411–414 (1992)
22. B.M. Laoide, N.S. Foulkes, F. Schlotter and P. Sassone-Corsi, The functional versatility of CREM is determined by its modular structure. *EMBO J.* 12: 1179–1191 (1993)
23. N.S. Foulkes, F. Schlotter, P. Pévet and P. Sassone-Corsi, Pituitary hormone FSH directs the CREM functional switch during spermatogenesis. *Nature* 362: 264–267 (1993)

24. V. Delmas, B.M. Laoide, D. Masquilier, R.P. de Groot, N.S. Foulkes and P. Sassone-Corsi, Alternative us-
     age of initiation codons in mRNA encoding the cAMP-responsive-element modulator (CREM) generates
     regulators with opposite functions. *Proc. Natl. Acad. Sci. U.S.A.* 89: 4226–4230 (1992)

25. C.A. Molina, N.S. Foulkes, E. Lalli and P. Sassone-Corsi, Inducibility and negative autoregulation of
     CREM: An alternative promoter directs the expression of ICER, an early response repressor. *Cell* 75:
     875–886 (1993)

26. J.H. Stehle, N.S. Foulkes, C.A. Molina, V. Simonneaux, P. Pévet and P. Sassone-Corsi, Adrenergic signals
     direct rhythmic expression of transcriptional repressor CREM in the pineal gland. *Nature* 365: 314–320
     (1993)

27. G.A. Gonzalez and M.R. Montminy, Cyclic AMP stimulates somatostatin gene transcription by phosphory-
     lation of CREB at Ser 133. *Cell* 59: 675–680 (1989)

28. C.Q. Lee, Y. Yun, J.P. Hoeffler and J.F. Habener, Cyclic-AMP-responsive transcriptional activation in-
     volves interdependent phosphorylated subdomains. *EMBO J.* 9: 4455–4465 (1990)

29. R.P. de Groot, J. den Hertog, J.R. Vandenheede, J. Goris and P. Sassone-Corsi, Multiple and cooperative
     phosphorylation events regulate the CREM activator function. *EMBO J.* 12: 3903–3911 (1993)

30. R.P. de Groot, R. Derua, J. Goris and P. Sassone-Corsi, Phosphorylation and negative regulation of the
     transcriptional activator CREM by p34cdc2. *Mol. Endocrinol.* 7: 1495–1501 (1993)

31. P. Sassone-Corsi, J. Visvader, L. Ferland, P.L. Mellon and I.M. Verma, Induction of proto-oncogene *fos*
     transcription through the adenylate cyclase pathway: characterization of a cAMP-responsive element.
     Genes Dev. 2: 1529–1538 (1988)

32. M. Sheng, G. McFadden and M.E. Greenberg, Membrane depolarization and calcium induce c-*fos* tran-
     scription via phosphorylation of transcription factor CREB. *Neuron* 4: 571–582 (1990)

33. P.K. Dash, K.A. Karl, M.A. Colicos, R. Prywes and E.R. Kandel, cAMP response element-binding protein
     is activated by Ca^{2+}/calmodulin- as well as cAMP-dependent protein kinase. *Proc. Natl. Acad. Sci. U.S.A.*
     88: 5061–5065 (1991)

34. D.D Ginty, D. Glowacka, D.S. Bader, H. Hidaka and J.A. Wagner, Induction of immediate early genes by
     Ca^{2+} influx requires cAMP-dependent protein kinase in PC12 cells. *J. Biol. Chem.* 266: 17454–17458
     (1991)

35. R.P. de Groot, L.M. Ballou and P. Sassone-Corsi, Positive Regulation of the cAMP-responsive Activator
     CREM by the p70 S6 Kinase: An Alternative Route to Mitogen-induced Gene expression. *Cell* 79: 81–91
     (1994)

36. A.J. Courey and R. Tjian, Analysis of Sp1 in vivo reveals multiple transcriptional domains, including a
     novel glutamine activation motif. *Cell,* 55, 887–898 (1989)

37. T. Williams, A. Admon, B. Luscher and R. Tjian, Cloning and Expression of AP-2, a cell-type-specific
     transcription factor that activates inducible enhancer elements. *Genes Dev.* 2: 1557–1569 (1988)

38. R.P. Rehfuss, K.M. Walton, M.M. Loriaux and R.H. Goodman, The cAMP- regulated enhancer-binding
     protein ATF-1 activates transcription in response to cAMP-dependent protein kinase A. *J. Biol. Chem.* 266:
     18431–18434 (1991)

39. M. Hagiwara, A. Alberts, P. Brindle, J. Meinkoth, J. Feramisco, T. Deng and M. Montminy, Transcriptional
     attenuation following cAMP induction requires PP-1- mediated dephosphorylation of CREB. *Cell* 70:
     105–113 (1992)

40. M. Nichols, F. Weih, W. Schmid, C. DeVack, E. Kowenz-Leutz, B. Luckow and G. Schutz, Phosphoryla-
     tion of CREB affects its binding to high and low affinity sites: implications for cAMP induced gene tran-
     scription. *EMBO J.* 11: 3337–3346 (1992)

41. I.M. Verma and P. Sassone-Corsi, Proto-oncogene *fos*: complex but versatile regulation. *Cell* 51: 513–514
     (1987)

42. T.E. Meyer, G. Waeber, J. Lin, W. Beckman and J. Habener, The promoter of the gene encoding 3' 5'-cy-
     clic adenosine monophopsphate (cAMP) response element binding protein contains cAMP response ele-
     ments: Evidence for positive autoregulation of gene transcription. *Endocrinology* 132: 770–777 (1993)

43. P. Sassone-Corsi, Rhythmic Transcription and Autoregulatory Loops: Winding up the Biological Clock.
     Cell 78: 361–364 (1994)

44. B. Jégou, The Sertoli-germ cell communication network in mammals. *Int. Rev. Cytol.* 147: 25–96 (1993)

45. V. Delmas, F. van der Hoorn, B. Mellström, B. Jégou and P. Sassone-Corsi, Induction of CREM activator
     proteins in spermatids: downstream targets and implications for haploid germ cell differentiation. *Mol. En-
     docrinol.* 7: 1502–1514 (1993)

46. M.K. Kistler, P. Sassone-Corsi and S.W. Kistler, Identification of a functional cAMP response element in
     the 5'-Flanking Region of the Gene for Transition Protein 1 (TP1), a basic Chromosomal Protein of Mam-
     malian Spermatids. *Biol. Reprod.* 51: 1322–1329 (1994)

47. Z. Sun, P. Sassone-Corsi and A. Means, Calspermin Gene Transcription is Regulated by two cyclic AMP response elements contained in an alternative Promoter in the Calmodulin Kinase IV gene. *Mol. Cell. Biol.* 15: 561–571 (1995)
48. L. Tamarkin, C.J. Baird and O.F.X. Almeida, Melatonin: A coordinating signal for mammalian reproduction? *Science*, 227: 714–720 (1985)
49. R.Y. Moore, Organization and function of the central nervous system circadian oscillator; the suprachiasmatic hypothalamic nucleus. *Federation Proc.* 42: 2783–2789 (1983)
50. B. Mellström, J.R. Naranjo, N.S. Foulkes, M. Lafarga and P. Sassone-Corsi, Transcriptional response to cAMP in brain: specific distribution and induction of CREM antagonists. *Neuron* 10: 655–65 (1993)
51. D.D. Ginty, J.M. Kornhauser, M. Thompson, H. Bading, K.E. Mayo, J.S. Takahashi and M. Greenberg, Regulation of CREB Phosphorylation in the suprachiasmatic Nucleus by Light and a circadian clock. *Science* 260: 238–241 (1993)

DISCUSSION

F. Rauscher: We have yet another protein that sticks to p53: Can you clarify a few things for me? What is the biological rationale for looking for p53 CREM association?

P. Sassone-Corsi: As I was just saying, in germ cells p53 and CREM are co-expressed. In the case of CREM this is important because this is the only place where there is a very large amount of CRE binding activator. There is no other tissue where there is such a high amount of CREM activator.

F. Rauscher: It sticks to CREM but not CREMτ you said?

P. Sassone-Corsi: No, it sticks to CREMτ.

F. Rauscher: Is that splicing different? Is this a glutamine rich region? The splicing difference, is this the glutamine rich region?

P. Sassone-Corsi: What I am saying is that by trying different kinds of CREM proteins the only way that CREM will not bind to p53 is when the glutamine rich regions are missing.

F. Rauscher: And how big is this glutamine rich region?

P. Sassone-Corsi: There are two of them. And each of them is about 60 amino acids.

F. Rauscher: And as GAL-4 fusions, are those glutamine rich regions themselves activators?

P. Sassone-Corsi: Yes.

F. Rauscher: Are they affected by p53?

P. Sassone-Corsi: Yes.

F. Rauscher: As GAL-4 fusions?

P. Sassone-Corsi: Yes.

M. Oren: Two questions: According to your very attractive model, you would predict that if you look at the p53 knockout mice and you look at the CREM transcriptional targets - like the ones you listed on the board - they will go up but will not go down?

P. Sassone-Corsi: Probably, yes. We are just looking for that. We are looking for the p53 knockout at that level - and other levels - but that is definitely one thing that we have to look at.

M. Oren: That would be a very nice closing of the circle.

P. Sassone-Corsi: Sure.

M. Oren: The other question is relating to the ICER. In principle in any tissue where you have a strong induction you are likely to activate the endogenous p2. In practice, you say this is very limited. What is the explanation for that and is there any evidence that activation of p2 ICER can serve a terminating role in other types of responses?

P. Sassone-Corsi: The answer is complex. Because we have found that there are differences within this model depending on which kind of system you are looking at. That is, in the pineal gland, that is definitely a place where we look in detail. We found that there are two possible modes depending on the photoperiod. This is kind of complex but I will try to explain it. You can super-impose to the normal day/night switch seasons, that is, long days and short nights or long nights and short days. It is important because it is a way to physiologically regulate very strictly an endocrine system. When you do that you put the gene in a supersensitive mode, that is, in a long day there will be no phosphorolation of the activators and no ICER. And as soon as the night starts (these are about three or four hour nights), phosphorylation of the activators goes up really fast and ICER then comes up and shuts off those activators right away. It is a very super-sensitive situation. In a long night instead we are going into the opposite situation, that is, the activators are constituitively phosphorylated and their oscillation is virtually none. Instead, ICER oscillation is very weak. What you are doing is weakly changing the balance between repressors and activators and that will give you this more shallow, dampened response. So, when you ask that question you get to understand that that depends a lot on the system which you are looking at. And that depends a lot on the endogenous level of activators with respect to repressors.

D. Livingston: Can you detect a stable CREM p53 complex?

P. Sassone-Corsi: We are just doing those experiments actually. In the very preliminary assay, I would say not. That is, apparently DNA binding is not required for that association. The association occurs without DNA binding. Instead what I can say is that the association is probably not very strong because when you do DNA binding first, then you add p53, there will be no change in CREM DNA binding.

D. Livingston: But, in non-denaturing, non-disruptive buffers are you able to detect a complex?

P. Sassone-Corsi: Using non-disruptive buffers is what we are just doing right now. And I believe the possibility we are going to see something.

D. Livingston: Suppose you do IPDOC on that, and go looking for released CREM or released p53 can you detect it?

P. Sassone-Corsi: We did not do that.

D. Livingston: Could you track such a complex as a DNA binding element; would that not be helpful?

P. Sassone-Corsi: Yes, that would be really nice. The only thing we did up to now is classical DNA binding. And we did not see anything at that stage. But possibly, it is also a matter of having the right technical tools. So we need to better do those experiments. But I agree with you. It would be nice to see what happens at the level of DNA binding.

D. Livingston: Two other questions: Can you detect CREM/CBP complexes as gel-shift complexes?

P. Sassone-Corsi: No, we did not do those experiments.

D. Livingston: Or ICER?

P. Sassone-Corsi: We do not do those experiments. The only thing I can say is since you are interested in CBP, the only time we did one experiment we could see that ICER would not bind CBP.

D. Livingston: *In-vitro*?

P. Sassone-Corsi: Yes. But I got to say that our CBP tools are not very good either.

D. Livingston: But you were able to detect CREM/CBP *in-vitro*?

P. Sassone-Corsi: CREMτ, yes.

D. Livingston: CREMτ/CBP *in-vitro*?

P. Sassone-Corsi: Yes.

D. Livingston: How about CREMτ p300, do you know?

P. Sassone-Corsi: We did not do that.

A. Nordheim: I have a question concerning the phosphorylation of CREM. You indicated that the 133 site could be phosphorylated by the Cdc2 kinase, and you indicated that this might serve a down regulatory function.

P. Sassone-Corsi: There are four sites for CDC-2.

A. Nordheim: And what is the evidence that this causes then a negative effect?

P. Sassone-Corsi: The evidence is based on the effects of transfection experiments using constitutively active CDC2 kinases on the transcriptional efficiency from a cAMP-inducible promoter. Similar results have also been obtained with the calcium calmodulin kinase which phosphorylates CREM at position Ser-142 and that results in down-regulation of PKA function. We did not perform the experiments to see whether CDC2 phosphorylation would block CREM-CBP association.

A. Nordheim: You indicated that in your model, when you also included cycloheximide, isosynthesis is prevented and therefore the ICER down regulatory effect is prevented. Under these circumstances did you look at the phosphorylation of CREB2; was that prolonged or affected in any way?

P. Sassone-Corsi: Yes, that is a good point. The answer to that is also complex. To simplify the situation I can say that apparently there is no direct effect of protein synthesis on the kinetics of phosphorylation of CREB or CREM. We have made cell lines where we expressed sense and anti-sense ICER. In those sense-antisense cell lines by overexpressing ICER or by blocking ICER expression, phosphorylation of the activators is not affected.

E. Nigg: Following up on Alfred's question: The CDC2 sites on one of your earlier slides were really highly heretical from a CDC2 point of view. What is the evidence that those sites get hit by CDC2?

P. Sassone-Corsi: We have clear *in-vitro* evidence. Also, we know that those sites are phosphorylated *in-vivo*, but we have no evidence that they are phosphorylated differentially during the cell cycle.

E. Nigg: Because there really is quite a lot of evidence on what constitutes a good CDC2 site. Yours looked like very poor candidates.

P. Sassone-Corsi: Yes, there are two other sites further in the c-terminal to those two that are more classical. But we failed to observe a cell cycle regulation in those sites.

E. Nigg: I seem to remember that many years ago, Stan McKnight, showed that it was impossible to actually boost PKA activity by simply overexpressing the catalytic subunit.

P. Sassone-Corsi: What Stan did was to overexpress the regulatory subunit. And that is how you dampened the catalytic subunit. You can overexpress catalytic subunit and have a very strong activation as I showed. That is well known.

M. Green: On the glutamine; do you think that the P53 interaction sites is the glutamine rich region? Is that correct?

P. Sassone-Corsi: Yes.

M. Green: Does it interact with CREB which also has a glutamine-rich region?

P. Sassone-Corsi: I showed that in one slide. Yes.

M. Green: So it does. I see. And the impression I got from your talk was that you thought that the glutamine rich region was really the activation domain, but I thought that the general view was that was the phosphopeptide serine-133 which then served as a docking site for CBP which was the primary activation domain?

P. Sassone-Corsi: If you take some CREB isoforms which contain phosphorylation sites but they do not contain glutamine-rich domains, they work as repressors. So the phosphorylation domain alone is not enough for transcriptional activation.

M. Green: Even though it binds CBP?

P. Sassone-Corsi: Absolutely, yes. You can transform them into activators if you provide tax, or provide some other transcriptional activation domain. Now what is important to say here is that the idea today is that you have phosphorylation at serine-133 and that will allow a better exposure of the glutamine-rich regions to CBP to interact with proteins such as TAF 110 for instance. But that interaction then requires CBP anyway, that is, it requires the phosphorylation. So the evidence we have today is that you need at least one glutamine-rich domain for activation. And, in fact, between the two domains, the first is better than the second. ATF-1, which contains only one of them, is a good transcriptional activator. So it is really the cooperation between the P-box and at least one glutamine rich region that allows for transcriptional activation.

M. Green: My final question: The repression you are observing in your co-transfection experiments - you do not think is the type of repression that Tom Shenk observes, for example, by sequestering TBP? And I presume the reason you think that is because of the VP-16 experiment?

P. Sassone-Corsi: Yes, absolutely.

M. Green: But the problem, as I saw it, the problem with the VP-16 experiment is that VP-16 starts out as a much better activator.

P. Sassone-Corsi: Yes of course we have done that also with other kinds of GAL-4 fusion transcriptional activators. I have shown VP-16 as a very well known trascriptional activator, but we have done that with jun-GAL-4 and things like that and nothing happened. The question you can ask instead is, do you need any kind of glutamine-rich domain, can you take the glutamine rich domain of SP-1 and do the same experiment? And that is what we are doing right now.

M. Green: But then are you thinking that p53 binds the glutamine-rich domain and masks its intrinsic activation potential - and that is why you see repressors?

P. Sassone-Corsi: Exactly.

P. Radice: Is there any evidence of an involvement of CREM in testicular germ cell tumors, and, the other question is, has the gene been mapped?

P. Sassone-Corsi: Yes, we mapped the gene in both a mouse and a human cell and whether it expresseed changes in tumors, yes, that is a very interesting question. We have been able to look at a couple of human testicular tumors, actually more than a couple, maybe six, and in all those CREM expression is absent. Although in a normal testicular human tissue it is very high just like in a mouse. We also had the chance to look at several mouse testicular tumors caused by trangenic expression of polyoma large T (mice from François Cuzin) and also in those, CREM expression disappears in the tumors. So, of course, this correlation is interesting.

P. Radice: So what is the location of the gene on the human genome?

P. Sassone-Corsi: Alright, you are testing my memory here. We published that two years ago. It is on chromosome 10 in humans and on chromosome 18 in the mouse.

9

MADS-DOMAIN TRANSCRIPTION FACTORS AND THEIR ACCESSORY PROTEINS (TCFS)

Nuclear Targets for Growth Control Signals

Michael A. Cahill, Henning Althöfer, and Alfred Nordheim

Institut für Molekularbiologie
Medizinische Hochschule Hannover
D-30623 Hannover, Federal Republik of Germany,

1. INTRODUCTION

Tightly regulated gene activity provides the molecular basis for ensuring properly controlled growth and division of eukaryotic cells. A comprehensive understanding of the regulatory mechanisms that direct gene activity of both proliferating and non-proliferating cells will provide important insight into the origin and causes of proliferative disorders in human pathology, including cancer.

The transition of non-proliferating, resting cells into active growth (i.e. the transition from the G0-to-G1 stages of the cell cycle) is accompanied by, and dependent upon, the rapid and transient activation of the class of immediate-early genes (IEGs) [1]. In this transition extracellular stimuli (e.g. growth factors) activate intracellular signalling cascades, involving the enzymatic activities of kinases and phosphatases, which eventually target the promoters of IEGs. Different MAPK (mitogen-activated protein kinase) pathways feature prominently in this mitogenic stimulation [2]. Transcription factor activity is modulated by these signalling events, thereby directing IEG transcriptional activity. In the proliferating mode, continuously dividing cells display a cell cycle-specific pattern of gene activity which again is subject to direct and indirect modulation by kinases, namely the cyclin-dependent kinases (CDKs) [3].

In the following we describe some of our findings regarding the involvement of a MADS-domain [4, 5] transcription factor (the serum response factor, SRF) and its accessory proteins (the ternary complex factors, TCFs) in directing IEG transcriptional control during the G0-G1 transition of mammalian cells. Different pathways of intracellular signalling are described that target these transcription factors and thereby regulate their

---

* Present address: California Institute of Technology, Division of Biology, Pasadena, California 91125, USA.

transcription activation potential. We further discuss recent results which indicate that in the budding yeast *Saccharomyces cerevisiae* ternary complexes containing the MADS-domain protein Mcm1, and an as yet unidentified accessory TCF partner, are involved in directing cell cycle-specific gene control during the G2 phase of the yeast cell cycle. This raises the intriguing possibility that in mammalian cells, as in yeast, MADS-domain proteins may direct cell cycle-dependent gene control during G2 as well as at the G0-G1 transition.

2. THE c-*fos* SRE: THE NUCLEATION SITE FOR TERNARY COMPLEX FORMATION

The c-*fos* gene is the IEG whose transcriptional control has been characterized most extensively [6, 7]. The plethora of extracellular stimuli which induce rapid and transient transcriptional activation of the c-*fos* gene is summarized in figure 1. This figure also shows that principally three major *cis*-elements (CRE, SRE, SIE) share the task of receiving these stimuli and converting them into a transcriptional response. The CRE (-60 element) and its cognate binding proteins (CREB, CREM, ATF-type factors) are targeted by kinases activated in response to elevated intracellular levels of either cAMP or Ca^{2+} [8]. Instead, the SIE receives activating signals via induced binding of a STAT transcription factor which is translocated into the nucleus subsequent to membrane receptor-mediated stimulation of individual members of the JAK family of kinases [6]. Our work has primarily focussed on the function of the SRE (serum response element) [9] and the role of the proteins bound to it. The SRE, a sequence displaying interrupted dyad symmetry, is bound di-

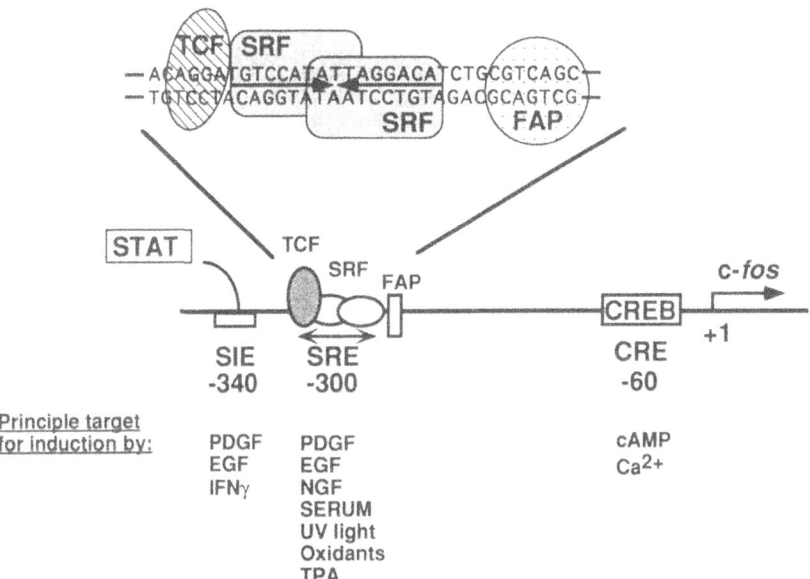

Figure 1. Schematic representation of the three main *cis*-elements (SIE, SRE, CRE) directing c-*fos* gene activity in response to the indicated extracellular signal activation. The sequence of the SRE and its *in vivo* protein occupance is shown enlarged in the upper part of the figure.

rectly and with high affinity by a homodimer of SRF [9, 10, 11]. In the SRE-SRF complex the DNA is strongly bent at the A/T stretch of the central CArG-box. This feature is revealed by the X-ray crystallographic structure of the SRE bound by the dimeric SRF core-domain which displays an overall DNA bending of $72°$ [12]. This X-ray analysis also identifies a novel protein structure within the DNA-binding core region of SRF, with three layers of protein subdomains (an anti-parallel coiled coil, a four-stranded antiparallel β-sheet, and an α-helical region composed of one helix from each dimer subunit) stacked on top of each other. DNA binding specificity of SRF is provided to a large extend by extensive minor groove contacts and the induced DNA bending of the SRE, as well as base-specific major groove contacts with the guanine bases of the consensus $CC(A/T)_6GG$ binding sequence. Phosphorylation of SRF increases the exchange rate of the SRE-SRF complex *in vitro*, however it is unclear what role this plays *in vivo* [13, 14].

The SRE-SRF binary complex was shown to recruit to the DNA an additional polypeptide, termed ternary complex factor (TCF), which alone was unable to bind to the c-*fos* SRE [15]. Once recruited into the complex, TCF specifically contacts the GGA sequence directly upstream of the SRF binding site (see figure 1). TCF activity was subsequently shown to be encoded by a subgroup of the family of Ets proto-oncoproteins [16, 17, 18, 19, 20] (see below). *In vivo* genomic footprinting revealed continuous occupance of the SRE by proteins whose methylation protection pattern was indistinguishable from the one generated by SRF-TCF *in vitro* [21, 22]. Whether rapid exchange of these proteins occurs *in vivo* is presently not understood. The genomic footprint also revealed the presence of a protein bound 3′ to the SRF (referred to as FAP in figure 1) whose identity and function is unknown at present.

The SRE-SRF-TCF ternary complex fulfils a crucial role in signal-induced activation of the c-*fos* gene (see below). It appears that both PKC- and MAPK-mediated activation strictly require TCF binding [15, 23, 24, 25], whereas serum activation of c-*fos* appears to involve additional signalling pathways that target the SRF and not TCF [26, 27, 28]. The signalling events mentioned lead to induced phosphorylation of TCF [29, 30, 31] and SRF [32] at identified sites (see below). These post-translational modifications are short-lived and the kinetics of TCF and SRF phosphorylation and subsequent dephosphorylation upon growth factor receptor activation correlate with the temporal pattern of c-*fos* transcriptional activation and down-regulation, respectively [31] (R. Zinck and A.N., unpublished). Interference with TCF dephosphorylation using inhibitors of serine/threonine phosphatase activities leads to prolonged c-*fos* expression [33]. It is presently not understood by what mechanism the phosphorylation of SRF and TCF contributes to the activation of c-*fos* transcription. It is conceivable that conformational changes in the ternary complex lead to altered protein-protein interactions that facilitate interactions with the basal transcriptional machinery. Such protein-protein interactions may involve the adaptor protein CBP [34] (R. Janknecht and A.N., unpublished). In addition to the c-*fos* gene, ternary complexes assembled at SREs have also been demonstrated to regulate other IEGs such as *egr-1* [33, 35] and *pip92* [36].

3. SRF AND Mcm1: MADS-DOMAIN PROTEINS

Transcription factors with homology to the SRF DNA binding domain exist in yeast [37, 38, 39], angiosperms [4, 40, 41, 42], insects [43] and vertebrates [10, 18, 44, 45, 46, 47, 48, 49, 50, 51]. This group of proteins has been called the MADS box family; named after the prototypical members Mcm1 from yeast, Agamous and Deficiens from plants, and SRF from humans [4, 5]. Agamous and Deficiens from plants are in turn prototypical members of multigene homeotic plant MADS subfamilies.

The existence of MADS proteins across the eukaryotic phylogenetic tree suggests the presence of related proteins in the unicellular ancestors of plants and animals, and therefore suggests a potential central role in eukaryotic cell biology. Molecular genetics on the yeasts *S. cerevisiae* and *Schizosaccharomyces pombe* has revealed a conserved mechanism of haplotype switching involving activation of a signal transduction cascade homologous to mammalian MAPK pathways [2, 52]. Mcm1 is one of the nuclear targets of this signal transduction cascade in *S. cerevisiae*, and is involved in the regulation of mating type genes which control the transition between haploid and diploid genotypes. As a heterodimer with the MADS protein Arg80, Mcm1 also contributes to arginine metabolism [53].

There are two haplotypes in *S. cerevisiae*, α and **a**, which differ at one locus, *MAT*. This locus encodes either the α1 and α2 proteins in α cells, or the **a**1 repressor in **a** cells, which are all homeodomain transcription factors. Mcm1 co-operates with α1, to activate α-specific genes, and with α2 to repress **a**-specific genes in α cells. Ste12 is additionally recruited by Mcm1 to **a**-specific genes in **a** cells. The **a**1 repressor has no known function in haploid cells. **a** cells express **a**-specific genes since they lack both the α2 repressor of **a**-specific genes, and the α1 activator of α-specific genes. However when **a** and α cells mate the **a**1 and α2 homeodomain proteins form a new dimeric factor which represses all **a**- and α-specific haploid transcription [54, 55]. The mode of ternary complex formation seems to be similar between Mcm1 and its accessory protein Ste12, and between SRF and the accessory mammalian TCF proteins, with similar MADS box residues required [56, 57]. Thus diploid-specific transcription is maintained via repression of haploid-specific genes, and Mcm1 regulates haploid-specific transcription in both haplotypes of *S. cerevisiae* by the differential recruitment of accessory proteins. In addition, by recruiting a protein called Swi Five Factor (Sff) to the *Swi5* promoter, Mcm1 is involved in conferring G2-specific transcription to that gene [58].

Vertebrates possess several proteins related to SRF, belonging to the RSRF/MEF2 family [49, 50, 51]. The DNA binding site consensuses for SRF, Mcm1 and RSRFs have been determined [49, 59, 60] and differ slightly, due primarily to the amino terminal region of the MADS box [59, 60, 61]. SRF and RSRF/MEF2s do not heterodimerize to form novel specificity transcription factors, and RSRF/MEF2s cannot recruit the TCFs associated with SRF [49]. Thus different suites of genes should be regulated by different MADS classes within one cell.

The known functions of mammalian SRF include regulation of a variety of immediate early genes, the IL-2Rα gene, and several muscle-specific genes [7]. Additionally, the protein has been shown by immunofluorescence to be present in the nucleus throughout the cell cycle, and microinjection of anti-SRF antibodies arrested cells in mid cycle [62]. Indeed SRF has been suggested to have a role in the G2 phase of the cell cycle [63]. Such functions would be probably independent of the TCFs associated with induction of the immediate-early response, and could represent transcriptional properties intrinsic to SRF itself, or the recruitment of different ternary complex factors such as SFF recruitment by Mcm1 in yeast.

4. MAMMALIAN TCFs FORM A SUBGROUP OF ETS FAMILY ONCO-PROTEINS

Ternary complex factor (TCF) activity is defined by a cooperative protein-protein interaction with MADS-domain factors leading to stable protein binding to DNA se-

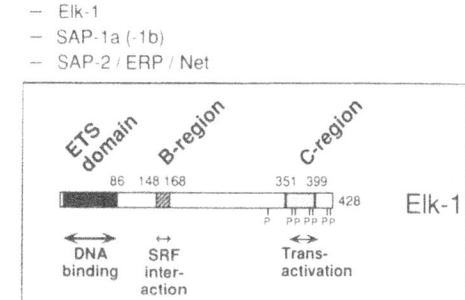

Figure 2. Structure of the presently known TCFs which form a subgroup of the·Ets family of transcription factors. The structure of Elk-1 is schematized inside the box. The three regions of homology (ETS domain, B-region, C-region) are shared by all TCFs, except for the splice variant Sap-1b lacking the complete C-region.

quences that otherwise can not be complexed by TCFs alone. The biochemical identification of such TCF activity at the c-*fos* SRE [15] led to the cDNA cloning of SRF accessory proteins with inherent TCF activity [18] and the realization that the TCF function is expressed by proteins belonging to the·family of Ets proto-oncoproteins [16, 18] (see below).

Ets proteins represent a group of transcription factors which share a region of homology, the ETS domain, encoding a protein domain of approximately 85 amino acids in length capable of specific DNA sequence recognition. Presently about 25 different Ets proteins have been identified and several recent reviews provide a detailed description of Ets protein characteristics [64, 65, 66]. All DNA sequences recognized by Ets proteins contain an almost invariant central $GGA^A/_T$ core sequence flanked by different juxtaposed nucleotides. The composition of the flanking sequences influences the DNA binding specificities of individual Ets proteins. Many Ets proteins have been shown to interact with other DNA-bound proteins at the protein-protein level, as described for example with Ets-1/AP-1, Ets-1/Sp1, Ets-1/PEBP2α [67] and PU.1/NF-EM5 [64].

The TCF subgroup of Ets proteins consists of the members Elk-1 [16, 18, 68], Sap-1a, Sap-1b [18], and Erp/Net/Sap-2 [17, 18, 19]. The TCFs are expressed in a broad range of tissues and cell types although some differential patterns of expression can be observed [69] (our unpublished data). All TCFs have their ETS domain positioned at the very N-terminus (see figure 2). In addition to the ETS domain, the TCFs also display two other regions of homology, namely Region B and Region C. Region B represents the domain enabling direct TCF interaction with SRF [70, 71, 72]. Region C contains a transcriptional activation domain with several serine/threonine phosphorylation sites for MAPK which are essential for kinase-induced stimulation of promoters activated by TCFs [6, 20] (see below).

5. SIGNALLING CASCADES TARGETING TCF/ELK-1

Transcriptional activation by Elk-1 has been shown by transient transfections to be responsive to growth factor-induced signalling [23, 24, 73]. The C-terminal activation domain of Elk-1 undergoes multiple phosphorylations following signal pathway activation [20], several of which are phosphorylated *in vitro* by the kinase ERK2, including serines which are critical for transactivation [23]. Induction of the pathway leading to activation of ERK2 [33, 74, 75] correlates not only with Elk-1 phosphorylation, but also with transcriptional activity of c-*fos* [31, 33, 75]. Thus ERK2 is discussed as being an activator of Elk-1 [76].

ERK2 belongs to the archetypical extracellular signal-regulated kinase (ERK) subgroup of MAPKs. These kinases are activated by dual specificity MAPK kinases

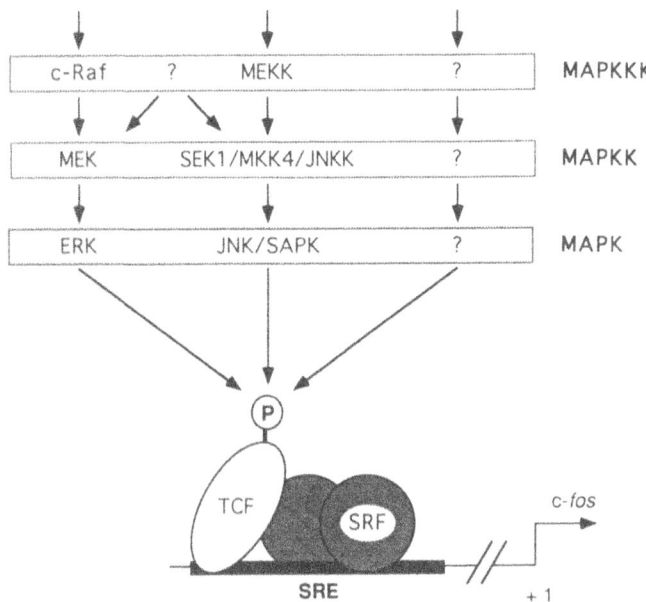

Figure 3. The TCF Elk-1 is a point of convergence for the ERK and JNK/SAPK pathways. Activators of c-Raf or MEKK activate the ERK and JNK/SAPK pathways respectively. Other MAPKKKs may activate these MAPK cascades, and other cascades may be found to target Elk-1.

(MAPKKs) which phosphorylate specific threonine and tyrosine residues in the regulatory motif T-X-Y near the catalytic site of MAPKs, where X represents an amino acid specific for MAPK/MAPKK classes. MAPKKs are in turn activated by MAPKK kinases (MAPKKKs). These kinase cascades have been conserved in evolution from unicellular eukaryotes to vertebrates [2, 52].

There are presently three categories of MAPK pathways characterized in vertebrates. The ERK subgroup consists of p44 ERK1 and p42 ERK2. MEK1 and MEK2 are the MAPKKs for the ERKs, and MEK activation is itself mediated by the Ras-activated MAPKKK Raf-1. The ERK pathway is activated through Ras by a variety of tyrosine kinase receptors and certain serpentine receptor-coupled G-proteins [7, 77].

The c-Jun kinases (JNKs) [78, 79] or stress activated protein kinases (SAPKs) [80] represent the second class of vertebrate MAPKs. This group consists of four genes; SAPKα, SAPKβ, JNK1, and JNK2/SAPKγ, with added complexity arising through differential splicing to give protein products between 45 kDa and 54 kDa. The reason for so many JNK/SAPK isoforms is presently unclear. A MAPKK differently known as SEK1 [81, 82], JNKK [83], or MKK4 [84] can activate JNK/SAPKs, which in turn is activated preferentially by MEKK, a MAPKKK [82, 85].

The third mammalian MAPK pathway involves a homolog of the *S. cerevisiae* protein Hog1p responsive to osmotic stress in yeast. The mammalian enzyme also functions in the osmotic stress response, and thus appears to be a direct functional homolog. It has been called p38, p40, Mpk2, reactivating kinase (RK), or cytokine-suppressive anti-inflammatory drug binding protein (CSBP) [86, 87, 88, 89], and can be activated by a specific MAPKK called MKK3 [84], as well as by SEK1/JNKK/MKK4 [83, 84].

JNK/SAPKs are potently induced by the protein synthesis inhibitor anisomycin in several cell types [80, 90]. The mechanism by which some protein synthesis inhibitors induce signal transduction cascades remains unclear [90, 91]. In mouse 10T1/2 cells anisomycin stimulated JNK/SAPKs but not ERKs, although the c-*fos* gene was strongly induced [90]. The observation that epidermal growth factor (EGF) stimulated not only ERK, but also JNK/SAPKs called into question the assumption that ERKs target Elk-1 *in vivo*, prompting speculation that JNK/SAPKs and not ERKs were responsible for Elk-1 activation and c-*fos* gene induction.

Other examples of differential activation of ERKs and JNK/SAPKs have been reported in several cell types [80, 90, 92, 93]. For instance in KB cells 45 kDa and 54 kDa isoforms of SAPKα were detected in cytoplasmic extracts of cells induced by the inflammatory cytokines interleukin 1 (IL-1) and tumor necrosis factor alpha (TNF-α) [93].

To study c-*fos* induction by protein synthesis inhibitors we examined the situation in HeLa cells [94]. Both cycloheximide and anisomycin induced kinases resembling ERKs and JNK/SAPKs in HeLa cells, in contrast to anisomycin treatment of mouse 10T1/2 cells [90]. Ultraviolet light (UVC) also induced ERKs and JNK/SAPKs, whereas phorbol esters (TPA) induced only ERKs, and EGF induced primarily ERKs with a small but reproducible induction of JNK/SAPKs [94]. Under all of these induction conditions Elk-1 was phosphorylated *in vivo*, and c-*fos* transcription was induced. The activation of all kinases was observed using the Elk-1 transactivation domain as the kinase substrate in in-gel kinase assays, suggesting that JNK/SAPKs might phosphorylate Elk-1 *in vivo*.

To assess whether JNK/SAPKs could activate c-*fos* by phosphorylating Elk-1, we sought conditions where JNK/SAPKs but not ERKs were activated. Anisomycin treatment of KB cells strongly induced Elk-1 phosphorylation, c-*fos* gene activity, and JNK/SAPK activation, with little if any activation of ERKs as measured by in-gel kinase assay. In addition, purified SAPKα catalyzed the similar transfer of ^{32}P to the Elk-1 transactivation domain as to c-Jun. The same purified SAPKα comigrated with a 54 kDa anisomycin-induced JNK/SAPK band in an in-gel kinase assay [94], and SAPKα is known to be strongly induced by anisomycin[80]. Taken together, this data suggests that JNK/SAPKs activate c-*fos* transcription by phosphorylating Elk-1. By contrast, TPA treatment of HeLa or KB cells activated ERKs but not JNK/SAPKs, which also correlated with Elk-1 phosphorylation and c-*fos* induction, indicating that the ERK pathway can also target c-*fos*. Indeed in our hands Elk-1 is much better substrate for ERKs than for JNK/SAPKs [94] (R. Zinck, M. Kracht, M.A.C, A.N.; unpublished). However the above series of results indicates that both pathways target Elk-1 *in vivo*, and therefore that Elk-1 provides a point of convergence for the ERK and JNK/SAPK pathways. This conclusion was als drawn by Whitmarsh et al., who found Elk-1 to be activated by IL-1-stimulated SAPK/JNKs in the absence of ERK activation [95].

It would not be surprising if other mammalian MAPK pathways additionally target Elk-1 or other TCFs. The transcription factor ATF2 provides another such convergence point for signal cascades between the SAPK/JNK and p38/RK/Hog MAPK pathways, and the protein kinase A pathway [92, 96, 97]. Therefore responsiveness to multiple signal pathways may be a feature of many transcription factors. Notably, Elk-1 regulates c-*fos*, while c-Jun and ATF2 bind the c-*jun* promoter as a heterodimer [98], so that the known transcription factor targets of the ERK and JNK/SAPK pathways lead to modulation of the transcription factor AP-1, which consists of heterodimers between Jun- and Fos-family members [99].

6. Mcm1 AND A TCF CONTROL CELL CYCLE-DIRECTED GENE EXPRESSION IN *S. CEREVISIAE*

As mentioned above, the *S. cerevisiae* transcription factor Mcm1, an essential DNA-binding protein of the budding yeast, recruits a variety of different accessory proteins (α1, α2, Ste12) to regulate both cell type-specific and pheromone -directed gene expression [100]. Another type of ternary complex factor, the Sff protein, has been shown to cooperate with Mcm1, and was implied as mediating the cell type-specific activation of the *Swi 5* gene during the G2 phase [58]. Recently, a more general role has been described for Mcm1-TCF complexes in directing G2-specific gene regulation [101, 102]. Using a conditional expression system for Mcm1 in yeast cells we demonstrated that several genes exhibiting a G2/M phase-specific expression pattern are under Mcm1 transcriptional control [102]. These include the genes encoding the mitotic cyclins Clb1 and Clb2, the M-phase specific kinase Cdc5, and the transcription factor Ace2. In this study Mcm1 was shown to be essential for cell cycle progression beyond the G2-M transition, providing a rationale for the lethal phenotype displayed by *mcm1* strains. A gene fusion that provided Mcm1 with a strong and constitutive transcriptional activation domain caused *SWI5*, *CLB1*, *CLB2*, and *CDC5* gene activities at inappropriate times of the cell cycle. However, wild-type Mcm1 alone was unable to direct activation of these genes. Instead, coordinated expression of G2-specific genes by Mcm1 was revealed to depend on an Sff-like ternary complex factor (also called TCF_{CLB2}), as indicated by *in vitro* binding studies as well as genomic footprinting and mutational analysis of the *SWI5* and *CLB2* promoters. Since these genomic footprints demonstrated continued presence of the Mcm1-directed ternary complexes throughout the cell cycle we speculated that ternary complex activity might be regulated by post-translational modification involving the Clb-Cdc28 kinase [102]. This would then identify a positive feed back loop to function in G2 control, i.e. Clb1/2 gene activation would be stimulated by Clb1/2-controlled Cdc28 kinase activity targeting the Mcm1-TCF ternary complex formed in the Clb1/2 gene promoters. Future biochemical characterization and genetic analysis of the postulated Sff-like ternary complex factor promises important new insight into the molecular mechanisms of G2-specific gene control in *S. cerevisiae*.

7. SUMMARY

MADS-domain proteins are transcription factors that are phylogenetically conserved from unicellular to multicellular eukaryotes, including plants and vertebrates [5]. They perform essential functions in directing cell type-specific and cell cycle-dependent gene activities. In doing so they function, in part, as genomic anchors for the recruitment to specific DNA sequences of accessory proteins, the ternary complex factors (TCFs). In mammalian cells the TCFs are encoded by a subgroup of the Ets family of transcription factors. The ternary complexes represent important nuclear gene regulatory structures, whereby the phosphorylation status of the proteins building ternary complexes strongly determines transcriptional activity of their target promoters. The phosphorylation status of these proteins is determined by kinase and phosphatase activities regulated during mitogenic stimulation and growth of cells.

7. ACKNOWLEDGMENT

The authors' work was funded by the Deutsche Forschungsgemeinschaft through grants No120/7–2 and No120/10–1.

8. REFERENCES

1. H.R. Herschman, Primary response genes induced by growth factors and tumor promoters. *Annu. Rev. Biochem.*, 60: 281–319 (1991)
2. C.J. Marshall, MAP kinase kinase kinase, MAP kinase kinase and MAP kinase. *Curr. Opin. Genet. Dev.*, 4: 82–89 (1994)
3. D.O. Morgan, Principles of CDK regulation. *Nature*, 374: 131–134 (1995)
4. Z. Schwarz-Sommer, P. Huijser, W. Nacken, H. Saedler and H. Sommer, Genetic control of flower development by homeotic genes in *Antirrhinum majus*. *Science*, 250: 931–936 (1990)
5. P. Shore and A.D. Sharrocks, The MADS-box family of transcription factors. *Eur. J. Biochem.*, 229: 1–13 (1995)
6. R. Janknecht, M.A. Cahill and A. Nordheim, Signal integration at the c-*fos* promoter. *Carcinogenesis*, 16: 443–450 (1995)
7. M.A. Cahill, R. Janknecht and A. Nordheim, Signal uptake by the c-*fos* serum response element. In: *Inducible Gene Expression* (Baeuerle, P. A., eds) Vol. 2, pp. 39–73, Birkhäuser Press, Boston (1995)
8. M. Sheng and M. Greenberg, The regulation and function of c-*fos* and other immediate early genes in the nervous system. *Neuron*, 4: 477–485 (1990)
9. R. Treisman, The serum response element. *Trends Biochem. Sci.*, 17: 423–426 (1992)
10. C. Norman, M. Runswick, R. Pollock and R. Treisman, Isolation and properties of cDNA clones encoding SRF, a transcription factor that binds to the c-*fos* serum response element. *Cell*, 55: 989–1003 (1988)
11. R. Treisman, Identification of a protein-binding site that mediates transcriptional response of the c-*fos* gene to serum factors. *Cell*, 46: 567–574 (1986)
12. L. Pellegrini, S. Tan and T.J. Richmond, Structure of serum response factor core bound to DNA. *Nature*, 376: 490–498 (1995)
13. R. Janknecht, R.A. Hipskind, T. Houthaeve, A. Nordheim and H.G. Stunnenberg, Identification of multiple SRF N-terminal phosphorylation sites affecting DNA binding properties. *EMBO J.*, 11: 1045–1054 (1992)
14. R.M. Marais, J.J. Hsuan, C. McGuigan, J. Wynne and R. Treisman, Casein kinase II phosphorylation increases the rate of serum response factor-binding site exchange. *EMBO J.*, 11: 97–105 (1992)
15. P.E. Shaw, H. Schröter and A. Nordheim, The ability of a ternary complex to form over the serum response element correlates with serum inducibility of the human c-*fos* promoter. *Cell*, 56: 563–572 (1989)
16. R.A. Hipskind, V.N. Rao, C.G.F. Mueller, E.S.P. Reddy and A. Nordheim, Ets-related protein Elk-1 is homologous to the c-*fos* regulatory factor p62[TCF]. *Nature*, 354: 531–534 (1991)
17. M. Lopez, P. Oettgen, Y. Akbarali, U. Dendorfer and T.A. Liberman, Erp, a new mwmber of the *ets* transcription factor/oncoprotein family: cloning, characterization, and differential expression during B-lymphocyte development. *Mol. Cell. Biol.*, 14: 3292–3309 (1994)
18. S. Dalton and R. Treisman, Characterization of SAP-1, a protein recruited by serum response factor to the c-*fos* serum response element. *Cell*, 68: 597–612 (1992)
19. A. Giovane, A. Pintzas, S.-M. Maria, P. Sobieszczuk and B. Wasylyk, Net, a new *ets* transcription factor that is activated by Ras. *Genes Dev.*, 8: 1502–1513 (1994)
20. R. Treisman, Ternary complex factors: growth factor regulated transcriptional activators. *Curr. Opin. Genet. Dev.*, 4: 96–101 (1994)
21. H. König, Cell-type specific multiprotein complex formation over the c-*fos* serum response element *in vivo*: ternary complex formation is not required for the induction of c-*fos*. *Nucl. Acids Res.*, 19: 3607–3611 (1991)
22. R.E. Herrera, P.E. Shaw and A. Nordheim, Occupation of the c-*fos* serum response element *in vivo* by a multi-protein complex is unaltered by growth factor induction. *Nature*, 340: 68–70 (1989)
23. R. Marais, J. Wynne and R. Treisman, The SRF accessory protein Elk-1 contains a growth factor-regulated transcriptional activation domain. *Cell*, 73: 381–393 (1993)
24. R. Janknecht, W.H. Ernst, V. Pingoud and A. Nordheim, Activation of ternary complex factor Elk-1 by MAP kinases. *EMBO J.*, 12: 5097–5104 (1993)
25. R. Graham and M. Gilman, Distinct protein targets for signals acting at the c-*fos* serum response element. *Science*, 251: 189–192 (1991)
26. F.-E. Johansen and R. Prywes, Two pathways for serum regulation of the c-*fos* serum response element require specific sequence elements and a minimal domain of serum response factor. *Mol. Cell. Biol.*, 14: 5920–5928 (1994)
27. C.S. Hill, J. Wynne and R. Treisman, The Rho family GTPases RhoA, Rac1, and CDC42Hs regulate transcriptional activation by SRF. *Cell*, 81: 1159–1170 (1995)

28. C.S. Hill, J. Wynne and R. Treisman, Serum-regulated transcription by Serum Response Factor (SRF): a novel role for the DNA binding domain. *EMBO J,* 13: 5421–5432 (1994)

29. C.S. Hill, R. Marais, S. John, J. Wynne, S. Dalton and R. Treisman, Functional analysis of a growth factor-responsive transcription factor complex. *Cell,* 73: 395–406 (1993)

30. H.G. Gille, A.D. Sharrocks and P.E. Shaw, Phosphorylation of transcription factor p62^{TCF} by MAP kinase stimulates ternary complex formation at the c-*fos* promotor. *Nature,* 358: 414–417 (1992)

31. R. Zinck, R.A. Hipskind, V. Pingoud and A. Nordheim, c-*fos* transcriptional activation and repression correlate temporally with the phosphorylation status of TCF. *EMBO J.,* 12: 2377–2387 (1993)

32. V.M. Rivera, C.K. Miranti, R.P. Misra, D.D. Ginty, R.-H. Chen, J. Blenis and M.E. Greenberg, A growth factor-induced kinase phosphorylates the serum response factor at a site that regulates its DNA-binding activity. *Mol. Cell. Biol.,* 13: 6260–6273 (1993)

33. R.A. Hipskind, M. Baccarini and A. Nordheim, Transient activation of RAF-1, MEK, and ERK2 coincides kinetically with ternary complex factor phoshorylation and immediate-early gene promoter activity in vivo. *Mol. Cell. Biol.,* 14: 6219–6231 (1994)

34. J. Arias, A.S. Alberts, P. Brindle, F.X. Claret, T. Smeal, M. Karin, J. Feramisco and M. Montminy, Activation of cAMP and mitogen responsive genes relies on a common nuclear factor. *Nature,* 370: 226–229 (1994)

35. M. Rim, S.A. Qureshi, D. Gius, J. Nho, V.P. Sukhatme and D.A. Foster, Evidence that activation of the Egr-1 promoter by v-Raf involves serum response elements. *Oncogene,* 7: 2065–2068 (1992)

36. B.V. Latinkic and L.F. Lau, Transcriptional activation of the immediate early gene *pip*92 by serum growth factors requires both Ets and CArG-like elements. *J. Biol. Chem.,* 269: 23163–23170 (1994)

37. T. Hayes, P. Sengupta and B. Cochrane, The human c-*fos* serum response factor and the yeast factors GRM/PRTF have related DNA-binding specificities. *Genes Dev.,* 2: 1713–1722 (1988)

38. E. Jarvis, K. Clark and G. Sprague, The yeast transcription activator PRTF, a homolog of the mammalian serum response factor, is encoded by the *MCM1* gene. *Genes Dev.,* 3: 936–945 (1989)

39. S. Passmore, R. Elble and B. Tye, A protein involved in minichromosome maintenance in yeast binds a transcriptional enhancer conserved in eukaryotes. *Genes Dev.,* 3: 921–935 (1989)

40. H. Sommer, J. Beltrán, P. Huijser, H. Pape, W. Lönnig, H. Saedler and Z. Schwarz-Sommer, *Deficiens,* a homeotic gene involved in the control of flower morphogenesis in *Antirrhinum majus*: the protein shows homolgy to transcription factors. *EMBO J.,* 9: 605–613 (1990)

41. M. Yanofsky, H. Ma, J. Bowman, N. Drews, K. Feldman and E. Meyerowitz, The protein encoded by the *Arabidopsis* homeotic gene *agamous* resembles transcription factors. *Nature.* 346: 35–39 (1990)

42. H. Ma, M.F. Yanofsky and E.M. Meyerowitz, AGL1-AGL6, an *Arabidopsis* gene family with similarity to floral homeotic and transcription factor genes. *Genes Dev.,* 5: 484–495 (1991)

43. M. Affolter, J. Montagne, U. Walldorf, J. Groppe, U. Kloter and M. LaRosa, The *Drosophila* SRF homolog is expressed in a subset of tracheal cells and maps within a genomic region required for tracheal development. *Development,* 120: 743–753 (1994)

44. L. Boxer, R. Prywes, R. Roeder and L. Kedes, The sarcomeric actin CArG binding factor is indistuinguishable from the c-*fos* serum response factor. *Mol. Cell. Biol.,* 9: 515–522 (1989)

45. K.T. Fujiwara, K. Ashida, H. Nishina, H. Iba, H. Miyajima, M. Nishizawa and S. Kawai, The chicken c-*fos* gene: cloning and nucleotide sequence analysis. *J. Virol.,* 61: 4012–4018 (1987)

46. Z. Liu, B. Moav, A. Faras, K. Guise, A. Kapuscinski and P. Hackett, Functional analysis of elements affecting expression of the β-actin gene of Carp. *Mol. Cell. Biol.,* 10: 3432–3440 (1990)

47. M. Taylor, R. Treisman, N. Garret and T. Mohun, Muscle-specific (CArG) and serum responsive (SRE) promoter elements are functionally interchangeable in *Xenopus* embryos and mouse fibroblasts. *Development,* 106: 67–78 (1989)

48. T.J. Mohun Chambers, A.E., Towers, N., Taylor, M.V., Expression of genes encoding the transcription factor SRF during development of Xenopus laevis: identification of a CArG box-binding activity as SRF. *EMBO J.,* 10: 933–940 (1991)

49. R. Pollock and R. Treisman, Human SRF-related proteins: DNA-binding properties and potential regulatory targets. *Genes Dev.,* 5: 2327–2341 (1991)

50. A.E. Chambers, S. Kotecha, N. Towers and T. Mohun, Muscle-specific expression of SRF-related genes in the early embryo of *Xenopus laevus. EMBO J.,* 11: 4981–4991 (1992)

51. Y.-Y. Yu, R.E. Breitbart, L.B. Smoot, Y. Lee, V. Mahdavi and B. Nadal-Ginard, Human myocyte-specific enhancer factor 2 comprises a group of tissue-restricted MADS box transcription factors. *Genes Dev.,* 6: 1783–1798 (1992)

52. G. Ammerer, Sex, stress and integrity: the importance of MAP kinases in yeast. *Curr. Opin. Genet. Dev.,* 4: 90–95 (1994)

53. M. de Rijka, S. Seneca, B. Punyammalee, N. Glansdorff and M. Crabeel, Characterization of the DNA target site for the yeast ARGR regulatory complex, a sequence able to mediate repression or induction by arginine. *Mol. Cell. Biol.*, 12: 68–81 (1992)

54. S.I. Reed, Pheromone signaling pathways in yeast. *Curr. Opin. Gen. Dev.*, 1: 391–396 (1991)

55. J.W. Dolan and S. Fields, Cell-type-specific transcription in yeast. *Biochim. Biophys. Acta*, 1088: 155–169 (1991)

56. P.E. Shaw, Ternary complex formation over the c-*fos* serum response element: p62^{TCF} exhibits dual component specificity with contacts to DNA and an extended structure in the DNA-binding domain of p67^{SRF}. *EMBO J.*, 11: 3011–3019 (1992)

57. C.G.F. Mueller Nordheim, A., A protein domain conserved between yeast MCM1 and human SRF directs ternary complex formation. *EMBO J.*, 10: 4219–4229 (1991)

58. D. Lydall, G. Ammerer and K. Nasmyth, A new role for MCM1 in yeast: cell cycle regulation of *SW15* transcription. *Genes Dev.*, 5: 2405–2419 (1991)

59. R. Pollock and R. Treisman, A sensitive method for the determination of protein-DNA binding specificities. *Nucl. Acids Res.*, 18: 6197–6204 (1990)

60. J. Wynne and R. Treisman, SRF and MCM1 have related but distinct DNA binding specificities. *Nucl. Acids Res.*, 20: 3297–3303 (1992)

61. A.D. Sharrocks, F. von Hesler and P.E. Shaw, The identification of elements determining the different DNA binding specificities of the MADS box proteins p67^{SRF} and RSRFC4. *Nucl. Acids Res.*, 21: 215–221 (1993)

62. C. Gauthier-Rouvière, J.-C. Cavadore, J.-M. Blanchard, N.J.C. Lamb and A. Fernandez, p67^{SRF} is a constitutive nuclear protein implicated in the modulation of genes required throughout the G1 period. *Cell Regulation*, 2: 575–588 (1991)

63. S.-H. Liu, H.-H. Lee, J.-J. Chen, C.-F. Chuang and S.-Y. Ng, Serum response element-regulated transcription in the cell cycle: possible correlation with microtubule reorganization. *Cell Growth and Differentiation*, 5: 447–455 (1994)

64. R. Janknecht and A. Nordheim, Gene regulation by Ets proteins. *Biochim. Biophys. Acta*, 1155: 346–356 (1993)

65. K. Macleod Leprince, D., Stehelin, D., The *ets* gene family. *Trends Biochem. Sci.*, 17: 251–256 (1992)

66. B. Wasylyk, S.L. Hahn and A. Giovane, The Ets family of transcription factors. *Eur. J. Biochem.*, 211: 7–18 (1993)

67. K. Giese, C. Kingsley, J.R. Kirschner and R. Grosschedl, Assembly and function of a TCRα enhancer complex is dependent on LEF-1-induced DNA bending and multiple protein-protein interactions. *Genes and Dev.*, 9: 995–1008 (1995)

68. V.N. Rao, K. Hueber, M. Isobe, A. Ar-Rushdi, C.M. Croce and E.S.P. Reddy, *elk*, tissue specific *ets*-related genes on chromosomes X and 14 near translocation breakpoints. *Science*, 244: 60–79 (1989)

69. M.A. Price, A.E. Rogers and R. Treisman, Comparative analysis of the ternary complex factors Elk-1, SAP-1a and SAP-2 (ERP/NET). *EMBO J*, 14: 2589–2601 (1995)

70. R. Janknecht and A. Nordheim, Elk-1 protein domains required for direct and SRF-assisted DNA-binding. *Nucl. Acids Res.*, 20: 3317–3324 (1992)

71. P. Shore and A.D. Sharrocks, The transcription factors Elk-1 and serum response factor interact by direct protein-protein contacts mediated by a short region of Elk-1. *Mol. Cell. Biol.*, 14: 3283–3291 (1994)

72. R. Treisman, R. Marais and J. Wynne, Spatial flexibility in ternary complexes between SRF and its accessory proteins. *EMBO J.*, 11: 4631–4640 (1992)

73. M. Kortenjann, O. Thomae and P.E. Shaw, Inhibition of v-raf-dependent c-fos expression and transformation by a kinase-defective mutant of the mitogen-activated protein kinase Erk2. *Mol. Cell. Biol*, 14: 4815–4824 (1994)

74. R.A. Hipskind, D. Büscher, A. Nordheim and M. Baccarini, Ras/MAP kinase-dependent and -independent signaling pathways target distinct ternary complex factors. *Genes Dev.*, 8: 1803–1816 (1994)

75. C. Sachsenmaier, A. Radler-Pohl, R. Zinck, A. Nordheim, P. Herrlich and H.J. Rahmsdorf, Involvement of growth factor receptors in the mammalian UVC response. *Cell*, 78: 963–972 (1994)

76. M. Karin, Signal transduction from the cell surface to the nucleus through the phosphorylation of transcription factors. *Curr. Opinion Cell Biol.*, 6: 415–424 (1994)

77. P. Crespo Xu, N., Simonds, W.F., Gutkind, J.S., Ras-dependent activation of MAP kinase pathway mediated by G-protein βγ subunits. *Nature*, 369: 418–420 (1994)

78. T. Kallunki, B. Su, I. Tsigelney, H.K. Sluss, B. Dérijard, G. Moore, R. Davis and M. Karin, JNK2 contains a specificity-determining region responsible for efficient c-Jun binding and phosphorylation. *Genes and Dev.*, 8: 2996–3007 (1994)

79. B. Dérijard, M. Hibi, I.-H. Wu, T. Barret, B. Su, T. Deng, M. Karin and R.J. Davis, JNK1: A Protein kinase stimulated by UV light and Ha-Ras that binds and phosphorylates the c-Jun activation domain. *Cell,* 76: 1025–1037 (1994)

80. J.M. Kyriakis, P. Banerjee, E. Nikolakaki, T. Dal, E.A. Ruble, M.F. Ahmad, J. Avruch and J.R. Woodgett, The stress-activated protein kinase subfamily of c-Jun kinases. *Nature,* 369: 156–160 (1994),

81. I. Sánchez, R.T. Hughes, B.J. Mayer, K. Yee, J.R. Woodget, J. Avruch, J.M. Kyriakis and L.I. Zon, Role of SAPK/ERK kinase-1 in the stress-activated pathway regulating transcription factor c-Jun. *Nature,* 372: 794–798 (1994)

82. M. Yan, T. Dal, J.C. Deak, J.M. Kyriakis, L.I. Zon, J.R. Woodgett and D.J. Templeton, Activation of stress-activated protein kinase by MEKK1 phosphorylation of its activator SEK1. *Nature,* 372: 798–800 (1994)

83. A. Lin, A. Minden, H. Martinetto, F.X. Claret, C. Lange-Carter, F. Mercurio, G.L. Johnson and M. Karin, Identification of a dual specificity kinase that activates the Jun kinases and p38-Mpk2. *Science,* 268: 286–290 (1995)

84. B. Dérijard, J. Raingeaud, T. Barret, I.H. Wu, J. Han, R.J. Ulevitch and R.J. Davis, Independent human MAP-kinase signal transduction pathways defined by MEK and MKK isoforms. *Science,* 267: 682–685 (1995)

85. A. Minden, A. Lin, M. McMahon, C. Lange-Carter, B. Dérijard, R.J. Davis, G.L. Johnson and M. Karin, Differential activation of ERK and JNK mitogen-activated protein kinases by Raf-1 and MEKK. *Science,* 266: 1719–1723 (1994)

86. N.W. Freshney, L. Rawlinson, F. Guesdon, E. Jones, S. Cowley, J. Hsuan and J. Saklatvala, Interleukin-1 activates a novel protein kinase cascade that results in phosphorylation of Hsp27. *Cell,* 78: 1039–1049 (1994)

87. J. Han, J.D. Lee, L. Bibbs and R.J. Ulevitch, A MAP kinase targeted by endotoxin and hyperosmolarity in mammalian cells. *Science,* 265: 808–811 (1994)

88. J.C. Lee, J.D. Laydon, P.C. McDonnell, T.F. Gallagher, S. Kumar, D. Green, D. McNulty, M.J. Blumenthal, J.R. Heys and S.W. Landvatter, A protein kinase involved in the regulation of inflammatory cytokine biosynthesis. *Nature,* 372: 739–746 (1994)

89. J. Rouse, P. Cohen, S. Trigon, M. Morange, A. Alonso-Llamazares, D. Zamanillo, T. Hunt and A.R. Nebreda, A novel kinase cascade triggered by stress and heat shock that stimulates MAPKAP kinase-2 and phosphorylation of HSP27. *Cell,* 78: 1027–1037 (1994)

90. E. Cano, C.A. Hazzalin and L.C. Mahadevan, Anisomycin-activated protein kinases p45 and p55 but not mitogen-activated protein kinases ERK-1 and -2 are implicated in the induction of c-*fos* and c-*jun. Mol. Cell. Biol.,* 14: 7352–7362 (1994)

91. L.C. Mahadevan and D.R. Edwards, Signalling and superinduction. *Nature,* 349: 747–748 (1991)

92. H. van Dam, D. Wilhelm, I. Herr, A. Steffen, P. Herrlich and P. Angel, ATF-2 is preferentially activated by stress-activated protein kinases to mediate c-*jun* induction in response to genotoxic agents. *EMBO J,* 14: 1798–1811 (1995)

93. M. Kracht, O. Truong, N.F. Totty, M. Shiroo and J. Saklatvala, Interleukin 1α activates two forms of p54α mitogen-activated protein kinase in rabbit liver. *J. Exp. Med.,* 180: 2017–2025 (1994)

94. R. Zinck, M.A. Cahill, M. Kracht, C. Sachsenmaier, R. Hipskind and A. Nordheim, Protein synthesis inhibitors reveal differential regulation of mitogen-activated protein kinase and stress-activated protein kinase pathways that converge on Elk-1. *Mol. Cell. Biol.,* 15: 4930–4938 (1995)

95. A.J. Whitmarsh, P. Shore, A.D. Sharrocks and R.J. Davis, Integration of MAP kinase signal transduction pathways at the serum response element. *Science,* 269: 403–407 (1995)

96. J. Raingeaud, S. Gupta, J.S. Rogers, M. Dickens, J. Han, R.J. Ulevitch and R.J. Davis, Pro-inflammatory cytokines and environmental stress cause p38 mitogen-activated protein kinase activation by dual phosphorylation on tyrosine and threonine. *J. Biol. Chem.,* 270: 7420–7426 (1995)

97. S. Gupta, D. Campbell, B. Dérijard and R.J. Davis, Transcription factor ATF2 regulation by the JNK signal transduction pathway. *Science,* 267: 389–393 (1995)

98. H. van Dam, M. Duyndam, R. Rottier, A. Bosch, L. de Vries-Smits, P. Herrlich, A. Zantema, P. Angel and A.J. van der Eb, Heterodimer formation of cJun and ATF-2 is responsible for induction of c-*jun* by the 243 amino acid E1A protein. *EMBO J.,* 12: 479–487 (1993)

99. P. Angel and M. Karin, The role of Jun, Fos, and the AP-1 complex in cell-proliferation and transformation. *Biochim. Biophys. Acta.,* 1072: 129–157 (1991)

100. R. Treisman and G. Ammerer, The SRF and MCM1 transcription factors. *Curr. Opin. Genet. Dev.,* 2: 221–226 (1992)

101. M. Maher, F. Cong, D. Kindelberger, K. Nasmyth and S. Dalton, Cell cycle-regulated transcription of the *CLB2* gene is dependent on Mcm1 and a ternary complex factor. *Mol. Cell. Biol.,* 15: 3129–3137 (1995)

102. H. Althöfer, A. Schleiffer, K. Wassmann, A. Nordheim and G. Ammerer, Essential function of MCM1 in G2 specific transcription in yeast. *Mol. Cell. Biol., in press.*, (1995)

DISCUSSION

M. Oren: Two questions: How similar are the DNA binding specificities of SRF and MCM-1? In other words, is there any chance that SRF can rescue an MCM-1 defect in the yeast? The other question is a more technical one: I thought that in one of your in-gel kinase assays you had a strong activation by anisomycin but not by cycloheximide - could you comment on that?

A. Nordheim: With regard to the DNA-binding specificities of SRF and MCM-1, I would like to point out that the two proteins bind similar sequences but not identical ones. In other words, many of the MCM-1 binding sites cannot be bound efficiently by SRF at all and vice versa, thus MCM1 and SRF have significantly different sequence recognition. This can be of practical importance in fact, i.e., SRF can be expressed in yeast cells and utilize cotransfected SRF binding sites without strongly interfering with endogenous promoters in the yeast chromosome that are normally under MCM-1 control.

With regard to the second question concerning in-gel kinase assays, I should qualify what these kinase assays are able to do and what they cannot be used for on the other hand. I think they are extremely powerful in revealing within a given cell extract the different types of kinase found in the active state. However, one also has to be aware of the drawbacks of this assay. For example, kinase unable to renature after gel separation cannot be identified. Also, if the kinase has subunits required for enzymatic activity, those would be separated in the gel and the enzymatic activity could not be revealed. Furthermore, if the wrong substrate is offered inside the gel a kinase of interest might not be detected. As long as one is aware of all these caveats and drawbacks in-gel kinase assays provide a very powerful way of detecting specific kinases present in active form in a given cell extract. So much for the technique itself and with regard to your specific question concerning kinase activation by anisomycin versus cycloheximide it is indeed the case that signaling seems to be activated more efficiently by anisomycin than by cycloheximide. For example, at concentrations at which protein biosynthesis is only inhibited to approximately 50% only very inefficient kinase activation is seen by cycloheximide whereas strong signaling is seen with anisomycin. At present, we do not know by which mechanism these agents initiate activation of signaling cascades, but future work will have to clarify this.

M. Oren: There is a possibility though, that perhaps what anisomycin is doing to activate the kinase is not through the block of protein synthesis but through some peculiar effect of anisomycin which has nothing to do with protein synthesis inhibition.

A. Nordheim: That is exactly my point. When investigators have previously employed the inhibitors of protein biosynthesis anisomycin and cycloheximide they very likely also activated intracellular signaling. Therefore, previous conclusions have to be treated with reservation since the signaling component excited by these substances was obviously not taken into consideration.

F. Rauscher: The ETS domain proteins the TCF factors bind when they are recruited to the complex, do they require their DNA binding domain? Or can they be recruited just by protein-protein interactions with SRF?

A. Nordheim: Yes. We, in our experiments, have never seen strong protein-protein interactions in the absence of DNA. Andy Sharrock's laboratory has reported conditions where he could see two proteins interact free in solution without DNA, but in our experiments we can certainly say that this is a very weak interaction, and for us, only measurable in the presence of DNA.

F. Rauscher: Is anything known of the phosphatases that down regulate the signal?

A. Nordheim: Yes, I did not comment on that, but the de-phosphorylation of TCF quite nicely correlates with down regulation of the c-fos promoter so we would then speculate that the event of de-phosphorylation is, sort of instrumentally, involved in down regulation. The phosphatases involved in-vivo are not identified, however, we could show that ocadaic acid in concentrations where it efficiently inactivates protein phosphatase 2A would prevent the de-phosphorylation of TCF and at the same time would cause the constitutively prolonged activity of the c-fos promoter.

M. Green: I am intrigued by the observations with the protein synthesis inhibitors. Do I understand you correctly, that you can get both increases and decreases of particular kinase with only one kind of inhibitor?

A. Nordheim: No, both types of protein synthesis inhibitors used lead to the activation of both MAPKs and SAPKs. However, the subsequent downregulation of these kinases is of interest. Whereas rapid deactivation of the MAPKs is seen even under conditions of full protein synthesis inhibition, the SAPKs are not downregulated when concentrations of protein synthesis inhibitors were used that were fully inhibitory to protein synthesis. This would suggest that phosphatases involved in MAPK downregulation are present, whereas phosphatase activity involved in downregulation of the SAPKs requires *de novo* protein synthesis.

M. Green: But at lower concentrations whether the inhibitors are activated; are the kinases activated?

A. Nordheim: They are activated.

M. Green: Were the cells first treated and then extracts prepared?

A. Nordheim: Of course.

M. Green: If you just took an extract first, or a purified kinase and added the inhibitors, would they have an effect? Because, I think you are suggesting that the effects you are seeing, at least part of them, are uncoupled from the ability of the drugs to inhibit protein synthesis.

A. Nordheim: That is what I am suggesting, however, we have not tried to reproduce the activation of kinases by anisomycin treatment of extracts.

M. Fried: Is there any cell specificity which TCF is used, as there are 4 or 5 different ones?

A. Nordheim: Yes. Richard Treisman just published a paper, where he basically argues that the 3 TCF's he looked at are fairly ubiquitously expressed, at least in all the cells he looked at, they were all three present. Which would then raise the question; what do they do? Why are there several of them? Do they perform different functions? Certainly they are not expressed identically in all different tissues, we have indication that, in the brain elk is much stronger than the other TCF's. This would now have to be investigated in much greater detail.

D. Housman: I wonder if I could return to the dephosphorylation: you mentioned that there is, in fact, a refractory period and I wonder how long the refractory period actually lasts? And how do you interpret the refractory period in terms of the dephosphorylation?

A. Nordheim: Well the refractory period could possibly be explained by the upstream kinase cascade i.e., by each individual step in the signaling pathway. The different pathways that form these individual steps might show this refractoriness in re-stimulation. Maybe once they are inactivated, supposedly by dephosphorylation, they cannot be reactivated again very rapidly. And different kinases may behave differently in that regard. We have not looked into that in great detail.

T. Graf: Does the activation of ternary complex factor by MAP kinase on the one hand and Jun kinase on the other, occur via the same phosphorylation targets?

A. Nordheim: To my knowledge, the accurate sites on TCF that are phosphorated by Jun kinase have not been mapped. Just phosphopeptide maps indicate that Map kinase phosphorylation and Sap kinase phosphorylation does not differ very dramatically. There might be subtle differences, but so far, we do not know whether there might be one individual site that is hit differently by the two types of kinase. If that were so, we would have missed it so far. We really have to map each individual position, mutate it, and then analyze the behavior of the mutant.

10

RETINOBLASTOMA PROTEIN, GENE EXPRESSION, AND CELL CYCLE CONTROL

Jane Clifford Azizkhan,[*] Shiaw Yih Lin, David Jensen,[†] Dusan Kostic, and Adrian R. Black

Department of Experimental Therapeutics
Grace Cancer Drug Center
Roswell Park Cancer Institute
Elm and Carlton Streets, Buffalo, New York 14263

INTRODUCTION

Regulation of cell proliferation is achieved by the tight control of the progression through the cell cycle which controls the transition of cells between quiescent and growing states. This regulation relies on the coordinated balance between inhibitory and stimulatory signals. The stimulatory factors (e.g., growth factors) and their receptors are often encoded by a class of genes called proto-oncogenes. Cells also contain several inhibitory proteins, encoded by tumor suppressor genes which act as either censors or pacers (Marx, 1994).

We have been studying the relationship between cell cycle control in the G_1/S phase and expression of cell growth promoting genes. A large subset of polymerase II promoters lacks the classical TATA box; these include several oncogenes, and several genes encoding growth factors, growth factor receptors, transcription factors, cyclins, and the housekeeping genes, so called because they encode proteins required for cellular metabolism (Azizkhan et al., 1993, for review). As a model of cell cycle regulated, TATA-less genes, we have been utilizing the hamster dihydrofolate reductase (DHFR) gene, the product of which reduces folates in the biosynthetic pathway for purines, thymidine and glycine (Hakala and Taylor, 1959). DHFR and many other TATA-less gene promoters are expressed at low or non-detectable levels in non-growing cells; however, when cells are induced to proliferate, e.g. by growth factor stimulation, transformation, or viral infection, transcription of these genes is stimulated (Pardee, 1989).

In the hamster DHFR promoter, the region from nucleotide position -210 to -23 has maximal constitutive activity and responds maximally to stimuli such as viral infection or

* Corresponding author.
† Present Address: Wistar Institute, 36th and Spruce Streets, Philadelphia, PA 19104.

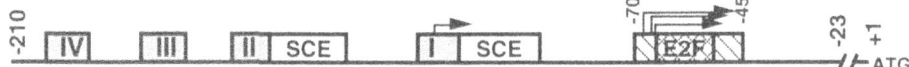

Figure 1. Diagrammatic representation of the hamster DHFR gene promoter. There are two overlapping binding sites for the transcription factor E2F (double cross-hatched box) within a larger conserved element designated the major initiation region (cross-hatched box), four binding sites for the transcription factor Sp1, called GC boxes (stippled boxes), and an element that flanks GC boxes I and II which we have designated the structural control element (SCE, open boxes). Transcription start sites are indicated by the arrows. All numbering is relative to +1 being the start of translation.

a growth signal (Swick et al., 1989). Within the -210 to -23 region of the hamster DHFR promoter (Fig. 1), there are four binding sites for the transcription factor Sp1 and two overlapping binding sites for E2F. These sites are highly conserved among the hamster, mouse and human DHFR promoters and are also found in promoters of several other promoters of TATA-less genes.

Transcription Factor Sp1

Transcription of DHFR cannot occur without Sp1 and more than one Sp1 binding site is required for efficient DHFR transcription *in vitro* and *in vivo* (Swick et al., 1989) . Sp1 binding is also involved in determining the relative usage of the two transcription start sites (Blake et al., 1990). A role for Sp1 in initiation of transcription in TATA-less promoters has also been demonstrated for Ha-ras (Lu et al., 1994), adenosine deaminase (Dusing and Wiginton, 1994), thymidylate synthetase (Jolliff et al., 1991) and in the human muscle phosphofructokinase P1 promoter (Johnson and McLachlan, 1994)

Sp1 was originally isolated from HeLa cell extracts as the transcription factor that binds to the GC rich sequences (GC boxes) of the SV40 early promoter (Dynan and Tjian, 1983). Binding of Sp1 to GC boxes is mediated by the three zinc fingers in the C terminal domain of the protein (Kadonaga et al., 1987). Transcriptional activation is mediated by a glutamine-rich transcription activation domain which has been proposed to interact with the general transcription machinery through the TATA-binding protein associated factor, TAF110 (Gill et al., 1994). Most of the mammalian TATA-less promoters reported in the literature appear to have multiple GC boxes which bind the transcription factor Sp1 and are essential for transcription.

Transcription Factor E2F

The conserved sequence element overlying the major initiation site of the DHFR promoters, TTTCGCGCCAAA, contains two partially overlapping binding sites for the transcription factor E2F, and is 100% conserved among mouse, human and hamster genes. Although the E2F sites in other E2F-containing genes are not located 3' to the mRNA cap site as in the DHFR gene, the dyad structure of the DHFR E2F site occurs frequently, e.g. in the cellular N-*myc*, c-*myc*, and E2F1 promoters and in eight different serotypes of the adenovirus E1A gene. A mutation that abolishes both E2F binding sites in the DHFR promoter reduces transcription 5- to 10-fold in log phase cells (Blake and Azizkhan, 1989). Mutation of either "half site", while preserving the ability to bind E2F, significantly increases the dissociation rate of E2F, and is functionally equivalent to abolishing both sites

(Wade et al., 1995). Many *TATA-less* promoters that regulate production of proteins essential for DNA synthesis, e.g., DHFR, DNA polymerase α, thymidylate synthase and thymidine kinase, contain E2F sites (Azizkhan et al., 1993). There are also E2F sites in the promoters of many genes implicated in cell cycle control, e.g., cyclins A and D1 (Henglein et al., 1994; Motokura and Arnold, 1993), p34cdc2 (Yamamoto et al., 1994), E2F1 (Li et al., 1994; Neuman et al., 1994), RB (Gill et al., 1994; Zacksenhaus et al., 1993), and PCNA (Lee et al., 1995).

E2F was first characterized as a human factor activated by the adenovirus immediate early protein, E1A, that binds to and transcriptionally activates the adenovirus E2 promoter (Kovesdi et al., 1986). E2F association with and dissociation from other cellular factors correlates with changes in its activity. The first E2F clone (E2F1) was isolated based on its ability to bind the product of the retinoblastoma tumor suppressor gene, pRb, and is characterized as a basic helix-loop-helix DNA binding protein with a leucine zipper dimerization region and an acidic transcription activation domain (Helin et al., 1992; Kaelin et al., 1992). E2F binds to DNA as a heterodimer with one of the three cloned members of the DP transcription factor family (Bandara et al., 1993). Four additional E2F clones have now been isolated, all of which recognize the same DNA binding motif but interact differently with other regulatory proteins (Beijersbergen et al., 1994; Ivey-Hoyle et al., 1993; Lees et al., 1993). For example, E2F-1, 2 and 3 interact with pRb, whereas E2F4 interacts with a related protein, p107 (Beijersbergen et al., 1994). The activity of E2F is regulated by association with and dissociation from other cell cycle regulated proteins. The hypophosphorylated form of pRb which is present during early G_1 can bind and mask the E2F activation domain and, in turn, suppress the expression of many cell growth promoting genes (Hiebert, 1993; Hiebert et al., 1992; Weintraub and Dean, 1992). Once the cells commit to enter S phase, pRb becomes hyperphosphorylated and releases E2F from the complex. The free E2F then activates the cell growth promoting genes and the cells can proceed into S phase. The hypophosphorylated form of pRb is also the form that is active in tumor suppression (Nevins, 1992). In mid to late G_1, E2F is associated with cyclin E and its associated kinase p33^{cdk2}, and upon entry into S phase, E2F associates with cyclin A/p33^{cdk2} (Mudryj et al., 1991). It has been proposed that one role for E2F is to localize the cyclin E/A related kinase p33^{cdk2} (Hunter and Pines, 1991). The role of E2F in growth control is emphasized by its oncogenic capacity and its ability to promote apoptosis (Johnson et al., 1994; Qin et al., 1994; Shan and Lee, 1994; Singh et al., 1994; Xu et al., 1995).

Retinoblastoma Protein

The protein product of the tumor suppressor retinoblastoma (RB) gene, is a nuclear phosphoprotein, pRb. pRb can activate Sp1-dependent expression of several promoters containing Sp1 binding sites, including DHFR (Kim et al., 1992; Udvadia et al., 1993). Although pRb activates Sp1-dependent transcription in several systems, association between Sp1 and pRb in cells has not been reported, although a weak and/or transient or indirect interaction may be difficult to detect. pRb may enhance the DNA binding activity of Sp1 by removing an inhibitor, or it may enhance transcriptional activation by Sp1 through removing an inhibitor bound to the trans-activation domain; two different putative inhibitors have been reported (Chen et al., 1994; Murata et al., 1994) . The C-terminal region of pRb, which is called the pocket domain because it mediates the interaction of pRb with other proteins, has limited homology to the general transcription factors, TATA-binding protein (TBP) and TFIIB (Gibson et al., 1994; Hagemeier et al., 1993). The homology between pRb and the general transcription factors raises the possibility that pRb may interact with the general transcription machinery, which in turn, could facilitate Sp1-dependent transcription by enhancing the interaction between Sp1 and the general machinery. Collectively, these data indicate that pRB is able to inhibit or stimulate transcription dependent on the transcription factor binding sites in the promoter.

The product of the wild type RB gene suppresses the growth and tumorgenicity of widely disparate types of RB-defective human tumor cell lines (Hiebert et al., 1992; Huang et al., 1992; Shan et al., 1994). pRb, is a nuclear phosphoprotein with an apparent molecular weight on SDS-PAGE between 105 kDa and 110 kDa, depending on its phosphorylation state (Lee et al., 1987). In cycling cells, the phosphorylation pattern of pRb oscillates through the cell cycle; the hypophosphorylated form is present from M phase to mid-late G_1 phase, and the hyperphosphorylated form is present from the G_1 check point to late M phase (Buchkovich et al., 1989; Chen et al., 1989). Viral oncoproteins (Ludlow et al., 1989) and the cellular transcription factor E2F (Chellappan et al., 1991) both interact exclusively with the hypophosphorylated form of pRb, indicating that this form mediates its repressive role. The interaction of these proteins is with the pRb pocket which is also the region most frequently mutated in transformed cells.

E2F and Sp1

In addition to several housekeeping genes [e.g., DHFR (Azizkhan et al., 1986); DNA polymerase α (Pearson et al., 1991); thymidine kinase (Ogris et al., 1993), thymidylate synthase (Liao et al., 1994), spermine/spermidine N1 acetyl transferase, uracil DNA glycosylase (Haug et al., 1994)], many of the known cell cycle regulatory gene promoters contain binding sites for **both** Sp1 and E2F; these include promoters for the genes encoding cyclin D1 (Motokura and Arnold, 1993), p34cdc2 (Yamamoto et al., 1994), human and mouse pRb (Gill et al., 1994; Zacksenhaus et al., 1993), and human and mouse E2F1 (Li et al., 1994; Neuman et al., 1994). The co-localization and common functional interaction of pRb with E2F and Sp1 strongly support the hypothesis that regulation of these genes is achieved by the balance of the interaction among these three proteins, which may also involve the transition between different cyclins and their cdk partners. Several oligonucleotides selected from among random oligonucleotide pools by their ability to bind pRb associated proteins show sequence identity to Sp1 and E2F binding sites (Chittenden et al., 1991; Ouellette et al., 1992), suggesting that Sp1 and E2F may interact.

RESULTS AND DISCUSSION

Induction of DHFR Promoter Activity in the G_0 to S Phase Transition

Transcriptional activity of the DHFR promoter is increased by serum stimulation of quiescent cells (Feder et al., 1990; Santiago et al., 1984), in a manner analogous to the late G_1 peak of transcription observed in cycling cells. This stimulation of DHFR promoter activity in NIH3T3 cells released into G_1 by addition of serum to serum-starved (G_0) cells has been attributed to the E2F sites in the mouse DHFR promoter (Means et al., 1992). We have tested serum induction of the hamster DHFR promoter in Balb/c 3T3 cells, and have found that CAT expression driven by the hamster DHFR promoter is very low in G_0 cells and increases 30- to 50-fold 24 hours after serum addition to cells that had been arrested in G_0 by serum deprivation (Fig. 2A). A co-transfection control, the metallothionein I promoter driving expression of

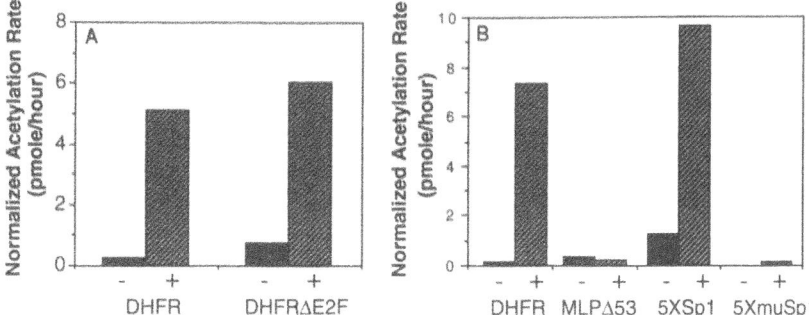

Figure 2. Activation of Sp1-dependent transcription in serum stimulated cells. Balb/c 3T3 mouse fibroblasts (3 X 10^5 cells per 10 cm plate) were transfected with 18 μg of each of the promoter-CAT constructs indicated and 2 μg of pXGH5 (as a transfection control; see Methods). Cells were then subjected to the serum starvation for 36 hours, followed by serum stimulation. Cells were harvested at the 24 hours after serum addition, lysates were prepared, and CAT activity was determined (Neumann et al., 1987). CAT activity values were normalized with respect to levels of GH expression from the co-transfected GH control plasmid (pXGH5). Data are representative of three separate experiments, all of which gave similar results. A) Cells were transfected with the wildtype DHFR promoter containing sequence from position -210 to -23 relative to ATG at +1. or with the same promoter bearing a double point mutation in the E2F site at positions -57/-56. B) Cells were transfected with the indicated promoter driving expression of CAT: MLPΔ53 contains major late promoter sequence from -53 to +33; 5XSp1 contains 5 copies of the consensus Sp1 binding site (oligonucleotide 5' GATCGGGGCGGGGC 3' and its complement ligated together) cloned into the multiple cloning region immediately 5' to MLPΔ53.

human growth hormone, was used in all of the experiments. To identify the element in the hamster DHFR promoter that mediates the serum response, we tested the induction of the DHFR promoter bearing a mutation in the E2F site. This promoter displayed 4-fold higher CAT activity in G_0 cells but was stimulated to the same level as the wild type DHFR promoter (Fig. 2A). The kinetics of activation were similar to those of the wild type DHFR promoter. Thus, the Sp1 binding sites are sufficient to mediate the serum response of the DHFR promoter. We then tested whether Sp1 sites confer serum inducibility on a heterologous promoter. A construct containing 5 Sp1 sites cloned 5' to the TATA box of a truncated adenovirus major late promoter (MLPΔ53) driving expression of CAT was transfected into Balb/c 3T3 cells which were then arrested in G_0 and subsequently induced to enter G_1. The artificial construct with 5 Sp1 sites upstream of a TATA box was stimulated to a high level, whereas MLPΔ53 or the MLPΔ53 construct with 5 copies of mutated Sp1 binding sequence that cannot bind Sp1 did not respond to serum (Fig. 2B).

We have found that Sp1 DNA binding activity in nuclear extracts obtained from serum stimulated cells is increased after serum stimulation and the increase is independent of protein synthesis. Two different post-translational modifications of Sp1 have been reported, O-linked glycosylation and phosphorylation (Jackson, 1992; Jackson et al., 1990). To determine whether changes in phosphorylation of Sp1 were involved in regulating its transcriptional activity, we first sought to determine whether the phosphorylation state of Sp1 changed during the G0 to S phase transition. We initially addressed this question using the Western blot procedure and found that the phosphorylated 105 kDa form of Sp1 was exclusively present 12 hours after release of Balb/c 3T3 cells from a G_0 block. We then examined phosphate incorporation into Sp1 and compared it to the rate of Sp1 synthesis, as measured by the incorporation of ^{35}S-methionine into immunoprecipitated Sp1. There is no difference in the rate of ^{35}S-methionine incorporation between the cells released from G_0 for 12 hours and those that remained in G_0. In contrast, there is a dramatic increase in ^{32}P incorporation into Sp1 in the serum stimulated cells. Thus, it would appear that the exclusive presence of the phosphorylated form of Sp1 12 hours after serum stimulation results from de novo phosphorylation of Sp1 and not from changes in the rate of Sp1 synthesis.

We then sought to perform these experiments in primary human cells to avoid the possible interference of viral gene products in immortalized rodent cells. Normal human diploid fibroblasts (NHDF) cells were synchronized by contact inhibition plus serum deprivation, then induced to re-enter the cell cycle by splitting the cells in a one to two ratio in 20% FCS. The cells were quiescent when starved and the onset of S phase was fairly synchronous at 16 hours determined by measuring thymidine incorporation which demonstrated a sharp increase at this time. To determine the Sp1 phosphorylation status from G_0 to S phase, NHDF cells arrested in G_0 were pulse-labeled in 2 hour intervals with ^{32}P-orthophosphate in the presence of 20% dialyzed fetal calf serum. Whole cell extracts from different time points were immunoprecipitated by polyclonal Sp1 antibody. After the pellet was resolved on 8% SDS PAGE, the phosphorylated Sp1 was visualized by autoradiography. The pulse-label experiment showed that phosphate incorporation into Sp1 initiated at 6 hours and continued to increase at 12 and 14 hours. This phosphorylation correlates with the onset of DHFR transcription, which further supports our hypothesis that phosphorylation of Sp1 modulates Sp1 activity.

A role for Sp1 in the control of proliferation has also been suggested in other systems. Sp1 expression correlates with proliferation in developing mouse embryos (Saffer et al., 1991) . Sp1 binding to DNA is induced in erythroleukemia cells in response to GM-CSF stimulation (Borellini and Glazer, 1993). Sp1 binding sites in the monocyte-specific CD14 gene mediate its tissue-specific expression, and preferentially bind the phosphorylated form of Sp1 upon differentiation (Zhang et al., 1994). Thus, although Sp1 has been classified as a constitutive transcription factor, these results, taken together with ours, suggest that Sp1 may have a role in growth control, and that this function may be modulated by the phosphorylation state of the protein.

The expression of many genes changes with the growth state and position of the cell in the cell cycle. Over the past few years, it has become clear that cyclins, cell cycle regulatory proteins that vary in concentration throughout the cell cycle, regulate not only critical transition points in the cell cycle but also modulate the expression and/or activity of many different targets. Cyclins are the regulatory subunits for cyclin-dependent kinases (cdks) whose activity thereby oscillates through the cell cycle, resulting in ordered phosphorylation of specific substrates which in turn regulate the activity of many different target genes. Perhaps the best characterized transcription factor that interacts with cdks is E2F. However, the change in the phosphorylation state of Sp1 in the cell cycle is consistent with its being a substrate for a cell cycle dependent kinase. Furthermore, Sp1 reportedly can be phosphorylated in vitro by cyclin A/cdk2 (Shao and Robbins, 1995). Sp1 can also be phosphorylated in vitro by the DNA-dependent protein kinase (DNA-PK) (Jackson et al., 1993); however, the DNA-PK binds to a double stranded DNA end and it must be co-localized with Sp1 on the same DNA molecule for phosphorylation to occur (Gottlieb and Jackson, 1993). This requirement makes DNA-PK an unlikely kinase in the context of transcription and induction in late G_1, but certainly supports a role during repair of DNA damage that may involve activation of Sp1.

Interaction of E2F1 and Sp1

The two major factors regulating the expression of the DHFR gene are Sp1 and E2F. Since both Sp1 and E2F are found in several different promoters, we suspected that they

Table 1. Synergistic -activation of the DHFR promoter by Sp1 and E2F

trans-activator	Average CAT Activity ± S.E.M.(pmole/hr/µg)
None	0.034 ± 0.011
E2F1	0.070 ± 0.041
Sp1	0.805 ± 0.083
E2F1+Sp1	2.531 ± 0.232

Plasmid expressing the DHFR promoter (-210/-23) driving expression of CAT (5 µg) was transfected into _Drosophila_ SL2 cells alone or with 100 ng of pPAC-Sp1 and/or with 5 µg CMV-E2F1 expression plasmid. The promoter activities were measured by CAT assay and normalized to the total amount of cellular protein. Values are the average CAT activity measured in three separate experiments ± the standard error of the mean (S.E.M.).

may functionally interact. To determine how Sp1 and E2F function to regulate the DHFR gene, we co-transfected Sp1 and E2F1 with DHFR-CAT into _Drosophila_ SL2 cells. This _Drosophila_ cell line was chosen to study the interaction between Sp1 and E2F1 (and pRb) because endogenous Sp1 and pRb are not known to be present, and the endogenous _Drosophila_ E2F (Dynlacht et al., 1994; Ohtani et al., 1994) is not able to efficiently activate E2F dependent expression of the exogenous hamster DHFR gene. E2F1 and Sp1 synergistically activated the wild type DHFR promoter (Table 1), as well as the DNA polymerase α promoter which also contains binding sites for both E2F and Sp1 (Table 2). Moreover, we also found that E2F1 could synergistically activate transcription of the DHFR promoter lacking the E2F site (Table 3), suggesting that E2F1 could functionally interact with Sp1. This kind of interaction is termed "superactivation" (Courey et al., 1989).

Since our functional data suggested that E2F1 and Sp1 may interact, we asked whether E2F was associated with Sp1 in cells. Cellular extract from U2OS cells was immunoprecipitated with E2F-1 antibody and co-immunoprecipitated proteins were analyzed for the presence of Sp1 by Western blot. Proteins were separated by SDS PAGE (8%). An Sp1 immunoreactive protein that comigrated with Sp1 was observed in the E2F1 immunoprecipitates, which indicated that an E2F1-Sp1 complex exists in these cells

Since E2F1 and Sp1 were apparently associated in cells, we asked whether Sp1 could bind to E2F1 in a cell free system. [35]S labeled Sp1 was incubated with different GST-E2F-1 fusion proteins, which include full-length E2F-1 and a variety of E2F-1 mu-

Table 2. Synergistic activation of the DNA polymerase α promoter by Sp1 and E2F

trans-activator	CAT Activity (pmole/hr/µg)	Fold Activation (Ave.) ± S.E.M
None	0.045	1.00 ± 0.00
E2F1	0.294	5.74 ± 1.58
Sp1	1.91	28.56 ± 8.92
E2F1 + Sp1	3.815	73.44 ± 13.47

Plasmid expressing the DNA polymerase α promoter driving expression of CAT (5 µg) was transfected into _Drosophila_ SL2 cells alone or with 100 ng of pPAC-Sp1 and/or with 5 µg CMV-E2F1 expression plasmid. The promoter activities were measured by CAT assay and normalized to the total amount of cellular protein. CAT activity for one of three experiments is in column 2 and values in column 3 are the average fold activation for three separate experiments ± the standard error of the mean (S.E.M.).

Table 3. Super-activation of the DHFR(ΔE2F) promoter by E2F and Sp1

trans-activator	Ave CAT Activity ± S.E.M.(pmole/hr/μg)
None	0.033 ± 0.0061
E2F-1	0.033 ± 0.0043
Sp1	0.187 ± 0.0220
E2F1 + Sp1	1.402 ± 0.2757

Plasmid expressing the DHFR promoter (-210/-23) bearing a double point mutation in the E2F binding site (pDHFRΔE2F) driving expression of CAT (5 μg) was transfected into *Drosophila* SL2 cells alone or with 100 ng of pPAC-Sp1 and/or with 5 μg CMV-E2F1 expression plasmid. The promoter activities were measured by CAT assay and normalized to the total amount of cellular protein. Values are the average CAT activity measured in three separate experiments ± the standard error of the mean (S.E.M.).

tants. We found that E2F1 binds to Sp1 in the cell free system. Furthermore, using deletion constructs of E2F1, we and others (E. Wintersberger, personal communication) have found that the interaction of E2F1 with Sp1 was mediated through the N-terminal region of E2F1 (aa 1–120).

Thus, Sp1 and E2F1 not only activate their cognate sites but also interact with each other to potentially regulate genes with binding sites for only one of the factors. A precedent for Sp1 interaction and synergistic activation with another transcription factor is found in studies of Sp1 and YY1 (Seto et al., 1993; Seto et al., 1991).

Activation of Transcription by pRb

DHFR gene expression in the cell cycle correlates closely with pRb function in terms of cell cycle progression. We have performed a series of transient transfection experiments in the *Drosophila* embryonic cell line (SL2) and the RB-defective SAOS-2 human osteosarcoma cell line. Endogenous Sp1 and pRb have not been detected in *Drosophila* cells. Although the best characterized mechanism of pRb is repressing transactivation by E2F, several groups have reported that pRb stimulates Sp1-dependent transcription (Kim et al., 1992; Udvadia et al., 1993). To test the effect of pRb on DHFR transcription, we co-transfected plasmids encoding Sp1, DHFR-CAT reporter construct, and different concentration of RB expression plasmids into *Drosophila* cells. After 48 hour incubation at room temperature, cells were harvested and the CAT activities were measured. We found that RB synergistically activated DHFR promoter activity when Sp1 was co-expressed, and this activation effect was pRb concentration dependent (Fig. 3). This result shows that pRb exerts a stimulatory effect on the DHFR promoter in a concentration-dependent manner. We also tested the specificity of this response for Sp1 by comparing reporter gene expression from the wild type DHFR promoter with one in which the E2F site has been mutated. When Sp1 was co-transfected, pRb activated the DHFR promoter with the E2F site mutated to essentially the same extent as that observed with the wildtype promoter. The negative control for this experiment was the co-transfection of the reporter construct and RB plasmid without the Sp1 expression plasmid. Very low activity was observed with this negative control, which further supported the conclusion that the pRb activity was through the Sp1 protein. In the same experiment, we tested two other members of the RB family, p107 and p130, which have significant homology with pRb, especially in the pocket region. The result shows that both of these proteins also activated Sp1-dependent transcription of this promoter, though the effect was not as dramatic as

Figure 3. Retinoblastoma protein activates Sp1-dependent transcription in *Drosophila* cells. 2 µg of DHFR-CAT was co-transfected with different concentration of RB expression plasmids (1.25 µg - 20 µg) into *Drosophila* SL2 cells with or without (bars 1,2) co-expression of 100 ng of pPAC-Sp1 plasmid. After 48 hours of transfection, cells were harvested and the DHFR promoter activity was determined by CAT assay. The CAT activity was normalized to the total amount of cellular protein. Data are representative of three separate experiments, all of which gave similar results.

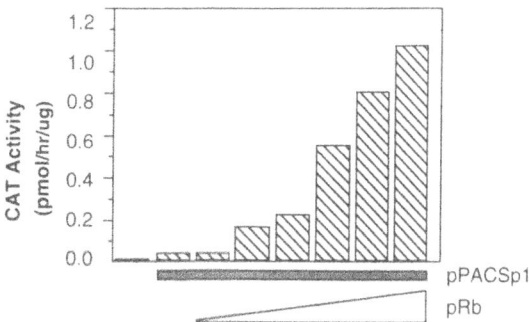

with pRb. Since the common feature of the RB family is the pocket domain, we suspect that the pocket might be the domain mediating this activation.

We also tested this interaction in SAOS-2 cells, an RB defective human osteosarcoma cell line. We co-transfected the RB plasmid with wild type DHFR-CAT or DHFR with the E2F site mutated (DHFRΔE2F-CAT). As shown in Figure 4, pRb repressed the wild type DHFR promoter but activated the mutant promoter. SAOS-2 cells are very sensitive to exogenous wild type pRb. It is reported that re-introduction of the wild type pRb into this cell line arrested the cells in the G_1 phase. When the reporter gene was under control of the wild type DHFR, exogenous pRb acted as a strong repressor on the E2F sites so the activation effect on the Sp1 sites was masked. However, when the E2F site on the promoter was mutated, pRb stimulated reporter gene expression, an effect presumably mediated by Sp1.

Summary

There are multiple levels of control of cell cycle progression and the precisely regulated involvement of specific transcription factors has been underscored in the recent literature. For example, recent work has shown that E2F transcription factor associates with proteins linked to both tumor suppression and cell cycle progression. pRb and cyclin A interact with the DHFR promoter through the E2F site, and there also is evidence that Sp1 sites are involved in growth stimulation, perhaps through interaction with Rb (Kim et al.,

Figure 4. Inhibition of transcription of the DHFR promoter in SAOS2 cells by pRB requires E2F binding. DHFR-CAT or DHFR(ΔE2F)-CAT (10 µg) was transfected into SAOS-2 cells with 20 µg of pRb. After 48 hours of transfection, cells were harvested and the DHFR promoter activity was determined by CAT assay. The CAT activity was normalized to the total amount of cellular protein.

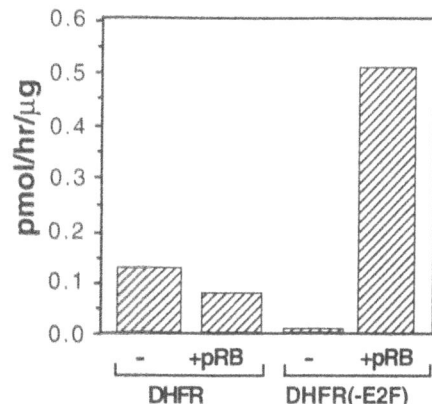

1992; Udvadia et al., 1993). Moreover, E2F and Sp1 can both physically and functionally interact. These multiprotein complexes interact with the DHFR promoter and those of other growth-regulated genes, probably at specific points in the cell cycle to either stimulate or repress transcription.

REFERENCES

Azizkhan, J. C., Jensen, D. E., Pierce, A. J. and Wade, M., 1993, Transcription from TATA-less promoters: dihydrofolate reductase as a model. *Critical Reviews in Eukaryotic Gene Expression* 3:229–254.

Azizkhan, J. C., Vaughn, J. P., Christy, R. J. and Hamlin, J. L., 1986, Nucleotide sequence and nuclease hypersensitivity of the Chinese hamster dihydrofolate reductase gene promoter region. *Biochemistry* 25:6228–6236.

Bandara, L. R., Buck, V. M., Zamanian, M., Johnston, L. H. and La Thangue, N. B., 1993, Functional synergy between DP-1 and E2F-1 in the cell cycle-regulating transcription factor DRTF1/E2F. *EMBO Journal* 12:4317–4324.

Beijersbergen, R. L., Hijmans, E. M., Zhu, L. and Bernards, R., 1994, Interaction of c-myc with the pRb-related protein p107 results in inhibition of c-Myc-mediated transactivation. *EMBO Journal* 13:4080–4086.

Beijersbergen, R. L., Kerkhoven, R. M., Zhu, L., Carlee, L., Voorhoeve, P. M. and Bernards, R., 1994, E2F-4, a new member of the E2F gene family, has oncogenic activity and associates with p107 in vivo. *Genes Dev.* 8:2680–2690.

Blake, M. C. and Azizkhan, J. C., 1989, Transcription factor E2F is required for efficient expression of the hamster dihydrofolate reductase gene in vitro and in vivo. *Mol. Cell. Biol.* 9:4994–5002.

Blake, M. C., Jambou, R. C., Swick, A. G., Kahn, J. W. and Azizkhan, J. C., 1990, Transcriptional initiation is controlled by upstream GC-box interactions in a TATAA-less promoter. *Mol. Cell. Biol.* 10:6632–6641.

Borellini, F. and Glazer, R. I., 1993, Induction of Sp1-p53 DNA-binding heterocomplexes during granulocyte/macrophage colony-stimulating factor-dependent proliferation in human erythroleukemia cell line TF-1. *J. Biol. Chem.* 268:7923–7928.

Buchkovich, K., Duffy, L. A. and Harlow, E., 1989, The retinoblastoma protein is phosphorylated during specific phases of the cell cycle. *Cell* 58:1097–1105.

Chellappan, S. P., Hiebert, S., Mudryj, M., Horowitz, J. M. and Nevins, J. R., 1991, The E2F transcription factor is a cellular target for the RB protein. *Cell* 65:1053–1061.

Chen, L. I., Nishinaka, T., Kwan, K., Kitabayashi, I., Yokoyama, K., Fu, Y. H., Grunwald, S. and Chiu, R., 1994, The retinoblastoma gene product RB stimulates Sp1-mediated transcription by liberating Sp1 from a negative regulator. *Mol. Cell. Biol.* 14:4380–4389.

Chen, P. L., Scully, P., Shew, J. Y., Wang, J. Y. and Lee, W. H., 1989, Phosphorylation of the retinoblastoma gene product is modulated during the cell cycle and cellular differentiation. *Cell* 58:1193–1198.

Chittenden, T., Livingston, D. M. and Kaelin, W. G., Jr, 1991, The T/E1A-binding domain of the retinoblastoma product can interact selectively with a sequence-specific DNA-binding protein. *Cell* 65:1073–1082.

Courey, A. J., Holtzman, D. A., Jackson, S. P. and Tjian, R., 1989, Synergistic activation by the glutamine-rich domains of human transcription factor Sp1. *Cell* 59:827–836.

Dusing, M. R. and Wiginton, D. A., 1994, Sp1 is essential for both enhancer-mediated and basal activation of the TATA-less human adenosine deaminase promoter. *Nucleic Acids Research* 22:669–677.

Dynan, W. S. and Tjian, R., 1983, Isolation of transcription factors that discriminate between different promoters recognized by RNA polymerase II. *Cell* 32:669–680.

Dynlacht, B. D., Brook, A., Dembski, M., Yenush, L. and Dyson, N., 1994, DNA-binding and trans-activation properties of Drosophila E2F and DP proteins. *Proc. Nat. Acad. Sci. USA* 91:6359–6363.

Feder, J. N., Guidos, C. J., Kusler, B., Carswell, C., Lewis, D. and Schimke, R. T., 1990, A cell cycle analysis of growth-related genes expressed during T lymphocyte maturation. *J. Cell Biol.* 111:2693–2701.

Gibson, T. J., Thompson, J. D., Blocker, A. and Kouzarides, T., 1994, Evidence of a protein domain superfamily shared by the cyclins, TFIIB and pRB/p107. *Nuc. Acids Res.* 22:946–952.

Gill, G., Pascal, E., Tseng, Z. H. and Tjian, R., 1994, A glutamine-rich hydrophobic patch in transcription factor Sp1 contacts the dTAFII110 component of the Drosophila TFIID complex and mediates transcriptional activation. *Proc. Nat. Acad. Sci. USA* 91:192–196.

Gill, R. M., Hamel, P. A., Jiang, Z., Zacksenhaus, E., Gallie, B. L. and Phillips, R. A., 1994, Characterization of the human RB1 promoter and of elements involved in transcriptional regulation. *Cell Growth & Differentiation* 5:467–474.

Gottlieb, T. M. and Jackson, S. P., 1993, The DNA-dependent protein kinase: requirement for DNA ends and association with Ku antigen. *Cell* 72:131–142.

Hagemeier, C., Bannister, A. J., Cook, A. and Kouzarides, T., 1993, The activation domain of transcription factor PU.1 binds the retinoblastoma (RB) protein and the transcription factor TFIID in vitro: RB shows sequence similarity to TFIID and TFIIB. *Proc. Nat. Acad. Sci. USA* 90:1580–1584.

Hakala, M. T. and Taylor, E., 1959, The ability of purine and thymidine derivatives and of glycine to support the growth of mammalian cells in culture. *J. Biol. Chem.* 234:126–128.

Haug, T., Skorpen, F., Lund, H. and Krokan, H. E., 1994, Structure of the gene for human uracil-DNA glycosylase and analysis of the promoter function. *FEBS Letters* 353:180–4.

Helin, K., Lees, J. A., Vidal, M., Dyson, N., Harlow, E. and Fattaey, A., 1992, A cDNA encoding a pRB-binding protein with properties of the transcription factor E2F. *Cell* 70:337–350.

Henglein, B., Chenivesse, X., Wang, J., Eick, D. and Brechot, C., 1994, Structure and cell cycle-regulated transcription of the human cyclin A gene. *Proc. Nat. Acad. Sci. USA* 91:5490–5494.

Hiebert, S. W., 1993, Regions of the retinoblastoma gene product required for its interaction with the E2F transcription factor are necessary for E2 promoter repression and pRb-mediated growth suppression. *Mol. Cell. Biol.* 13:3384–3391.

Hiebert, S. W., Chellappan, S. P., Horowitz, J. M. and Nevins, J. R., 1992, The interaction of RB with E2F coincides with an inhibition of the transcriptional activity of E2F. *Genes Dev.* 6:177–185.

Huang, S., Shin, E., Sheppard, K. A., Chokroverty, L., Shan, B., Qian, Y. W., Lee, E. Y. and Yee, A. S., 1992, The retinoblastoma protein region required for interaction with the E2F transcription factor includes the T/E1A binding and carboxy-terminal sequences. *DNA Cell Biol.* 11:539–548.

Hunter, T. and Pines, J., 1991, Cyclins and Cancer. *Cell* 68:1071–1074.

Ivey-Hoyle, M., Conroy, R., Huber, H. E., Goodhart, P. J., Oliff, A. and Heimbrook, D. C., 1993, Cloning and characterization of E2F-2, a novel protein with the biochemical properties of transcription factor E2F. *Mol. Cell. Biol.* 13:7802–7812.

Jackson, S., Gottlieb, T. and Hartley, K., 1993, Phosphorylation of transcription factor Sp1 by the DNA-dependent protein kinase. *Adv Second Messenger Phosphoprotein Res* 28:279–286.

Jackson, S. P., 1992, Regulating transcription factor activity by phosphorylation. *Tr. Cell Biol.* 2:104–108.

Jackson, S. P., MacDonald, J. J., Lees-Miller, S. and Tjian, R., 1990, GC box binding induces phosphorylation of Sp1 by a DNA-dependent protein kinase. *Cell* 63:155–165.

Johnson, D. G., Cress, W. D., Jakoi, L. and Nevins, J. R., 1994, Oncogenic capacity of the E2F1 gene. *Proc. Nat. Acad. Sci., USA* 91:12823–12827.

Johnson, J. L. and McLachlan, A., 1994, Novel clustering of Sp1 transcription factor binding sites at the transcription initiation site of the human muscle phosphofructokinase P1 promoter. *Nuc. Acids Res.* 22:5085–5092.

Jolliff, K., Li, Y. and Johnson, L. F., 1991, Multiple protein-DNA interactions in the TATAA-less mouse thymidylate synthase promoter. *Nuc. Acids Res* 19:2267–2274.

Kadonaga, J. T., Carner, K. R., Masiarz, F. R. and Tjian, R., 1987, Isolation of cDNA encoding transcription factor Sp1 and functional analysis of the DNA binding domain. *Cell* 51:1079–1090.

Kaelin, W. G., Krek, W., Sellers, W. R., DeCaprio, J. A., Ajchanbaum, F., Fuchs, C. S., Chittenden, T., Li, Y., Farnham, P. J., Blanar, M. A., Livingston, D. M. and Flemington, E. K., 1992, Expression cloning of a cDNA encoding a retinoblastoma binding protein with E2F-like properties. *Cell* 70:351–364.

Kim, S. J., Onwuta, U. S., Lee, Y. I., Li, R., Botchan, M. R. and Robbins, P. D., 1992, The retinoblastoma gene product regulates Sp1-mediated transcription. *Mol. Cell. Biol.* 12:2455–2463.

Kovesdi, I., Reichel, R. and Nevins, J. R., 1986, Identification of a cellular transcription factor involved in E1A trans-activation. *Cell* 45:219–228.

Lee, H. H., Chiang, W. H., Chiang, S. H., Liu, Y. C., Hwang, J. and Ng, S. Y., 1995, Regulation of cyclin D1, DNA topoisomerase I, and proliferating cell nuclear antigen promoters during the cell cycle. *Gene Expression* 4:95–109.

Lee, W. H., Shew, J. Y., Hong, F. D., Sery, T. W., Donoso, L. A., Young, L. J., Bookstein, R. and Lee, E. Y., 1987, The retinoblastoma susceptibility gene encodes a nuclear phosphoprotein associated with DNA binding activity. *Nature (London)* 329:624–645.

Lees, J. A., Saito, M., Vidal, M., Valentine, M., Look, T., Harlow, E., Dyson, N. and Helin, K., 1993, The retinoblastoma protein binds to a family of E2F transcription factors. *Molecular & Cellular Biology* 13:7813–25.

Li, Y., Slansky, J. E., Myers, D. J., Drinkwater, N. R., Kaelin, W. G. and Farnham, P. J., 1994, Cloning, chromosomal location, and characterization of mouse E2F1. *Mol. Cell. Biol.* 14:1861–1869.

Liao, W. C., Ash, J. and Johnson, L. F., 1994, Bidirectional promoter of the mouse thymidylate synthase gene. *Nuc. Acids Res.* 22:4044–4049.

Lu, J., Lee, W., Jiang, C. and Keller, E. B., 1994, Start site selection by Sp1 in the TATA-less human Ha-ras promoter. *J. Biol. Chem.* 269:5391–402.

Ludlow, J. W., DeCaprio, J. A., Huang, G.-M., Lee, W.-H., Paucha, E. and Livingston, D. M., 1989, SV40 large T antigen binds preferentially to an underphosphorylated member of the retinoblastoma suxceptibility gene product family. *Cell* 56:57–65.

Marx, J., 1994, *Science* 264: 344–345.

Means, A. L., Slansky, J., E., McMahon, S. L., Knuth, M. W. and Farnham, P. J., 1992, The HIP1 binding site is required for growth regulation of the dihydrofolate reductase gene promoter. *Mol. Cell. Biol.* 12:1054–1063.

Motokura, T. and Arnold, A., 1993, PRAD1/cyclin D1 proto-oncogene: Genomic organization, 5' DNA sequence, and sequence of a tumor-specific rearrangement breakpoint. *Genes, Chromosomes, and Cancer* 7:89–95.

Mudryj, M., Devoto, S. H., Hiebert, S. W., Hunter, T., Pines, J. and Nevins, J. R., 1991, Cell cycle regulation of the E2F transcription factor involves an interaction with cyclin A. *Cell* 65:1243–53.

Murata, Y., Kim, H. G., Rogers, K. T., Udvadia, A. J. and Horowitz, J. M., 1994, Negative regulation of Sp1 trans-activation is correlated with the binding of cellular proteins to the amino terminus of the Sp1 trans-activation domain. *J. Biol. Chem.* 269:20674–20681.

Neuman, E., Flemington, E. K., Sellers, W. R. and Kaelin, W. G., Jr., 1994, Transcription of the E2F-1 gene is rendered cell cycle dependent by E2F DNA binding within its own promoter. *Mol. Cell. Biol.* 14:6607–6615.

Neumann, J. R., Morency, C. A. and Russian, K. O., 1987, A rapid fluor diffusion assay for detection of chloramphenicol acetyl transferase activity. *Biotechniques* 5:444–448.

Nevins, J. R., 1992, E2F: A link between the Rb tumor suppressor protein and viral oncoproteins. *Science* 258:424–429.

Ogris, E., Rotheneder, H., Mudrak, I., Pichler, A. and Wintersberger, E., 1993, A binding site for transcription factor E2F is a target for trans activation of murine thymidine kinase by polyomavirus large T antigen and plays an important role in growth regulation of the gene. *J. Virol.* 67:1765–1771.

Ohtani, K., Nevins, J. R., Dou, Q. P., Zhao, S., Levin, A. H., Wang, J., Helin, K. and Pardee, A. B., 1994, Functional properties of a Drosophila homolog of the E2F1 gene G1/S-regulated E2F-containing protein complexes bind to the mouse thymidine kinase gene promoter. *Mol. Cell. Biol.* 14:1603–1612.

Ouellette, M. M., Chen, J., Wright, W. E. and Shay, J. W., 1992, Complexes containing the retinoblastoma gene product recognize different DNA motifs related to the E2F binding site. *Oncogene* 7:1075–1081.

Pardee, A. B., 1989, G1 events and regulation of cell proliferation. *Science* 246:603–608.

Pearson, B. E., Nasheuer, H.-P. and Wang, T. S.-F., 1991, Human DNA polymerase a hene: Sequences controlling expression in cycling and serum-stimulated cells. *Mol. Cell. Biol.* 11:2081–2095.

Qin, X. Q., Livingston, D. M., Kaelin, W. G., Jr. and Adams, P. D., 1994, Deregulated transcription factor E2F-1 expression leads to S-phase entry and p53-mediated apoptosis. *Proc. Nat. Acad. Sci. U.S.A.* 91:10918–10922.

Saffer, J. D., Jackson, S. P. and Annarella, M. B., 1991, Developmental expression of Sp1 in the mouse. *Mol. Cell. Biol.* 11:2189–2199.

Santiago, C., Collins, M. and Johnson, L. F., 1984, In vitro and in vivo analysis of the control of dihydrofolate reductase gene transcription in serum-stimulated mouse fibroblasts. *J. Cell. Physiol.* 118:79–86.

Seto, E., Lewis, B. and Shenk, T., 1993, Interaction between transcription factors Sp1 and YY1. *Nature* 365:462–464.

Seto, E., Shi, Y. and Shenk, T., 1991, YY1 is an initiator sequence-binding protein that directs and activates transcription in vitro. *Nature* 354:241–245.

Shan, B., Chang, C. Y., Jones, D. and Lee, W. H., 1994, The transcription factor E2F-1 mediates the autoregulation of RB gene expression. *Mol. Cell. Biol.* 14:299–309.

Shan, B. and Lee, W. H., 1994, Deregulated expression of E2F-1 induces S-phase entry and leads to apoptosis. *Mol. Cell. Biol.* 14:8166–8173.

Shao, Z. and Robbins, P. D., 1995, Differential regulation of E2F and Sp1-mediated transcription by G1 cyclins. *Oncogene* 10:221–228.

Singh, P., Wong, S. H. and Hong, W., 1994, Overexpression of E2F-1 in rat embryo fibroblasts leads to neoplastic transformation. *EMBO Journal* 13:3329–3338.

Swick, A. G., Blake, M. C., Kahn, J. W. and Azizkhan, J. C., 1989, Functional analysis of GC element binding and transcription in the hamster dihydrofolate reductase gene promoter. *Nucleic Acids Res.* 17:9291–9304.

Udvadia, A. J., Rogers, K. T., Higgins, P. D., Murata, Y., Martin, K. H., Humphrey, P. A. and Horowitz, J. M., 1993, Sp-1 binds promoter elements regulated by the RB protein and Sp-1-mediated transcription is stimulated by RB coexpression. *Proc. Nat. Acad. Sci. USA* 90:3265–3269.

Wade, M., Blake, M. C., Jambou, R. C., Helin, K., Harlow, E. and Azizkhan, J. C., 1995, An inverted repeat motif stabilizes binding of E2F and enhances transcription of the dihydrofolate reductase gene. *J. Biol. Chem.* 270:9783–9791.

Weintraub, S. J. and Dean, D. C., 1992, Interaction of a common factor with ATF, Sp1, or TATAA promoter elements is required for these sequences to mediate transactivation by the adenoviral oncogene E1a. *Mol. Cell. Biol.* 12:512–517.

Xu, G. F., Livingston, D. M. and Krek, W., 1995, Multiple members of the E2F transcription factor family are the products of oncogenes. *Proc. Nat. Acad. Sci., USA* 92:1357–1361.

Yamamoto, M., Yoshida, M., Ono, K., Fujita, T., Ohtani-Fujita, N., Sakai, T. and Nikaido, T., 1994, Effect of tumor suppressors on cell cycle regulatory genes: RB suppresses p34cdc2 expression and normal p53 suppresses cyclin A expression. *Experimental Cell Research* 210:94–101.

Zacksenhaus, E., Bremner, R., Phillips, R. A. and Gallie, B. L., 1993, A bipartite nuclear localization signal in the retinoblastoma gene product and its importance for biological activity. *Mol. Cell. Biol.* 13:4588–4599.

Zhang, D. E., Hetherington, C. J., Tan, S., Dziennis, S. E., Gonzalez, D. A., Chen, H. M. and Tenen, D. G., 1994, Sp1 is a critical factor in monocyte specific expression of human CD14. *J. Biol. Chem.* 268:11425–11434.

DISCUSSION

F. Rauscher: Did you map the region on Sp1 required for E2F interaction?

J. Azizkhan: No, we have not yet. Those experiments are underway.

F. Rauscher: And can you find in a nuclear extract an E2F-Sp1 complex by gel shift that is super-shiftable by either antibody?

J. Azizkhan: We cannot find a complex in cells containing both proteins that will bind to DNA. I think this is probably a situation of finding the right binding conditions. E2F and Sp1 gel shifts are done under dramatically different conditions. What we can do is, do an Sp1 gel shift, add excess E2F-1 and super-shift the Sp1 gel shift with E2F-1. So the proteins are capable of interacting on DNA. Surprisingly - and I did not show the data but - the reciprocal experiment has also been done where Sp1 can super activate a promoter containing only E2F cites.

P. Sassone-Corsi: Did you say that a single Sp1 site can provide serum inducibility?

J. Azizkhan: No, we have multiple Sp1 sites in all of our constructs. I do not think a single Sp1 site clone would be induced.

P. Sassone-Corsi: Do you know whether other genes which have multiple Sp1 cites are serum inducible?

J. Azizkhan: Most of them are.

P. Sassone-Corsi: Is the SV40 promoter serum inducible?

J. Azizkhan: The SV40 promoter is serum inducible.

P. Sassone-Corsi: Do you know whether for the interaction you need Sp1 phosphorylation?

J. Azizkhan: We think we need Sp1 phosphorylation. We have had a problem de-phosphorylating Sp1. We had many phosphatases and we have still got a 105 kilo dalton Sp1.

P. Sassone-Corsi: What is the *in vivo* relevance of these results?

J. Azizkhan: What I showed you was an *in vivo* preliminary experiment.

P. Sassone-Corsi: I am talking about in-vivo as in a tissue - what is the ratio between normal Sp1 and RB and E2F in tissues?

J. Azizkhan: Sp1 is present in excess of E2F. As the E2F family grows, I am not sure that will necessarily be true. And in terms of RB, there is certainly plenty of RB - you do not find free E2F with high frequency in Rb$^+$ cells.

P. Sassone-Corsi: I was just wondering what is the significance *in vivo* of this observation in terms of transcriptional regulation in a tissue?

J. Azizkhan: We have not really looked at that carefully enough to answer that.

D. Livingston: Can you do the experiment reversing things, taking the DHFR promoter of hamster and killing the Sp1 sites?

J. Azizkhan: Most of our experiments are done in Drosophila to get the background down.

D. Livingston: No, but for the serum dependence?

J. Azizkhan: Oh, for the serum dependence, we do it in either primary, fibroblast or Balb/c 3T3 cells.

D. Livingston: With calcium?

J. Azizkhan: Yes.

D. Livingston: If you simply transfect that reporter into a cell - is it serum activated?

J. Azizkhan: It is serum activated but to a very low level. And the reason for the very low level may well be that you have essentially inactivated the promoter. Without the Sp1 cites you get extremely low level transcription. I showed you an experiment using the E2 promoter where you have just the E2F sites with the ATF site mutated and that is serum inducible.

D. Livingston: And if you replicate the number of E2F sites in that setting? Does one see enhanced power?

J. Azizkhan: We have not done that. That should be done. The problem with the DHFR is that the Sp1 sites are probably fixing the start site of transcription. When we actually map the start in our promoter, in which we have eliminated the Sp1 sites, we see heterogeneous initiation over a large region and very low promoter inactivity.

D. Livingston: Is there Sp1 protein in those cells under those conditions for example? How come you do not get cooperation such as you suggested might be the case?

J. Azizkhan: Yes, There is Sp1 protein. In DHFR, you do not see that because you need the Sp1 sites for basal activity. In the E2 promoter, you do see cooperation. We have not actually tried pulling out the Sp1 to see if you would lose it; transcriptional activation may well be the cooperation between Sp1 and E2F.

D. Livingston: If you micro inject monoclonal antibody to Sp1 into serum arrested cells, will they come out?

J. Azizkhan: We need to do those experiments.

P. Sassone-Corsi: If you look at the endogenous gene in RB-minus cells, that gene will be better induced by serum?

J. Azizkhan: We have not done that experiment.

P. Sassone-Corsi: And do you know anything about the kinetics of induction by serum of the endogenous gene?

J. Azizkhan: The kinetics of induction of an endogenous gene are virtually identical to what I showed you.

P. Sassone-Corsi: But that changes in RB-minus cells?

J. Azizkhan: We have not done that experiment.

T. Taniguchi: Let me ask about the function of this DHFR in controlling cell cycles; if you constitutively express DHFR, what happens in the cell?

J. Azizkhan: Actually, nothing. Adding DHFR or tetrahydrofolate does not feedback at all. I am not sure how important the control of DHFR per se is. I do not think there are any consequences at all.

D. Livingston: How do you reconcile these results with those of Peggy Farnham, who has observed a rather dramatic E2F-1 dependent activation of DHFR in acutely transfected cells?

J. Azizkhan: I have not been able to reconcile these differences. I have sent her my clones but have not received the results obtained in her system. But we need to resolve the differences. I can reconcile her failure to see Sp1 dependent activation because she has put the Sp1 sites with no initiator or TATA sequence.

D. Livingston: Is there RB protein in these cells?

J. Azizkhan: Yes, there is, absolutely.

D. Livingston: And can you detect, for example, RB-E2F gel shift activity during the exit period?

J. Azizkhan: It comes up.

11

CYCLIN A-KINASE BINDING TO AND REGULATION OF THE FUNCTION OF A GROWTH-PROMOTING TRANSCRIPTION FACTOR

Wilhelm Krek,[*] Gangfeng Xu, and David M. Livingston

The Dana-Farber Cancer Institute and
The Harvard Medical School
Boston, Massachusetts 02115

INTRODUCTION

Cyclin A function is required for a successful S phase of the mammalian cell cycle(Girard et al., 1991; Pagano et al., 1992; Zindy et al., 1992). In this role, it functions in complex with its cdk partner, cdk2 (Pines and Hunter, 1990), and it is the cyclin A-cdk2-dependent phosphorylation of selected target proteins at the appropriate time in the cell cycle which translates into the successful prosecution of its S phase function. This notwithstanding, there has been no clear understanding of the nature of critical cyclin A-cdk2 targets. Thus, the identification and functional characterization of physiologically relevant substrates of this enzyme remains a major problem, which must be solved if one is to understand, in detail, how cyclin A controls S phase progression.

THE E2F FAMILY OF TRANSCRIPTION FACTORS

In mammalian cells, the E2F family of transcription factors includes at least seven members. Five, termed E2F 1–5, are related by the existence of homologous N-terminal DNA binding domains, abutted on their C-terminal sides by hydrophobic heterodimerization domains, and homologous transactivation units at their C-termini. Within the latter are short peptide sequences necessary for the binding of the retinoblastoma gene product (pRB) and the related 'pocket' proteins, p107 and p130. The other two members are termed DP proteins - DP 1 and 2. They, too, contain N-terminal DNA binding domains, homologous to those of the E2F-like proteins, as well as adjoining hydrophobic heterodi-

* Present Address: Friedrich Miescher Institut Maulbeerstrasse 66 CH-4058 Basel Switzerland.

merization domains with which they heterodimerize with the relevant E2F-like partner. However, unlike the E2F family members, they lack potent transactivation and 'pocket' protein binding domains.

Naturally occurring E2F complexes that are detected in cell extracts of various cell lines are heterodimers composed of a polypeptide encoded by an E2F gene and a polypeptide encoded by a DP gene. Indeed, E2F 1–5 are relatively weak DNA binding and transactivation elements. By contrast, E2F-DP heterodimers are powerful DNA binding and transactivating elements. Therefore, DP binding to a given E2F polypeptide licenses the transcription activation function of the latter.

E2F-DP heterodimers are negatively regulated at the level of transactivation by 'pocket' proteins, which bind efficiently to the above-noted 'pocket' protein binding sequence. Indeed, there is strong evidence suggesting that when an E2F and a DP species heterodimerize, there is not only enhancement of both E2F DNA binding and E2F transactivation, but also marked facilitation of 'pocket' protein binding to the heterodimer. This observation underscores the importance of negative regulation of E2F action by a 'pocket' protein. Indeed, it is now known that pRB regulation of E2F 1,2, and 3 function contributes, in a major way, to the control of progression towards S. Included in the effects of pRB binding to its E2F target(s) is the conversion of the latter into a transcriptional repressor. This function is likely essential to the G1 arrest function of pRB, which, at least in part, depends upon the ability of pRB to block the expression of certain E2F-dependent genes, the products of which promote G1 exit and S phase entry and progression.

CYCLIN A-KINASE REGULATION OF E2F FUNCTION

Of the 5 E2F-like species known, we have shown that E2F-1 (in complex with DP-1) binds cyclin A-cdk2 directly and in a stable manner (Krek et al., 1994, 1995). We have also shown that stable cyclin A-cdk2/E2F-1 complexes exist during S phase and that these complexes contain kinase activity. Where studied, this activity was found to be cell cycle-dependent and to result in the phosphorylation of DP-1, a normal heterodimerization partner of E2F-1. Phosphorylation in this case was on a single serine residue and depended upon proper binding of cyclin A-cdk2 to a specific N-terminal, 41 amino acid segment of E2F-1, which was shown to be the specific cyclin A-cdk2 binding site on that protein.

More to the point, we found that the DNA binding activity of E2F-1 was lost following DP-1 phosphorylation by cyclin A-cdk2. Furthermore, cyclin A-kinase modulation of E2F-1-dependent DNA binding function is also cell cycle specific, with DNA binding activity present in G1, reaching a maximum around G1/S, and then declining as the culture passed into S phase. Thus, as shown in Figure 1, the regulation of E2F-1 function as a transcription factor begins in G1 where it forms heterodimeric complexes with DP-1. Heterodimer formation greatly facilitates pRB binding, which, in turn, inhibits E2F-1 transactivation function and represses certain E2F-1-dependent genes (Weintraub et al, 1992; Sellers et al, 1995). As pRB phosphorylation begins, E2F-1 is freed of 'pocket' protein regulation and certain E2F-dependent genes, previously inhibited, are activated. This process may well be a critical event in the decision of a cell to enter S phase.

As cells move into S phase, free E2F-1 is subject to negative control exerted by the action of a specifically bound, cyclin A-cdk2 complex, which leads to the phosphorylation of a specific serine on DP-1 and loss of E2F-1/DP-1 DNA binding activity. One possible outcome of this effect is diminished activation of the above-noted promoters.

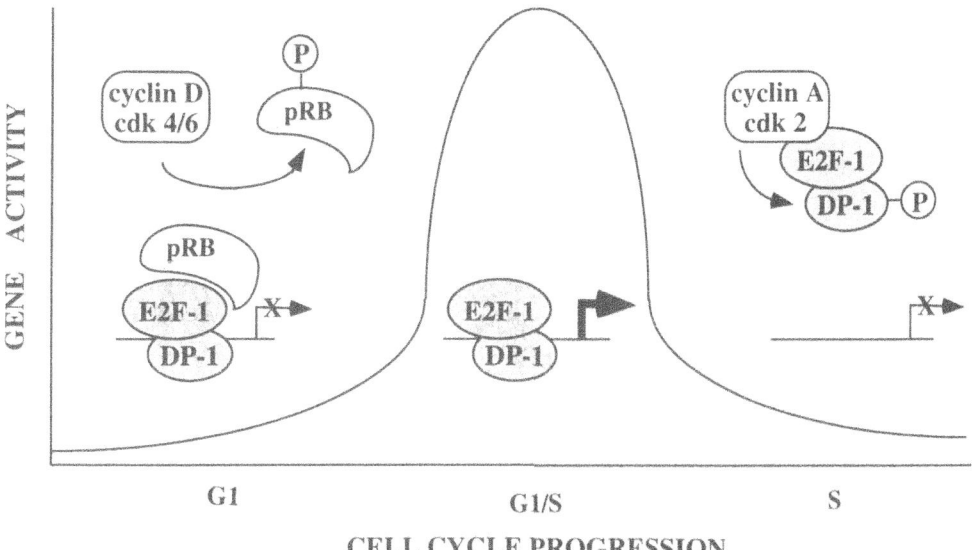

Figure 1. Regulation of E2F-1 Function During Cell Cycle Progression. According the model depicted here, during most of G1, the E2F-1 (in complex with DP-1) is bound to pRB and thus, exists in an transcriptionally inactive, but DNA binding competent state. It is suggested that concomitant with the decision of a cell to enter S phase, the E2F-1 is activated through the action of G1-cyclin-dependent kinases (e. g. cyclin D-cdk4 or 6), which initiate pRB phosphorylation thereby releasing the heterodimer from the inhibitory constraints of pRB. A direct consequence of this series of events is the time-dependent activation of this transcription complex in mid-late G1, which in turn triggers the activation of genes whose products are required for S phase entry and progression. As cells move into S phase, active cyclin A-cdk2 complexes accumulate, bind stably to the E2F-1-DP-1 transcription factor complex. Complex formation leads to specific phosphorylation of the DP-1 subunit with concomitant loss of E2F-1-dependent DNA binding activity. Consequently, certain promoters, previously activated, are again grossly inhibited. Thus, time-dependent interactions of E2F-1-DP-1 heterodimers with proteins that inhibit its function limits the activity of this transcription complex, and by extension gene activity, to a pulse at G1/S.

These findings clearly implied that DP-1 is a physiological important substrate of the S phase specific cyclin A-kinase - the first such protein substrate identified at the time (Krek et al., 1994).

BIOLOGICAL EFFECTS OF CYCLIN A-KINASE BINDING TO E2F-1 AND OF DP-1 PHOSPHORYLATION

More recently, the question of the biological value of cyclin A-kinase phosphorylation of DP-1 has arisen. While the story is far from complete, there are certain clues which are worthy of consideration.

Introduction of mutants of E2F-1 which are selectively unable to bind to cyclin A-kinase can now be achieved using high titer retroviral vectors generated following the technique of Baltimore's group (Pear et al., 1993). These vectors can be produced, alike, with wt and cyclin A-kinase mutant alleles of E2F-1. The effect is an ability to generate approximately equivalent titers of E2F-1 wt and mutant viruses and, then, to acutely infect cultures of NIH-3T3 cells which, then, producie equivalent quantities of the relevant gene products.

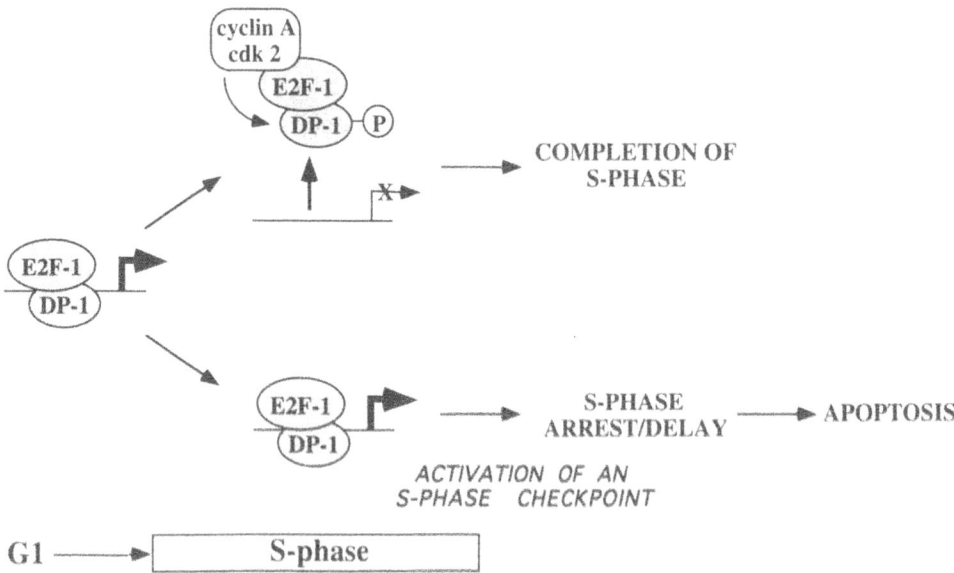

Figure 2. A Possible Participation of E2F-1 in an S phase Checkpoint. Under normal conditions, activation of E2F-1 (in complex with DP-1) in mid-late G1 is followed by the development of active cyclin A-cdk2 which extinguishes E2F-1-dependent DNA binding activity in S phase, thus promoting normal progression through S phase. When regulation of E2F-1 DNA binding activity by cyclin A-cdk2 fails, E2F-1 would remain bound to DNA resulting in the activation of a specific S phase checkpoint. Following this argumentation, it is tempting to speculate that there is a cellular monitoring system that is, in part, able to monitor the absence or presence of E2F-1 on DNA in S. Thus, it seems that it is important to confine the presence of E2F-1 on specific DNA sequences to specific cell cycle intervals otherwise S phase is delayed/arrested and a cell death program is activated.

Our results (Krek et al, 1995) suggest two outcomes of overproducing two different cyclin A-kinase binding-defective mutant species of E2F-1 in these cells. Specifically, these cells both arrested in S phase and died by apoptosis. This death differs from that induced in rodent and monkey cells by overproducing wt E2F-1 under conditions of serum deprivation (Qin et al, 1994, Wu and Levine, 1994). There, the cells died after forced exit from G1 and passage through S. In the case of death resulting from overproduction of the cyclin A-kinase mutants, serum deprivation was not essential to the process. Therefore, the mechanisms resulting in the two phenomena appear to be different.

How cyclin A-kinase phosphorylation of DP-1 during S phase contributes to passage through what seems to be a specific S phase checkpoint remains to be determined. However, one possibility is that cells monitor whether or not E2F-1 remains bound to the chromosome during S phase (Figure 2; see also Krek et al., 1995). If it does, one outcome might well be cell cycle arrest and, in the right circumstance, death. The potential biological value of such a checkpoint remains to be determined, but integrity of a diploid genome seems a possibility worthy of speculation. It is at least worth noting that failure to maintain absolute diploidy is a characteristic of cancer cells. It would be no surprise, then, if this S phase checkpoint were violated in certain cycling tumor cells. If so, the mechanisms underlying such an event might well be fundamental to the evolution of genome plasticity which, in turn, might contribute to certain steps in the tumor development process.

REFERENCES

Girard, F., Strausfeld, U., Fernandez, A. and Lamb, N. J. C. (1991). Cyclin A is required for the onset of DNA replication in mammalian fibroblasts. Cell. 67, 1169–1179.

Krek, W., Xu, G. and Livingston, D. M. (1995). Cyclin A-kinase regulation of E2F-1 DNA binding function underlies suppression of an S phase checkpoint. Cell 83, 1149–1158.

Krek, W., Ewen, M. E., Shirodkar, S., Arany, Z., Kaelin, W. G. and Livingston, D. M. (1994). Negative regulation of the growth-promoting transcription factor E2F-1 by a stably bound cyclin A-dependent protein kinase. Cell 78, 161–172.

Pagano, M., Pepperkok, R., Verde, F., Ansorge, W. and Draetta, G. (1992). Cyclin A is required at two points in the human cell cycle. EMBO J. 11, 961–971.

Pear, W. S., Nolan, G. P., Scott, M. L. and Baltimore, D. (1993). Production of high-titer helper-free retroviruses by transient transfection. Proc. Natl. Acad. Sci. USA. 90, 8392–8396.

Pines, J. and Hunter, T. (1990). Human cyclin A is adenovirus E1A associated protein p60 and behaves differently form cyclin B. Nature 346, 760–763.

Qin, X-Q, Livingston, D., Kaelin Jr., W., and Adams, P. (1994) Deregulated transcritpion factor E2F-1 expression leads to S-phase entry and p53-mediated apoptosis. Proc Nat Acad Sci USA 91, 10918–10922.

Sellers, W., Rodgers, J., and Kaelin Jr., W. (1995) A potent transrepression domain in the retinoblastoma protein induces a cell cycle arrest when bound to E2F sites. Proc Nat Acad Sci USA, 92, 11544–11548.

Weintraub, S., Prater, C., and Dean, D. (1992) Retinoblastoma protein switches the E2F site from positive to negative element Nature, 358, 259–261.

Wu, X. and Levine, A. (1994) p53 and E2F-1 cooperate to mediate apoptosis. Proc Nat Acad Sci USA 91, 3602–3606.

Zindy, F., Lamas, E., Chenivesse, X., Sobczak, J., Wang, J., Fesquet, D., B., H. and Brechot, C. (1992). Cyclin A is required in S phase in normal epithelial cells. Biochem. Biophys Res. Commun. 182, 1144–1154.

DISCUSSION

M. Fried: If I understood you, the cell stops for a while, but then in the next cycle it does not stop again? Does it slow down?

D. Livingston: That is right. We have no evidence that it slows down.

M. Fried: So the question I would ask is: Have you re-isolated the E2F to see if it is really the same one that you initially used--I mean, has it mutated, has it changed in some way?

D. Livingston: The only thing we can say is the following: the E2F that is in those cells in G1 still has the ability to bind to DNA; the E2F-1 in those cells is of the right size; the E2F-1 in those cells is of the same abundance as a mutant that could not bind to DNA intrinsically which was introduced at the same time.

M. Fried: But you have not re-isolated the virus and seen if that virus does the same thing a second time?

D. Livingston: No, that is a good experiment.

F. Rauscher: Could you simply argue that the sniffer or the monitor is simply the output from the target genes?

D. Livingston: It is entirely possible.

F. Rauscher: It is the most likely.

D. Livingston: The question that was asked, is whether the sniffer simply sniffs the output of the target genes. Maybe, but you remember the dl24 transactivation minus mutant also stops the show. And that mutant cannot activate certain genes, just as if it were discharged by cyclin-A kinase phosphorylation from the DNA.

F. Rauscher: So you would argue that there is something else that is recognizing the DNA-bound E2F-DP1 complex?

D. Livingston: There is the testable possibility that, the cell can tell the difference between whether or not certain E2F sites are loaded at the right or the wrong time in S.

G. Evan: Do you know if the apoptotic transcriptional program that E2F elicits arises as a result of the conflict, or is it there whenever E2F is expressed, actively suppressed until there is a cyclin A defect?

D. Livingston: I do not know the answer to that question. The one thing we know is that the NIH-3T3 cells in which these experiments took place are almost certainly p53 plus-minus. So whatever the death mechanism is, it probably does not run through p53.

E. Nigg: There were two members of E2F which do not bind the cyclin-A kinase. Those are the ones that bind to p107, is that right?

D. Livingston: One of them binds p107, and two of them bind p130.

E. Nigg: And those proteins, p107 and p130, in contrast to Rb, they directly bind cyclin-A kinase, themselves.

D. Livingston: They bind cyclin-A kinase but they do so on their pocket spacer elements.

E. Nigg: I know that, but is there a link? Is there a reason why some E2F's would bind directly to cyclin A-cdk2, whereas others would bind via the spacers of p107 and p130?

D. Livingston: It has not escaped our attention that transcription factor binding to certain recognition sites helps certain viral origins of replication to fire. Therefore, are there E2F sites in certain cellular origins?

E. Mihich: There is a restriction point within S. Is there a qualitative difference in DNA synthesis machinery before the restriction point and after, or is machinery completely dissociable from the progression mechanisms? In other words, there is a restriction point in terms of progression or it recognizes a qualitative change in the characteristics of DNA synthesis?

D. Livingston: I cannot tell you in this case, but people have argued for years that there are families of cellular origins that fire at different times in S and that not all origins fire at the beginning of S. So, we would like to try to learn whether the timing of activation of certain origins is altered as a result of failure of cyclin A kinase to bind to a mutant that is defective in transactivation.

G. Evan: Back to my old chestnuts here. So it is described that when you de-regulate the expression of E2F you get p53 dependent apoptosis?

D. Livingston: Yes, and that phenomenon, we think, is different from this one. This phenomenon occurs in high or low serum. Non-cyclin A linked E2F-1 dependents death only occurs in low serum.

G. Evan: When does the latter occur in the cell cycle?

D. Livingston: Death occurs after completion of S and before mitosis.

G. Evan: I am just wondering, if you could invert the argument. So whenever E2F is expressed, an apoptotic program is active - a lá myc. Can you now think of it in terms of things that would be repressing that and which during the course of your experiment, become depressed. So, for example, cyclin-A might be repressing the apoptotic program that is already there, or turning it off by some mechanism. Do these sorts of arguments work?

D. Livingston: Well, I cannot say, but there is a substantial difference between cyclin A deficient and E2F-1 overproduction/low serum death in that a) it appeared to be p53 dependent, b) it occurred somewhere around G2, and, c) there was no S phase arrest.

G. Evan: I will just finish that. But it just seems to me, can you be sure that this apoptosis is not occurring when it is occurring, because you have crippled it.

D. Livingston: Well, the only thing I can say is that it is definitely DNA-binding dependent. That is clear. To kill the protein must be able to bind DNA and to transactivate.

T. Taniguchi: What do you think about the death-inducing and cell cycle control behavior of different E2F family members?

D. Livingston: We have not done cell cycle arrest and control experiments with E2F-2 or 3. We have shown that, like E2F-1, intact E2F-2 and E2F-3 are also oncogenes and that their transforming function is suppressed, in part, by pocket protein binding.

Y. Xiong: What is the evidence that Cyclin A kinase phosphorylation of DP-1 is the key step in preventing the activation of your S phase checkpoint?

D. Livingston: The evidence, one way or the other, should come from experiments performed with a mutant of DP-1 unable to be phosphorylated by E2F-1 bound cyclin A kinase.

M. Oren: A little bit of paraphrasing on Evan's question - You could still argue that cells which are hung up in S because they do not have the transactivation function, are more prone to undergo apoptosis, but they need some kind of push - have you looked at whether those cells can be induced to undergo apoptosis by certain exposures which will not kill normal cells?

D. Livingston: No.

12

HOMEOSTATIC MECHANISMS GOVERNING THE GO PHASE AS DEFINED BY THE *gas* GENES

Claudio Schneider,[*] Giannino Del Sal, Claudio Brancolini, Elisabetta Ruaro, and Sandro Goruppi

Laboratorio Nazionale C.I.B. (Consorzio Interuniversitario per le Biotecnologie
Area Science Park, 99 Padriciano, 34012 Trieste Italy

SUMMARY

Control of proliferation in animal cells is defined by the possible alternative fates that can be chosen, namely differentiation, apoptosis, cell division cycle or Go reversible growth arrest. Here we consider the known biological activities of a set of genes named *gas* (growth arrest specific) that are expressed during Go in NIH3T3 fibroblasts thus identifying an intrinsic genetic program involved in the maintenance of Go.

The products of the *gas* genes show activities that interfere both positively and negatively with the potential of Go cells to re-enter the cell division cycle or to undergo apoptosis thus demonstrating that Go is quite a dynamic state.

INTRODUCTION

The homeostasis of cell proliferation is presently considered as the balance among the following alternative states:

1. RESIDENCE in cell division cycle (CDC)
2. RESIDENCE in Go (REVERSIBLE "OUT OF CYCLE")
3. DIFFERENTIATION
4. APOPTOSIS

Each fate is defined by an *intrinsic control program*, that is a specific genetic program responsible for the coordination and maintenance of the various stages required

---

* Corresponding author. phone (40) 398985; fax (40) 398979.

Cancer Genes, edited by Mihich and Housman
Plenum Press, New York, 1996

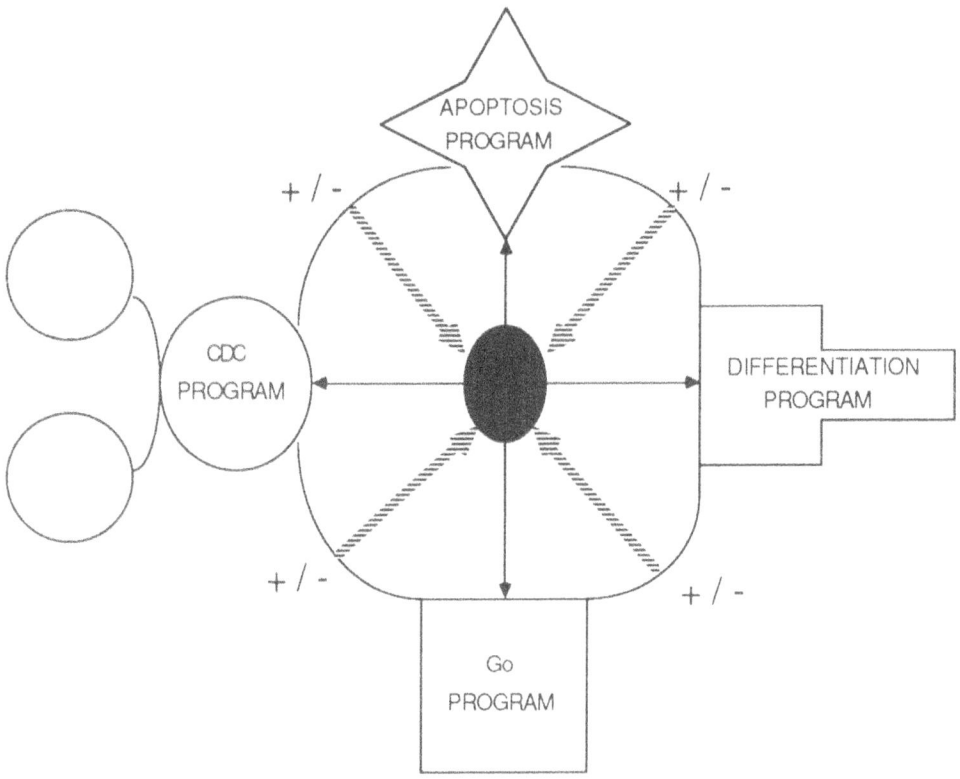

Figure 1. Control of cell proliferation is accomplished by the choice of the various fates as represented here. Each fate corresponds to an autonomous *intrinsic genetic program* (CDC is the abbreviation for Cell Division Cycle). (+/-) represent the *extrinsic factors* necessary either to induce or repress the transition from one fate to another. Shadowed arrows represent the signal transduction pathways and all the changes that take place during the transition from one fate to another (see also fig.2). The black circle represents the signal converting/integrating system whose output sets the final choice commitment.

within the respective fates (for instance, the various phase transitions during the cell division cycle).

Together, these fates define the complex equation of cell proliferation control, the net fraction of dividing cells within a tissue representing the final result among all these available options. The choice among the different fates, as defined by the specific *intrinsic control program*, is governed by *extrinsic controls* ([+]/- in fig.1) the most relevant being:

    1. SELECTIVE SIGNALS: growth factors/survival factors
    2. INSTRUCTIVE SIGNALS: differentiation factors - cytokines
    3. ADHESION TO ECM (extracellular matrix)
    4. CELL-CELL CONTACT - COMMUNICATION
    5. "DAMAGING" agents (physical/chemical)

It is generally accepted that cellular responses are determined both by the total input of extrinsic factors and the actual cellular context (as defined by the intrinsic control program) rather than by a single factor causing an invariant response regardless of the actual context (1,2). Thus, between the extrinsic control elements and the intrinsic control program there lies a shared and complex signal transducing-integrating system (black circle in fig.1). In addition each intrinsic program expresses a specific set of effector elements that feed information through the signal transducing-integrating system, thus conditioning the final response. For instance, given a successful transduction response to a differentiation factor (cytokine), the differentiation program will not necessarily be activated, this being dependent on the effector elements expressed by the former intrinsic program that determine the cellular responsive state (2).

The study of cellular oncogenes has set the framework for the dissection of the extrinsic control and transducing elements while the study of cell cycle control provides us with an understanding of the elements that control and coordinate the different transitions within the intrinsic cell cycle program.

Here we focus on the intrinsic genetic program characterizing Go/reversible growth arrest *in vitro* as exemplified by the study of *gas* (growth arrest specific) genes.

The *gas* (Growth-Arrest-Specific) Genes

When cultured fibroblasts are exposed to external conditions that are restrictive for growth namely diminished growth factor concentration or high cell density, the expression of *gas* genes is increased. On the other hand, when growth restricting conditions are removed (by adding back growth factors and/or decreasing cell density), growth arrested cells re-enter the cell division cycle and concomitantly the expression of the *gas* genes is rapidly downregulated (3). This latter response was in fact the selection imposed to isolate the *gas* genes by subtractive hybridization between growth-arrested versus serum-stimulated NIH3T3 cells. Thus *gas* genes define the existence of a gene repression program that is complementary to the well characterized induction program during the Go to G1 transition (fig.2). Their biological roles more likely reflect a Go maintenance program rather than the actual induction of exit from cell cycle, where an important function seems to be played by different cyclin-dependent kinase (cdk)inhibitory proteins that control the activity of the cell cycle regulatory elements (4).

The following points strenghten this conclusion:

1. the kinetics of *gas* gene induction in response to external growth restrictions is not fast (i.e. occurring within a few hours) but takes at least 12 hours.

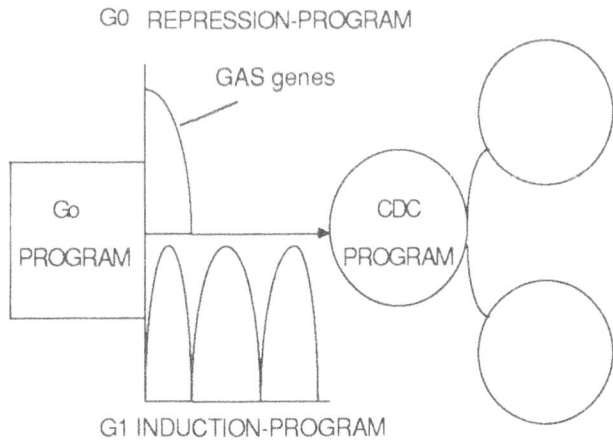

Figure 2. Representation of the genetic changes taking place during the Go to G1 transition. In general during the transitions from a program into another, it is expected that the transduction pathways set up both a "repression program" for genes that were expressed in the previous phase and an "induction program" for genes that are required to set the stage for the final decision (start).

2. with the only exception of *gas1*, the expression of *gas* genes is mainly post transcriptionally controlled (5,6), thus suggesting that their induction is the consequence of a more general and earlier induction mechanism for commitment to
growth arrest.

Similarly to what happens during the various phases of the cell division cycle where
cyclin destruction or cdk inactivation is a prerequisite for entry into next cell cycle phase
(7) we could anticipate that the *gas* gene repression program may represent the required
clearing of the Go program thus allowing the alternative programs to take place. .

With these considerations in mind we will now analyze the known biological activities of the *gas* genes that have been studied so far in our laboratory.

RESULTS

gas 1

The protein product of *gas1* cDNA has an apparent molecular weight of 40 kD. It is
a glycosylated membrane protein that faces the extracellular side of the plasma membrane
(8) to which it is linked via a GPI anchor (Stebel et al, submitted). When the steady state
analysis of the protein level is performed at different growth conditions, the protein expression pattern parallels exactly the mRNA behaviour (8), namely high relative expression at Go, low expression in exponentially dividing cells or during the Go to G1
transition. Cloning of the human *gas1* homologue led to the chromosomal localization of
the *gas1* gene on 9q21.3–22.1 in a region which is involved in myeloid neoplasias and
also in bladder carcinomas. Alignment between the protein products of human and mouse
gas1 revealed 82 % of amino acid identity (9).

Expression analysis of the human and murine Gas1, in resting versus proliferating
normal fibroblasts and in transformed cells, invariably shows that its down-modulation
correlates with the transition from the resting to the activated state, in untransformed cells,
or from the normal to the transformed state. The involvement of Gas1 as a putative negative regulator of cell growth was therefore suggested.

We addressed the question of the biological effects caused by ectopic expression of
gas1 under conditions where the endogenous *gas1* product is not expressed, namely: i)
during the Go-->S phase transition of untrasformed murine fibroblasts ii) in cells growing
asynchronously and iii) in the same cells transformed with various oncogenes.

A detailed microinjection analysis showed that overexpression of *gas1* in quiescent
cells abrogates their ability to enter S phase after serum addition. However, this block in
G1 is not the result of a defective early serum response, since the induction of *c-fos* and *c-
jun* was normal. Single oncogene transformed cell lines (*v-fos*, *v-myc*, *v-ras* and *v-src*) are
also growth arrested by *gas1* overexpression, suggesting that these cells, although unable
to regulate the endogenous *gas1* and the quiescence program, nevertheless retain the ability to respond to Gas1 reintroduction. All this evidence suggests that the putative effector
for the proliferation block induced by *gas1* may be constitutively expressed in all the
tested cells. However, cells transformed with SV40-LT and with the Adenovirus type 5
were unresponsive to Gas1 reintroduction (8). The lack of response in these cell lines, together with the lack of response later observed also in the SAOS2 cell line (9), suggested
that the inactivation of RB and /or p53 could play a role in the *gas1* mediated growth arrest.

In fact, by using various cell lines transformed with LT mutants defective in the RB/p107 or the p53 binding, we have been able to demonstrate that Gas1 blocks cell proliferation only in the presence of p53 (10). This result was confirmed by extending the analysis also in cell lines transformed with the oncogene products of the human papilloma virus type 16 and in fibroblasts derived from the p53 -/- null mice.

The role of p53 in growth control is well established and in this context its transactivating functions seem to play a major role (11). By using various p53 mutants defective in its DNA binding (p53 AV135 or p53KH215) or in its transactivating functions (p53 double mutant LQ24WS25) we found that the latter function is dispensable for mediating the *gas1* growth inhibitory effect (10.). Since the DNA binding of p53 is, however, still required to allow the *gas1*-mediated growth arrest the p53 function required could involve either its reported transcription repression activity or its association with other transcription factors to repress or indirectly induce genes responsible for the *gas1* growth arrest. These genes may not necessarily coincide with those induced directly by p53 and, in fact, we have not observed induction of *waf1* which is probably more relevant in the G1 arrest directly induced by p53(10)

These results point to the existence of a still uncharacterized gas1-dependent signaling pathway from the membrane to p53 causing growth arrest consequent to unbalanced growth conditions as represented by the unscheduled expression of the growth arrest specific gene *gas1*.

gas2

gas2 gene encodes a protein of 36 kd (3) which is a component of the microfilament system predominantly located at the cell border of growth arrested mouse and human fibroblasts (12). Upon treatment of growth arrested cells with different mitogenic stimuli such as serum, PDGF, LPA and PMA, Gas2 biosynthesis is downregulated, but, since the half-life of the Gas2 product is longer than 12 hours, the total amount of protein does not change appreciably during growth stimulation. Indeed a remarkable difference can be observed in the level of phosphorylation: Gas2 is rapidly phosphorylated within the first minutes of the Go->G1 transition (13).

Whether Gas2 phosphorylation is an important switch to regulate its activity is still unknown. However, its kinetics of phosphorylation is temporally coupled to changes in microfilament system organization as observed during Go->G1 transition. In fact, Gas2 relocalizes at the membrane ruffling following treatment of growth arrested cells with different mitogenic stimuli. Moreover, the specific relationship between Gas2 phosphorylation and membrane ruffling formation is strengthened by the fact that stimuli able to elicit membrane ruffling formation (such PDGF, or PMA) trigger Gas2 phosphorylation, while mitogenic stimuli unable to elicit membrane ruffling formation, such as LPA, are unable to hyperphosphorylate Gas2 (13).

Membrane ruffling is drastically inhibited in serum-starved and contact inhibited cells, conditions that normally induce *gas2* expression. Conversely cellular transformation by various oncogenes is accompanied by an increased membrane ruffling (14), and these cells fail to induce *gas2* expression (12). Thus, if any correlation exists between Gas2 and membrane ruffling, this would uncover a negative controlling function of Gas2 on the formation of membrane ruffling which could be circumvented by its phosphorylation.

Reorganization of the microfilament system is a consensus requirement during Go->G1 transition together with the activation of motility: these changes are regulated by the small GTP-binding protein rho and rac (15).

Conversely, cellular responses dependent on the microfilament systems, become dramatically restricted in quiescent cells and in analogy with *gas2*, also increased expression of MARCKS (myristoylated alanine rich protein kinase C substrate), a protein involved in cross-linking actin filaments to plasma membrane (16), has been observed (17).

Involvement of Gas2 in the organization of the microfilament system was clearly shown by overexpression of a deleted derivative lacking the carboxyl-terminal region (gas2 Δ276–314) which, in contrast to overexpression of the wild-type gas2, induces dramatic changes in actin architecture and cell shape as shown in figure 3. These effects were shown to be ascribed to a gain of function since no interference by the wild-type product could be found (18).

If the Gas2 had a role in the organization of microfilament system by restricting cell motility, the uncovering of such a potent activity in a deleted derivative called for a candidate function of Gas2 in the other two alternative fates, that is differentiation and apoptosis. In both cases reorganization of the microfilament system takes place and involvement of Gas2 could be predicted if a strictly controlled biochemical mechanism generating such a carboxyl-terminal deletion could exist. By serendipity we have been able to demonstrate that during apoptosis the carboxy terminal domain of Gas2 is specifically removed by proteolytic cleavage resulting in a protein that is similar in size to the ar-

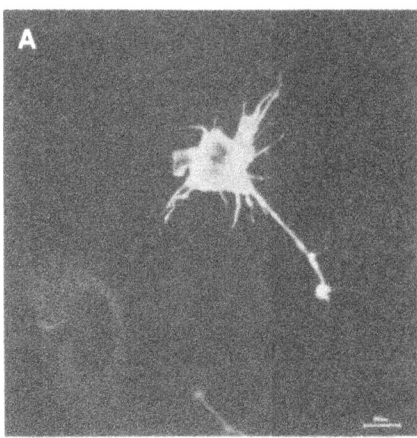
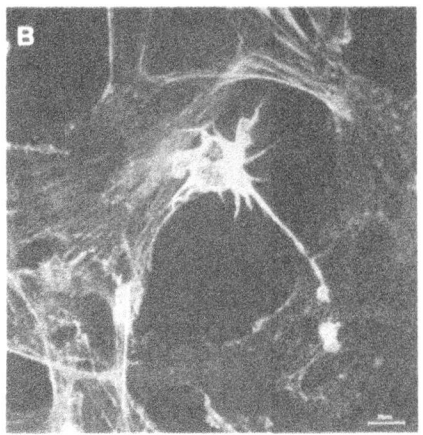

Figure 3. Immunofluorescence analysis of NIH3T3 cells overexpressing *gas2* COOH-terminal deleted derivative. NIH3T3 cells 24 hours after seeding were microinjected with an eukaryotic expression vector containing *gas2* COOH deleted derivative (100ng/μl). After 20 hours cells were fixed and processed for immunofluorescence analysis to visualize Gas2 (A) and stained with phalloidin-TRITC to visualize actin filaments (B). Bar 25 μm.

tificially deleted product showing such striking morphological effects. By using in vitro mutagenesis we have clarified that the in vivo apotosis-associated processing is dependent on an aspartic residue at position 279 of the Gas2 thus indicating the possible involvement of an ICE-like protease (18)

It is worth to note that the apoptotic phenotype should depend on a fine orchestration between different regulators and effectors each responsible for the distinct changes taking place in the various cellular compartments . In this respect the ICE-like dependent proteolytic cleavage of Gas2 represents the first example of a mechanism coupling apoptosis with the changes in the microfilament system. It remains to be understood if Go is generally characterized by increased susceptibility to apoptosis thus possibly explaining the accumulation of an apoptotic effector such as Gas2 in a preactivated state. In addition, by a choice for economy, two different functions could coexist in the Gas2 : a growth-arrest function related to its increased level and an apoptotic function dependent on its proteolytic cleavage at the carboxy-terminal domain. Both functions should involve regulation of the microfilament system as related to the different requirements of reversible growth-arrest or apoptosis.

gas3

gas3 gene encodes a 22 kD integral membrane glycoprotein (6). Two other groups studying gene expression during peripheral nerve regeneration, have independently isolated the rat homologue of *gas3*, named *PMP22* (peripheral myelin protein) (19,20).Nerve injury leads to proliferation of Schwann cells with the accompanying downregulation of mRNA and protein levels of Gas3/PMP22 (21). These results suggested similar regulatory mechanisms dependent on *gas3* expression in NIH3T3 *in vitro* and in Schwann cells *in vivo*. Genetic defects in both the *Trembler* (Tr) and TrJ mutant mice, characterised by increased proliferation of Schwann cells and hypomyelination, were shown to depend on point mutations within the transmembrane domains of Gas3/PMP22 (22). The human peripheral neuropathys Charcot-Marie Tooth type 1A (CMT1A) and Dejerine-Sottas syndrome are also characterized by point mutations within *gas3/PMP22* (23,24)with dominant type of inheritance while in HNPP-tomaculous neuropathy a mutation within gas3/PMP22 has been shown to segregate as a recessive trait.(24). Other cases of CMT1A have been accounted by large duplications of the short arm of chromosome 17 containing the *gas3/PMP22* gene while in the case of HNPP by a deletion of the same chromosomal region(24). These studies give clear evidence that a variety of genetic alterations, such as point mutations, amplifications and deletions of the *gas3/PMP22* gene result in a pathological phenotype, suggesting that both gene dosage and gene function are critical for the correct control of Schwann cell proliferation during differentiation to myelin.

Although the Gas3/PMP22 protein is expressed at highest levels in differentiated Schwann cells, its reported expression in non-neuronal tissues and in growth-arrested NIH-3T3 fibroblasts (25) indicates a more general function that is uncoupled to myelin structure. We have shown that *wt-gas3/PMP22* overexpression in NIH-3T3 cells leads to an apoptotic phenotype which is efficiently suppressed by antioxidants and characterized by typical membrane blebbing, rounding-up and chromatin condensation but with no evidence of DNA fragmentation.(25 and figure 4). When the dominant behaving alleles of CMT1A or the recessive allele associated with HNPP were similarly overexpressed in NIH-3T3 cells a significant reduced ability in inducing the apoptotic phenotype was noticed. By coexpressing the different mutants with the wild-type, thus reproducing a heterozygous condition, we have provided evidence that the dominant mutations behave as

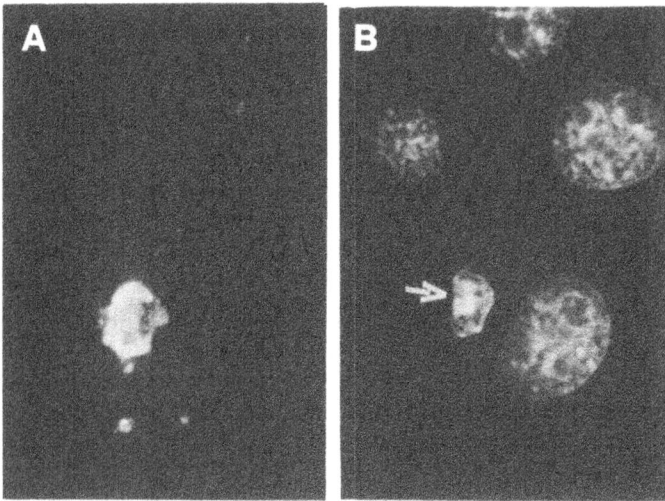

Figure 4. Confocal generated overlay of NIH3T3 cells overexpressing *gas3*. NIH3T3 cells 24 hours after seeding were microinjected with an eukaryotic expression vector containing *gas3* (100ng/µl). After 20 hours cells were fixed and processed for immunofluorescence analysis to visualize Gas3 (green) and stained with propidium iodide to visualize nuclei (red). Images were overlaied using a Zeiss confocal microscope and are displayed in pseudocolors. Bar 25 µm.

dominant negative with respect to the apoptotic phenotype induced by the wild type whereas the recessive mutant behaves as recessive under the same coexpression experiments (25).

We can thus speculate that the regulation of susceptibility to apoptosis by Gas3/PMP22 could play a relevant role in the control of Schwann cell-differentiation. Here again control of Schwann cell renewal *in vivo* should reflect the balance of the various alternative fates namely continued cellular division, Go, differentiation into myelin or apoptosis. Defects in modulating cellular responsiveness to apoptosis as evidenced in the Gas3/PMP22 mutants could thus explain continued proliferation and a cosequent lack of correct differentiation as found in the pathological conditions. However, as previously hypothesised for Gas2, this function of Gas3/PMP22 does not exclude a second ,more specialized, structural role in myelin formation or maintenance. This second function should only be compatible with suppression of its apoptotic modulatory function which in turn depends on the actual intrinsic cellular responsiveness. The case of a dual function, both as a regulator of apoptosis and as structural component in a given differentiation pathway, could be evolutionary economical and logical. A similar dual function has also been claimed for the structurally related myelin protein of the central nervous system PLP (proteolipid protein). Mutations in PLP gene are responsible for the Pelizaeus-Merzbacher disease characterized by degeneration and premature cell death of oligodendrocytes with associated hypomyelination. In this case particular mutations (rumpshaker mouse) have led to a clear dissection between a constitutive function of PLP in myelin and a control function for survival of oligodendrocytes (26) In non neuronal tissues, where gas3/PMP22 is also expressed, only the antiproliferative activity as related to its apoptotic effector function should be considered. Apoptosis should in fact be considered as part of the homeostatic balance that regulates Go where Gas3/PMP22 expression is increased. Withdrawal from the cell cycle after growth factor deprivation increases cellular sensitivity towards apoptosis : increased expression of Gas3/PMP22 should therefore represent a logical consequence.

gas6

Gas6 is a secreted glycoprotein, member of the vitamin K-dependent protein family with a clear homology to the human serum protein S (44% of amino acid identity) (27), a negative co-regulator in the blood coagulation cascade. Both murine and human *gas6* cDNA were isolated and shown to code for highly conserved proteins (81% amino acid sequence identity). Similarly to protein S (28), Gas6 consists of several defined structural motifs : an extensively γ-carboxylated amino terminal domain (Gla-domain), four EGF like repeats and a long carboxy terminal domain with similarity to steroid binding globulin. This domain is the most divergent from protein S showing different gaps within the sequence alignement. We suggested that, despite the significant homology of Gas6 with protein S, the function of Gas6 *in vivo* is likely to be different from that of protein S, at least for the control of blood coagulation and complement proteolytic cascades. This is confirmed by the different pattern of expression of *gas6* with respect to protein S, whose expression is most abundant in liver, while *gas6* is widely expressed in many tissues both in mouse and human.

Using a cell based autophosphorylation assay, Gas6 was recently identified from conditioned media of cultured cells as the ligand for the orphan growth factor receptor Axl (29). Axl is a tyrosine kinase receptor (TKR) involved in cell transformation (30,31) with an extracellular domain consisting of two fibronectin type III repeats linked with two immunoglobulin like domains. Axl is the founder of a growing family of TKR whose members recognize related ligands. Recently the Axl related Tyro TKR has been demonstrated to specifically interact with bovine ProteinS (32) thus possibly explaining the role of humanProteinS as a mitogen for vascular smooth muscle cells(33). The transforming activity of Axl indicates that it should be able to drive cellular proliferation. Consistently we have demonstrated that Gas6 behaves as a growth factor stimulating cell cycle re-entry of NIH3T3 growth arrested by low serum(34) and that such mitogenic effect is ascribed to Axl-Gas6 interaction. Moreover, as could be anticipated, the mitogenic activity coincides with activation of Axl tyrosine kinase and consequent MAPK cascade. In addition to this mitogenic activity we have shown that Gas6 can efficiently protect serum starved NIH3T3 fibroblasts from cell death as induced by complete factor removal(34). Gas6 survival factor activity was in fact biochemically assessed by its ability to prevent Gas2 proteolytic processing as specifically related to apoptosis. We have also been able to uncouple the mitogenic from survival activity since growth-arrested NIH3T3 cells fail to enter S-phase after complete factor removal in the presence of Gas6 while efficiently re-entering the cell cycle in the presence of bFGF(34). Therefore Gas6 can display separate activities during growth arrest induced by low serum starvation: cell proliferation and cell survival. The apparent paradox of enhanced expression at growth arrest of *gas6*, a mitogenic growth factor, should therefore be explained by considering its distinct survival factor function as uncovered after complete serum removal from NIH3T3 cells. When considering the G0 state as a "out of cycle" situation where cells can decide for different options such as proliferation or apoptosis, the regulated expression of Gas6 should be viewed within the respective homeostatic control for maintaining such options open.

DISCUSSION

Go as a Dynamic "State"

Each cellular fate involved in the control of cell proliferation (fig.1) represents by itself a fine homeostasis governed both by the extrinsic factors and by the intrinsic program (expressed effector elements) feeding their specific information into the signal transducing-integrating system. The decision whether to stay within the same program or to choose an alternative fate is taken once all incoming signals have been processed and integrated .

Functional analysis of the *gas* gene products has indicated that Go is to be considered as a homeostatic balance whereby the products of Go intrinsic program,the gas genes,are both able to restrict and promote cellular responses leading to the alternative choices allowed from Go .

When considering the interface between Go and the cell division cycle program, Gas1 shows a clear growth suppressing activity while Gas6 shows growth promoting activity. These two activities, determined by the intrinsic Go program, could therefore work as a homeostasic mechanism for maintaining the reversible option to enter the cell division cycle program as alternative to Go.

When considering the interface of Go with the apoptosis program, both *gas2* and *gas3* seem to act as " apoptotic effectors" at distinct subcellular domains. In fact the processed product of *gas2*, as produced during activation of the apoptotic program by the ICE-like upstream effectors, is sufficient to organize the microfilament dependent changes in morphology that accompany apoptosis. Gas3, when reaching a critical level of expression, seems to be involved in the compaction of the plasmamembrane that typically takes place in apoptosing cells, as well as during myelin formation (35). On the other side Gas6 should act here as a potent survival factor, thus establishing the relevant homeostatic loop.

The activities of the *gas* gene products, relative to their involvement in the homeostatic mechanisms here hypothesized, are schematically represented in figure 5.

The hypothesis that some products of the Go maintenance program are to be considered as potential apoptotic effectors poses an obvious paradox: why should Go prime for the apoptosis program?

It has been established (1) that withdrawal from the cell cycle after growth factor deprivation increases cellular susceptibility toward apoptosis : increased expression both Gas2 and Gas3 should represent an expected consequence. Moreover when we consider *gas* gene downregulation during cell cycle reentry and differentiation, both fully viable alternative choices with respect to apoptosis, active neutralization of the apoptotic effectors intrinsic to Go program should become a necessary requirement to be overcome by the extrinsic factors. If the external conditions are non optimal, apoptosis might represent the best and only choice.

In a wider perspective downregulation of *gas* genes and/or neutralization of their products should thus be considered as a "checkpoint" to pass before the 'start' of other programs. In this light the growth suppressing function of *gas1* should also be a checkpoint identifying an unbalanced growth condition as defined by the unscheduled expression of a growth arrest specific gene during the 'in cycle' program. In line with this hypothesis, the cell cycle checkpoint function of p53 has been shown to transduce the *gas1*-dependent arrest. We cannot rule out that under defined conditions also *gas1* might be involved in the homeostasis Goapoptosis due to its ability to activate p53 functions . In this respect it has been reported that tissues undergoing programmed cell death, such as

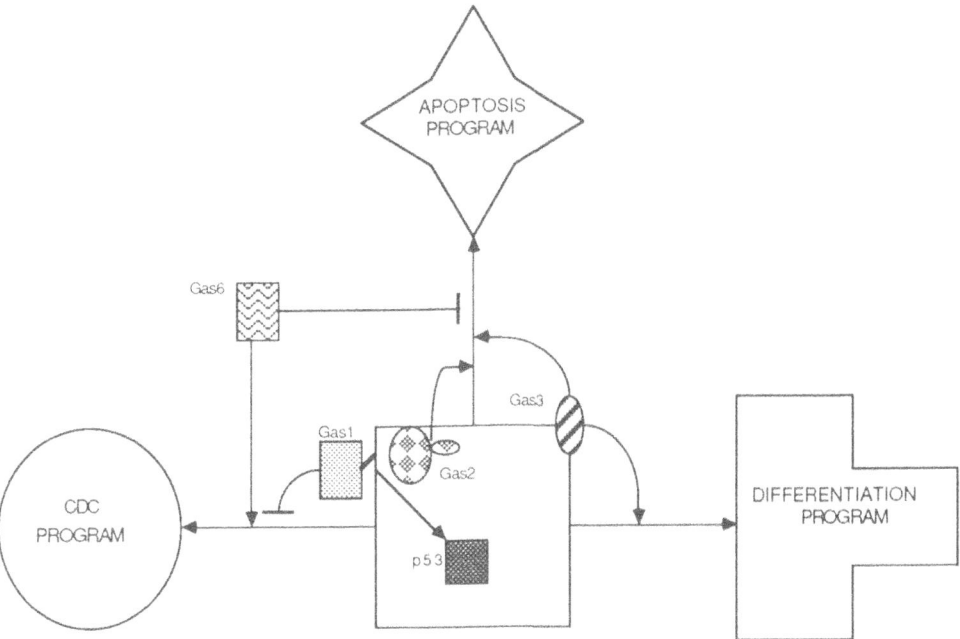

Figure 5. Summary of the known and hypothesized functions for the *gas* gene products analyzed in relation to the alternative programs available from the reversible growth arrest Go state. Arrows indicate activation or stimulation while lines with blunt arrowheads indicate repression or inhibition.

uterus (36) and both prostate and mammary epithelium (R. Friis, pers. comm.) show a marked increase in the expression of *gas1* during organ involution.

Finally, when considering the interface Go/differentiation, active neutralization of the potential apoptotic effector functions could be used as a selection step in some differentiation pathways for conditional survival, whenever the same gene product serves a dual function both as a regulator of apoptosis and as a structural component within a specific differentiative program. This is best exemplified by the expression of *gas3* during myelin formation in Schwann cells where refractoriness to Gas3 apoptotic function could become intrinsically coupled to its putatively required constitutive function for membrane compaction.

In conclusion, *gas* gene products seem to act within Go to either restrict or promote alternative fates thus defining the Go homeostasis. They also seem to fulfill the role of checkpoints in regulating the transitions into the alternative fates as driven by the extrinsic factors .

Transformed cells are by definition unable to obey growth restrictions by exiting cell cycle and reaching Go. In agreement no induction of *gas* gene expression has been observed in transformed cells upon serum starvation (3,6,8). This is likely to be a consequence of the intrinsic defects in inducing the Go program that characterize transformed cells. However we have clearly shown that transformed cells are still responsive to the growth suppressing activity of Gas1 as long as they express a functional p53. In addition we can envisage that uncoupled *gas* gene expression might even prime transformed cells for apoptosis. Obviously the transformation process selects against mechanisms making available such fates (Go or apoptosis), as extensively shown by the high incidence of mutations found in the p53 gene (37), and lack of *gas* gene expression thus appears to be necessary consequence.

ACKNOWLEDGMENTS

We would like to thank dr. Margherita Zanetti for carefully reading the manuscript. Work in this laboratory has been supported by funds from AIRC (Associazione Italiana per la Ricerca sul Cancro) and Telethon to C.S.

REFERENCES

1. Raff, M.C. (1992). Social controls on cell survival and cell death. *Nature(London)* **356,** 397–399.
2. Jessen, K.R. and Mirsky, R. (1994). Fate diverted. *Current Biology* **4,** 824–827.
3. Schneider, C., King, R.M. and Philipson, L. (1988). Genes specifically expressed at growth arrest of mammalian cells. *Cell* **54,** 787–793.
4. Peter, M. and Herskowitz, I. (1994). Joining the complex: Cyclin-dependent kinase inhibitory proteins and the cell cycle. *Cell* **79,** 181–184.
5. Ciccarelli, C., Philipson, L. and Sorrentino, V. (1990). Regulation of expression of growth arrest specific genes in mouse fibroblasts. *Mol. Cell. Biol.* **10,** 1525–1529.
6. Manfioletti, G., Ruaro, M.E., Del Sal, G., Philipson, L. and Schneider, C. (1990). A growth arrest-specific (*gas*) gene codes for a membrane protein. *Mol. Cell. Biol.* **10,** 2924–2930.
7. Hartwell, L.H. and Weinert, T.A. (1989). Checkpoints: controls that ensure the order of cell cycle events. *Science* **246,** 629–634.
8. Del Sal, G., Ruaro, M.E., Philipson, L. and Schneider, C. (1992). The growth arrest specific gene, gas 1, is involved in growth suppression. *Cell* **70,** 595–607.
9. Del Sal, G., Collavin, L., Ruaro, M.E. Edomi, P., Saccone, S., Della Valle, G. and Schneider, C. (1994). Structure, function, and chromosome mapping of the growth suppressing human homologue of the murine gas1 gene. *Proc. Natl. Acad. Sci. USA* **91,** 1848–1852.
10. DelSal, G., Ruaro, M.E., Utrera, R., Cole, C.N., Levine, A.J. and Schneider, C. (1995) Gas1 induced growth suppression requires p53 independently of its intrinsic transactivation function. submitted *Mol.Cell Biol.*
11. Zambetti, G.P. and Levine, A.J. (1993). A comparison of the biological activities of wild-type and mutant p53.*FASEB J.* **7,** 855–865.
12. Brancolini, C., Bottega, S. and Schneider, C. (1992). Gas2, a growth arrest-specific protein, is a component of the microfilament network system. *J. Cell Biol.* **117,**1251–1261.
13. Brancolini, C. and Schneider, C. (1994). Phosphorylation of the growth arrest specific protein Gas2 is coupled to actin rearrangements during Go-> G1 transition in NIH 3T3 cells. *J. Cell Biol.* **124,** 743–756.
14. Ridley, A.J. (1994). Membrane ruffling and signal transduction. *BioEssays.* **16,** 321–327.
15. Nobes, C. and Hall, A. (1994). Regulation and function of the Rho subfamily of small GTPase. *Curr. Opin. Gen. Dev.* **4,** 77–81.
16. Hartwig, J. H., Thelen, M., Rosen, A., Janmey, P.A., Nairn, A.C. and Aderem, A. (1992). MARCKS is an actin filament crosslinking protein regulated by protein kinase C and calcium-calmodulin. *Nature (London)* **356,** 618–622.
17. Herget, T., Brooks, S.F., Broad, S. and Rozengurt, E. (1993). Expression of the major protein kinase C substrate, the acidic 80-kilodalton myristoylated alanine-rich C kinase substrate, increases sharply when Swiss 3T3 cells move out of cycle. *Proc. Natl. Acad. Sci. USA.* **90,** 2945–2949.
18. Brancolini, C., Benedetti, M. and Schneider, C. (1995) Microfilament reorganization during apoptosis: the role of Gas2, apossible substrate for ICE-like proteases *EMBO J.* in the press
19. Spreyer, P., Kuhn, G., Hanemann, C.O., Gillen, C., Schaal, H., Kuhn, R., Lemke, G. and Muller, H.W. (1991). Axon-regulated expression of a Schwann cell transcript that is homologous to a "growth arrest-specific" gene. *EMBO J.* **10,** 3661–3668.
20. Welcher, A.A., Suter, U., De Leon, M., Snipes, G.J. and Shooter, E.M. (1991). A myelin protein is encoded by the homologue of a growth arrest-specific gene. *Proc. Natl. Acad. Sci. USA* **88,** 7195–7199.

21. Snipes, G.J., Suter, U., Welcher, A.A. and Shooter, E.M. (1992). Characterization of a novel peripheral nervous system myelin protein (PMP-22/SR13). *J. Cell Biol.* **117**, 225–238.

22. Suter, U., Welcher, A.A., Ozcelik, T., Snipes, G.J., Kosaras, B., Francke, U., Billings-Gagliardi, S., Sidman, R.L. and Shooter, E.M. (1992). Trembler mouse carries a point mutation in a myelin gene. *Nature(London)* **356**, 241–244.

23. Valentijn, L.J., Baas, F., Wolterman, R.A., Hoogendijk, J.E., Van Den Bosch, N.H.A., Zorn, I., Gabreels-Festen, A.A.W.M., De Visser, M. and Bolhuis, P.A. (1992). Identical point mutations of PMP-22 in Trembler-J mouse and Charcot-Marie-Tooth disease type 1A. *Nature Genet.* **2**, 228–291.

24. Patel, P.J. and Lupski, J.R. (1994). Charcot-Marie-Tooth disease: a new paradigm for the mechanism of inherited disease. *TIG.* **10**, 128–133.

25. Fabbretti, E., Edomi, P., Brancolini, C. and Schneider, C. (1995) Apoptotic phenotype induced by overrepression of wild-type *gas3/PMP22* : its relation to the demyelinating peripheral neuropathy CMT1A. *Genes & Develop.* in the press

26. Schneider, A., Montague, P., Griffiths, I., Fanarraga, M., Kennedy, P., Brophy, P., and Nave, K.A. (1992). Uncoupling of hypomyelination and glial cell death by mutation in the proteolipid protein gene. *Nature (London)* **358**, 758–761.

27. Manfioletti, G., Brancolini, C., Avanzi, G. and Schneider, C. (1993). The protein encoded by a growth arrest specific gene (gas6) is a new member of the vitamin K-dependent proteins related to protein S, a negative coregulator in the blood coagulation cascade. *Mol. Cell. Biol.* **13**, 4976–4985.

28. Lundwall, A., Dackowski, W., Cohen, E., Shaffer, M., Mahr, A., Dahlbäck, B., Stenflo, J. and Wydro, R. (1986). Isolation and sequence of the cDNA for human protein S, a regulator of blood coagulation. *Proc. Natl. Acad. Sci. USA* **83**, 6716–6720.

29. Varnum,B.et al. (1995) Axl receptor tyrosine kinase stimulated by the vitamin K-dependent protein encoded by growth-arrest-specific gene 6 *Nature*, **373**,623–626

30. O'Bryan, J.P., Frye, R.A., Cogswell, P.C., Neubauer, A., Kitch, B., Prokop, C., EspinosaIII, R., Le Beau, M.M., Earp, H.S. and Liu, E.T. (1991). Axl, a transforming gene isolated from primary human myeloid leukemia cells, encodes a novel receptor tyrosine kinase. *Mol. Cell. Biol.* **11**, 5016–5031.

31. Janssen, J.W.G., Schultz, A.S., Steendoorden, A.C.N., Schmidberger, M., Strehl, S., Ambros, P.F. and Bartram, C.R. (1991). A novel putative tyrosine kinase receptor with oncogenic potential. *Oncogene* **6**, 2113–2120.

32. Stltt, T.N. et al. (1995) The anticoagulant factor proteinS and its relative, Gas6, are ligands for the Tyro3/Axl family of receptor tyrosine kinases *Cell*,80, 661–670

33. Gasic, P., Arenas, C.P., Gasic, T.B. and Gasic, G.J. (1992). Coagulation factors X, Xa, and protein S as potent mitogens of cultured aortic smooth muscle cells. *Proc.Natl.Acad.Sci. USA* **89**, 2317–2320.

34. Goruppi,S., Ruaro,M.E. and Schneider,C. (1995) Gas6, the ligand of Axl tyrosine kinase receptor, has mitogenic and survival activities for serum starved NIH3T3 fibroblasts. Submitted *Oncogene*

35. Doyle, J.P. and Colman, D.R. (1993). Glial-neuron interactions and the regulation of myelin formation. *Curr. Opin. Cell Biol.* **5**, 779–785.

36. Ferrero, M. and Cairo, G. (1993). Estrogen-regulated expression of growth arrest specific gene (gas1) in rat uterus. *Cell Biol. International* **17**, 857–862.

37. Hollstein, M., Sidransky, D., Vogelstein, B. and Harris, C.C. (1991). p53 Mutations in human cancers. *Science* **253**, 49–53.

DISCUSSION

G. Draetta: You are putting these gas genes, in that picture, as if they belonged to the same cell type but in fact you do see differences in expression.

C. Schneider: Yes.

G. Draetta: So the effects that you see in induction of apoptosis could be, for example, in the case of gas-3, due to the heterologous expression of the gene and have nothing to do with the fact that this gene is normally involved in the regulating apoptosis?

C. Schneider: As I have shown for REF52 cells which do not express any endogenous gas3, they do not respond to overexpression of gas3 in terms of apoptosis. In this case my interpretation is that REF52 cells also lack the downstream mechanisms required for inducing the described phenotypic alterations as seen in NIH3T3 cells. Obviously it is important in this respect to bear in mind that within various differentiation pathways or within a given pathway it is expected to find different responses towards apoptotic regulators.

P. Comoglio: I am a little confused as to why gas-6 is a gas gene, because it looked to me like a growth factor; it is expressed by cells, it activates the RAS pathway and kinases, and under peculiar conditions does not induce proliferation but only survival. This is sort of a common feature for other growth factors. Did I miss some critical point? Why is it a gas gene?

C. Schneider: It is a "gas" gene because it is produced by growth arrested cells and not by growing cells.

P. Comoglio: 99% of growth factor are produced by non-growing cells.

C. Schneider: I agree, but in the case of gas 6, it is specifically induced when cells are growth arrested. Actually, I did not show the slide demonstrating that gas 6 becomes dramatically and specifically accumulated in the conditioned medium of serum starved human fibroblasts. In fact, gas 6 was identified as the ligand of Axl from conditioned medium of human fibroblasts serum starved for one week. So, it is specifically produced when cells are growth arrested. If it turns out to have professional growth factor activity for NIH3T3 cells, this could only be dependent on its demonstrated ability to turn on, albeit not dramatically, the ras/mapk pathway in these very cells. Its real biological function should anyway be transduced through other yet unidentificated and not Ras depending signaling pathway that we are trying to characterize. In the context of homeostatis at growth arrest its elected function should be anyway suppression of apoptosis as I have shown. In fact, when serum starved NIH3T3 cells are treated with gas 6 in serum free medium they happily survive (up to 24 hours) without entering S phase (as in the case of bFGF). I can therefore conclude that in this case also in NIH3T3 gas 6 does not activate the Ras/mapK pathway. In addition, I expect that gas 6 should also induce specific differentiation functions in fibroblasts or in general stromal cells where axl receptor is expressed. As shown from the 2D pattern of proteins induced by gas6 there are clear differences from the pattern induced by PDFG. In conclusion, gas6 is not a professional growth factor and its response should at the moment be envisaged in terms of its functional role at growth arrest.

T. Sutter: Did you examine these genes also in benign and malignant tumors from patients with neurofibromatosis?

C. Schneider: We have not looked at those.

13

THE *TEL* GENE AND HUMAN LEUKEMIAS

Todd R. Golub, George F. Barker, Kimberly Stegmaier, and D. Gary Gilliland

Division of Hematology/Oncology
Department of Medicine
Brigham and Women's Hospital and Children's Hospital
Harvard Medical School, Boston, Massachusetts 02115

1. INTRODUCTION

Chromosomal translocations have provided valuable insights into the molecular mechanisms of leukemogenesis in humans. Examples of genes implicated in pathogenesis of hematologic malignancy by virtue of involvement in translocation breakpoints include the PML-RARa fusion associated with t(15;17) acute promyelocytic leukemia (APML, refs. 1–3), the AML1-ETO fusion associated with t(8;21) acute myeloid leukemia (AML, ref.4), the CBFß-MYHII fusion associated with inv(16) acute myelomonocytic leukemia and eosinophilia (5), and MLL fusions at 11q23 breakpoints with various fusion proteins associatcd with acute myeloid leukemias (6).

Evidence which supports a role for these fusion proteins in pathogenesis of acute myeloid leukemia includes the invariant association of chromosomal translocations with specific disease phenotypes and the striking conservation of translocation breakpoints. For example, all leukemias associated with 11q23 translocations have highly conserved breakpoints within the MLL (ALL-1, HRX) gene (6). Similar conservation of breakpoints is seen in patients with APML. Patients with APML invariably have translocations involving the retinoic acid receptor-a (RAR-a) gene. The vast majority of these have t(15;17), and t(15;17) is invariably associated with the phenotype of APML but not with other subtypes of AML. The consequence of t(15;17) is fusion of the PML and RARa genes; the breakpoint occurs within the same intron of RARa in all patients, and occurs in one of two introns within the PML gene. All of the resultant fusions preserve the same functional domains of PML-RARa . Similar conservation of functional domains and association with specific phenotypes is seen in chromosomal translocations associated with the other subtypes of AML noted above.

Although these data provide convincing evidence that chromosomal translocations are necessary for manifestation of the leukemic phenotype, there is equally convincing evidence that leukemia, like other human cancers, requires more than one molecular genetic abnormality. Multistep pathogenesis of leukemia is supported first by rare but informative families with inherited propensity to develop leukemia (7) As for pedigrees with inherited forms of breast cancer and colon cancer, it is likely that affected members of pedigrees with inherited leukemia carry a germ line mutation which predisposes to the acquisition of a second mutation in somatic tissue, which in turn gives rise to the malignant phenotype. One example is the inheritance of a mutant DNA repair gene, MSH2, which predisposes affected members of hereditary non-polyposis coli pedigrees to the development of colon cancer (8). A second observation which supports multistep pathogenesis of AML is the phenomenon of clonal remission (9). Clonal remission occurs infrequently after induction of remission from AML using chemotherapeutic agents. Patients with clonal remission meet all diagnostic criteria for remission including normal blood counts and differential, normal morphology and normal cytogenetics, but can still be documented to have clonal hematopoiesis by X-chromosome inactivation based assays. These findings are consistent with persistent somatic mutation which gives rise to a clonal proliferative advantage, but is not sufficient to give rise to the clinical phenotype of AML.

A third argument in support of multistep pathogenesis of AML are the myelodysplastic syndromes (MDS). MDS are a heterogeneous group of hematologic disorders characterized by pancytopenia and dysplastic growth of hematopoietic progenitors, and can be considered a transition state between normal hematopoiesis and leukemia. Patients with MDS have clonal hematopoiesis as evidenced by X-chromosome inactivation based assays, and by clonal karyotype abnormalities including del 5q, del 7q, del 12p, and del 20q among others. MDS may be indolent for months to years, but frequently progresses to AML associated with acquisition of additional cytogenetic abnormalities. Thus, at least two molecular genetic abnormalities appear to be necessary for the development of the malignant phenotype in these cases.

Cloning and characterizing the genes responsible for familial leukemia and myelodysplastic syndromes should provide insight into the early molecular genetic events that govern the transition from normal hematopoiesis to acute leukemia. However, there are few pedigrees large enough for generalized linkage analysis of familial leukemia, and myelodysplastic syndromes have proven difficult to analyze due to the large size of the deletions commonly associated with MDS.

In order to characterize early molecular genetic abnormalities in the multistep pathogenesis of AML, we have focused attention on molecular genetic abnormalities in myelodysplastic syndromes. In particular, we have analyzed rare patients with MDS who have translocations rather than large deletions as a mechanism for pinpointing the genomic localization of genes involved in pathogenesis of MDS.

2.0 RESULTS AND DISCUSSION

2.1 The Tel-PDGFRß fusion associated with t(5;12) CMML

2.1.1 The Platelet-Derived Growth Factor Receptor β (PDGFRβ Is Involved in the T(5;12) Chromosomal Translocation Associated with Chronic Myelomonocytic Leukemia (CMML). CMML, one of the FAB subtypes of MDS, is characterized by dysplastic proliferation of monocytes, and progression to AML. A recurring translocation in CMML occurs between chromosome bands 5q33 and 12p13. t(5;12)(q33;p13) is of particular interest because it occurs in regions of chromosome 5q and 12p13 which are abnormal in a significant number of patients with hematologic malignancy. For example, approximately 10% of cases of acute lymphoblastic leukemia (ALL) of childhood are associated with 12p13 deletions (10, 11). Since ALL is the most common cancer of children (del) (12p) is perhaps the most frequent cytogenetic abnormality in pediatric malignancy. The t(5;12)(q33;12p13) may therefore serve to localize genes involved in CMML, as well as in other hematologic malignancies.

We identified a patient with t(5;12)(q33;p13) and CMML, who subsequently developed AML associated with acquisition of t(8;21)(q22:q22) in addition to t(5;12). The t(8;21) is identical at the cytogenetic level to t(8;21) seen in <u>de novo</u> AML. t(5;12) thus appears to satisfy criteria for an early molecular genetic abnormality which gives rise to AML by virtue of its recurring association with CMML. In this specific example, t(5;12) appears to be an early mutation antedating development of t(8;21) associated AML.

The t(5;12) breakpoint was cloned without benefit of a cell line or patient cDNA library (12). Limitations in available clinical material led us to consider strategies which would maximize the blood and bone marrow specimens available. Fluorescence-in-situ-hybridization (FISH) was performed with ordered chromosome 5q cosmid probes to localize the breakpoint between the genes encoding c-fms and ribosomal protein S14. PCR primers specific for c-fms and RPS14 were used simultaneously to screen the CEPH megaYAC Library, and identified a 600Kb YAC 745d10 containing both c-fms and RPS14. 745d10 spanned the translocation by FISH, confirming the localization of the breakpoint and delineating a 600Kb genomic region within which the breakpoint must lie. Long range genomic maps were prepared by pulsed-field gel electrophoresis, and localized the breakpoint within the platelet-derived growth factor ß (PDGFRß) gene. Ribonuclease protection assays (RPA) were then used to localize the breakpoint with PDGFRß RNA using PDGFRß specific probes on patient bone marrow RNA. RNA analysis localized a partial transcript for the 3' end of the PDGFRß gene, beginning near the transmembrane domain of PDGFRß and extending through the tyrosine kinase domains. Northern blot analysis of patient bone marrow using PDGFRß probes showed a single 5 Kb transcript, which was larger than would be predicted by a partial PDGFRß transcript, consistent with a PDGFRß fusion partner derived from chromosome 12p13 (12).

2.1.2 A Novel ETS-Like Gene, Tel, Is Fused to PDGFRß in T(5;12) CMML. Anchored PCR on patient marrow RNA was performed using nested PDGFRß primers to obtain a partial cDNA for the chromosome 12 fusion partner. Involvement of the partial cDNA in the t(5;12) translocation was confirmed by RPA of patient bone marrow, and the partial cDNA was used to screen a human K562 cDNA library to obtain a full length cDNA.

The PDGFRß fusion partner is a novel ets-like gene, *TEL*. TEL is a predicted 452 aa protein which contains two functional domains: (i) a 3' DNA binding domain which defines ETS family members, and (ii) a 5' predicted helix-loop-helix (HLH) domain which is shared by approximately one third of ETS family members (Fig 1). The TEL HLH domain is conserved among other ets family members, including ets-1 and fli-1, and the Drosophila gene yan/pok, a transcriptional repressor.

The consequence of the t(5;12) translocation is a fusion transcript whose expression is driven by the *TEL* promoter, and results in fusion of the TEL HLH domain in frame to the PDGFRß transmembrane and tyrosine kinase domains (Fig. 2).

Figure 1. TEL is a member of the ets family of transcription factors, and contains a 3' helix-loop-helix (HLH) domain and a 5' DNA binding domain.

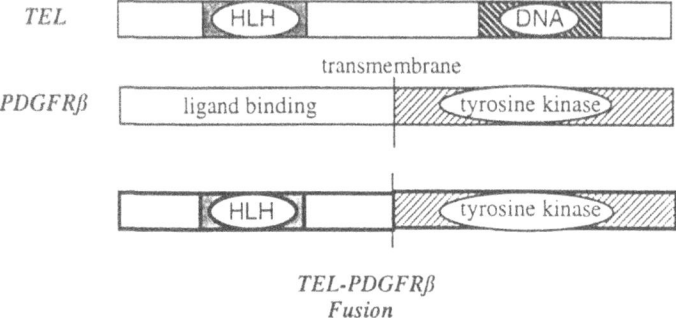

Figure 2. The consequence of the t(5;12) associated with CMML is fusion of the TELHLH domain to the transmembrane and tyrosine kinase domains of the PDGFRß.

2.1.3 Mechanism of Transformation of the TEL-PDGFRß Fusion. The structure of the TEL-PDGFRß fusion suggests several possible mechanisms of transformation. Wildtype PDGFRß is known to signal a variety of cellular responses, including mitogenesis, on binding to its dimeric ligand, PDGF. PDGF mediates dimerization of PDGFRß, which activates the tyrosine kinase leading to autophosphorylation of the receptor on tyrosine residues. Phosphorylated tyrosines on the PDGFRß serve as docking sites for a number of proteins which initiate signal transduction cascades, including src, syp/Grb2, PI3 kinase, and PLCg. It is plausible based on the known function of wildtype PDGFRß that the HLH domain of TEL-PDGFRß mediates dimerization and constitutive activation of the PDGFRß tyrosine kinase domain.

The TEL-PDGFRß fusion was first tested for transforming activity in cultured mammalian cell lines. TEL-PDGFRß confers factor independent growth to the IL-3 dependent hematopoietic cell line, Ba/F3. Consistent with a model of PDGFRß tyrosine kinase activation, TEL-PDGFRß is constitutively phosphorylated in factor independent Ba/F3 cells transfected with TEL-PDGFRß.

Another possible model for TEL-PDGFRß transforming activity is that TEL has tumor suppressor activity, and that TEL-PDGFRß interferes with wildtype function. In this model, the TEL HLH domain would mediate heterodimerization between TEL-PDGFRß and wild type TEL, leading to TEL loss of function. Indirect evidence which supports TEL loss of function in pathogenesis of malignancy is provided below, and includes translocations involving TEL in which the other TEL allele is deleted, such as the TEL-AML1 fusion. In these cases, there is no functional TEL in the leukemic cells: one TEL allele is deleted and the other is disrupted by translocation (13). Other data supporting a role for TEL loss of function in hematologic malignancy is frequent loss of heterozygosity at the TEL gene locus in ALL (14).

2.2 TEL Is Frequently Involved in Translocations Involving Human Chromosome band 12p13

One rationale for cloning the t(5;12) translocation breakpoint was to determine whether the translocation would identify genes in other translocations involving chromosome 12p13. To test this possibility, additional patients with cytogenetic evidence of 12p13 rearrangements were analyzed for evidence of involvement of the TEL gene locus.

Yeast artificial chromosomes (YACs) containing the TEL gene were used to analyze patients with cytogenetic evidence of 12p13 abnormalities (15). The majority of patients (26/34) were shown to have abnormalities at the TEL gene locus. RPA was used to map to translocation breakpoints within TEL, and disclosed an unusual distribution of breakpoints within the TEL gene (Fig 3). As noted earlier, translocation breakpoints within a given gene are usually highly conserved, even when different fusion partners have been identified. For example, the MLL gene at chromosome band 11q23 is associated with AML and has numerous fusion partners. However, the breakpoint with MLL is highly conserved, regardless of the fusion partner. In contrast, there are at least three different breakpoints within the TEL gene which give rise to fusion products which express different functional domains of TEL.

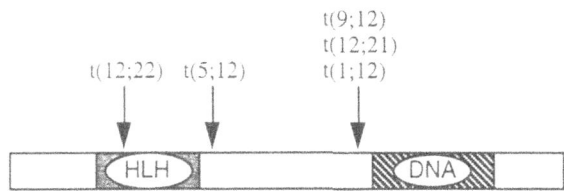

Figure 3. Diverse translocation breakpoints in TEL mapped by ribonuclease protection assays.

For example, in contrast with the structure of the TEL-PDGFRß which involves the TEL HLH domain, patients evaluated in our laboratory with the t(12;22) showed evidence of abnormal expression of the TEL DNA binding domain driven by the promoter of a chromosome 22 gene. The t(12;22) breakpoint has been cloned by Grosveld et al and gives rise to a fusion transcript containing the MNI gene fused in frame to the TEL DNA binding domain (16). The MN1-TEL fusion is analogous in structure to the EWS-fli1 fusion associated with t(11;22) Ewing's sarcoma (17), and the TLS-ERG fusion associated with t(16;21) leukemia (18), in which an ETS-family DNA binding domain is abnormally expressed.

2.3 The Consequence of t(9;12;14) in Acute Undifferentiated Leukemia Is Fusion of TEL to the Protooncogene ABL

RPA was used as described above to delineate a breakpoint within the TEL gene in a patient with a complex t(9;12;14) translocation and acute undifferentiated leukemia with

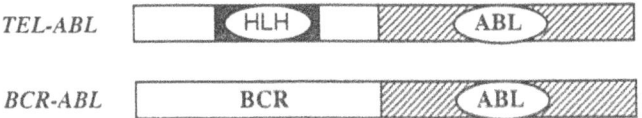

Figure 4. T TEL-ABL and BCR-ABl fusions associated with t(9;12) and t(9;22) translocations, respectively. In each case, fusion occurs in frame at exon 2 of ABL.

myeloid markers (AMoL). Anchored PCR with nested TEL primers was used to clone the TEL fusion partner, the ABL protooncogene on chromosome 9q34. The consequence of the translocation is fusion of the TEL HLH domain inframe to exon 2 of ABL (Fig 4).

The TEL-ABL fusion has several interesting features. TEL-ABL is similar in structure to the well characterized BCR-ABL fusion associated with chronic myelogenous leukemia (CML) and t(9;22). TEL is the only other fusion partner that has been identified for ABL, and has important similarities and differences from BCR. For example, BCR contains a 5' predicted coiled-coil interaction motif which is necessary for tyrosine kinase and transforming activity of BCR-ABL. The coiled-coil motif BCR and the putative HLH domain of TEL may both therefore serve dimerization or multimerization functions as a mechanism for constitutive activation of tyrosine kinase activity. The theme of dimerization leading to constitutive tyrosine kinase activity and transformation might then be shared by TEL-PDGFRß, TEL-ABL and BCR-ABL. Consistent with this hypothesis, TEL-ABL transforms Rat1 fibroblasts and is constitutively phosphorylated when stably expressed in these cells. In addition, like TEL-PDGFRß, TEL-ABL is capable of conferring IL-3 independent growth to Ba/F3 cells.

As another example of the usefulness of new fusion genes to elucidate functional domains which are relevant to transforming activity, TEL-ABL lacks a Grb2 binding site on the TEL moiety. BCR-ABL contains a Y177 Grb2 binding site on the BCR portion of the fusion, whose role in transformation has been debated (19). Since TEL-ABL lacks a Grb2 binding site, at a minimum it can be stated that transformation of cultured mammalian cells mediated by ABL fusions does not require a functional Grb2 binding site.

2.4 Tel Is Fused to the Transcription Factor AML1 in t(12;21) Acute Lymphoblastic Leukemia (ALL)

As noted above, another TEL breakpoint involving the TEL HLH domain was identified in patients with ALL and t(12;21). The translocation breakpoint was cloned using anchored PCR with TEL specific primers. Based on our previous experience with cloning of TEL-PDGFRß and TEL-ABL, one might have predicted a tyrosine kinase fusion partner for TEL. However, in the case of t(12;21), TEL is fused inframe to the transcription factor AML1 (13), (Fig 5). The AML1 gene on chromosome 21q22 was first cloned by virtue of its involvement with t(8;21) and t(3;21) associated with de novo AML and therapy-related AML, respectively (20). AML1 contains two functional domains; (i) a DNA binding domain with homology to the Drosophila pair-rule gene *runt*, and (ii) a 3' transcriptional activation domain. The TEL-AML1 fusion consists of the TEL HLH domain fused in frame to AML1 at intron 2, with expression of both the AML1 DNA binding domain and the AML1 transcriptional activation domain.

TEL-AML1 is fascinating from several perspectives. First, it suggests that the TEL HLH domain can contribute to pathogenesis of leukemia when fused either to a tyrosine

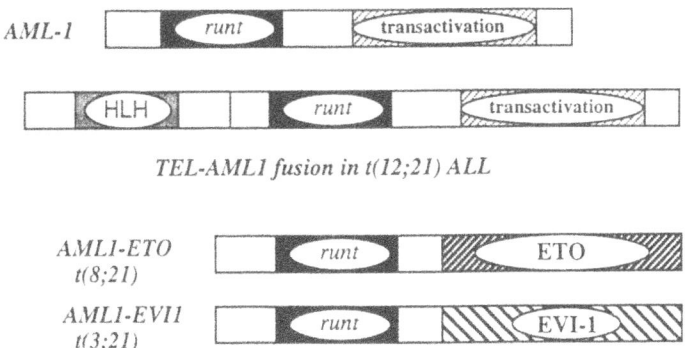

Figure 5. The TEL-AML1 fusion associated with t(12;21) differs from other AML1 fusions: TEL-AML1 is associated with ALL rather than AML, and involves expression of both the runt and transactivation domains of AML1.

kinase or to a transcription factor. Second, the structure of the TEL-AML1 fusion differs significantly from the AML1 fusions involved in t(8;21) and t(3;21) translocations. In these translocations, the 5' end of the AML1 gene including the DNA binding domain, is fused to one of several partners just 3' of the *runt* domain (Fig 5). Fusion partners include ETO in t(8;21), and various partners in t(3;21) including EVI-1, EAP and MDS 1. In each of these fusions, the AML1 transactivation domain is lost. In contrast, in the TEL-AML1 fusion, the full length AML1 gene is expressed, including the *runt* and transactivation domains. AML1 had previously only been associated with myeloid leukemias (hence the name of the gene). In two cases of TEL-AML1 reported from our laboratory, and two cases subsequently reported by Romana et al, have been associated with lymphoid leukemias (21). In part, the difference in lineage specificity of TEL-AML1 versus other AML1 fusions can be explained by the t(8;21) and t(3;21) AML1 fusions being driven by the AML1 promoter, whereas the TEL-AML1 fusion is driven by the TEL promoter. However, at a minimum it is clear that AML1 can contribute to the pathogenesis of both myeloid and lymphoid malignancies. Fourth, in each case of TEL-AML1 fusions characterized thus far (13), the other TEL allele is deleted. Thus, in these leukemic cells, there is no functional TEL: one TEL allele is deleted and the other is disrupted by translocation. Based in part on this observation, the possibility that TEL loss of function might contribute to pathogenesis of leukemia was evaluated in ALL patients, as described in the next section.

2.5 Loss of TEL Function May Contribute to Pathogenisis of Human Leukemias

To evaluate the possibility that TEL loss of function might contribute to pathogenesis of leukemia, a patient population was chosen for analysis that has frequent deletions in the 12p13 region. Approximately 10% of pediatric ALL cases have 12p13 deletions. Since the most common childhood malignancy is ALL, del(12p13) is among the most common molecular genetic abnormality of childhood cancer.

To determine whether the loss of TEL function could be implicated in pathogenesis of ALL, we first determined the frequency of loss of heterozygosity (LOH) at the TEL gene locus. Genomic DNA was prepared from 81 pediatric patients at the time of diagno-

Table 1. Loss of heterozygosity (LOH) at the *TEL* locus in pediatric ALL

Marker	No. patients	No informative	Patients with LOH
D12S89	81	63/81 (78%)	9/63 (14%)
D12S98	81	53/81 (65%)	9/53 (17%)

sis of ALL. Polymorphic microsatellite markers, D12S89 and D12S98 which flanked the TEL gene, were then tested for LOH. LOH of two microsatellite markers which flank the TEL gene would provide convincing evidence for LOH at the TEL locus. As controls to confirm that ALL patients with a single microsatellite band had loss of heterozygosity, rather than simply being homozygous for that marker, paired leukemia and remission samples were analyzed. Patients were considered informative only when remission samples documented that the patient was heterozygous at that locus. As seen in Table 1, approximately 15% of ALL patients had LOH at the TEL gene locus (14).

Of note, only one of the 9 patients with TEL LOH had cytogenetic evidence of 12p13 loss. This is in consonance with most studies of LOH in malignancy in which cytogenetic analysis underestimates LOH at most loci. Taken together, these findings suggest that TEL LOH may occur in as many as 20–25% of ALL patients.

To further delineate the region of LOH on 12p13, additional microsatellite markers telomeric and centromeric to TEL were evaluated. The region of LOH includes TEL, but extends to the centromere and also invariably includes the gene KIP1, encoding for the protein p27. p27 is a cyclin-dependent kinase (CDK) inhibitor which regulates the G1/s transition in the cell cycle. Other CDK inhibitors, such as p15 and p16, have been strongly implicated in pathogenesis of cancer through loss of function. p27 is thus a superb candidate for loss of function in ALL. Sequence analysis of the residual alleles for TEL and KIP1 are underway in these patients, as well as efforts to identify other transcription units in this region.

3.0 CONCLUSIONS

TEL contributes to pathogenesis of leukemia by remarkably diverse molecular genetic mechanisms. We have presented evidence that in t(5;12) CMML, the *TEL* gene is fused in frame to the receptor tyrosine kinase PDGFRß in a manner which appears to confer constitutive kinase activity to PDGFRß. We have further demonstrated that TEL is fused to the protooncogene ABL in acute undifferentiated leukemia, providing a second example of possible constitutive activation of a tyrosine kinase, similar to that seen in the BCR-ABL fusion associated with t(9;22) CML. Finally, and somewhat surprisingly, we have documented that the TEL HLH domain may be fused to the transcription factor AML1 in lymphoid malignancies.

In contrast to these examples in which the TEL HLH domain is fused a various partners, the TEL DNA binding domain may be abnormally expressed in t(12;22) leukemias in a manner analogous to other ETS DNA binding domain fusions, such as EWS-fli1 and TLS-ERG. Finally, we have presented indirect evidence that TEL loss of function may contribute to pathogenesis of leukemia. Data in support of this hypothesis includes complete loss of functional TEL in t(12;21) ALL, and LOH at the TEL locus on 12p13 in a significant proportion of cases of pediatric ALL.

The diversity of molecular genetic mechanisms by which TEL can be transforming suggests an important role for TEL in cell growth and differentiation. Further analysis of TEL, and its related oncogenic fusion genes, may provide further insight into the role of TEL in normal physiology of mammalian cells.

REFERENCES

1. de The H, Chomienne C, Lanotte M, Degos L, Dejean A. 1990. The t(15;17) translocation of acute promyelocytic leukaemia fuses the retinoic acid receptor a gene to a novel transcribed locus. **Nature** 347:558–561.
2. de The H, Lavau C, Marcio A, Chomienne C, Degos L, Dejean A. 1991. The PML-RAR-alpha fusion mRNA generated by the t(15;17) translocation in acute promyelocytic leukemia encodes a functionally altered RAR. **Cell 66**:675.
3. Warrell RP, de The H, Wang Z-Y, Degos L. 1993. Acute promyelocytic leukemia. **New England Journal of Medicine 329**:177–189.
4. Erickson P, Gao J, Chang KS, Look T, Whisenant E, Raimondi S, Lasher J, Rowley J, Drabkin H. 1992. Identification of breakpoints in t(8;21) acute myelogenous leukemia and isolation of a fusion transcript, AML1/ETO, with similarity to Drosophila segmentation gene, runt. **Blood 80**:1825–1831.
5. Liu P, Tarle SA, Hajra A, Claxton DF, Marlton P, Freedman M, Siciliano MJ, Collins FS. 1993. Fusion between transcription factor /PEBP2B and a myosin heavy chain in acute myeloid leukemia. **Science 261**:1041–1044.
6. Thirman MJ, Gill HJ, Burnett RC, Mbangkollo D, McCabe NR, Kobayashi H, Ziemin-van der Poel S, Kaneko Y, Morgan R, Sandberg AA, Chaganti RSK, Larson RA, Le Beau MM, Diaz MO, Rowley JD. 1993. Rearrangement of the MLL gene in acute lymphoblastic and acute myeloid leukemias with 11q23 chromosomal translocations. **New England Journal of Medicine 329**:909–914.
7. Dowton SB, Beardsley D, Jamison D, Blattner S, Li FP. 1985. Studies of a familial platelet disorder. **Blood 65**:557–563.
8. Bronner CE, Baker SM, Morrison PT, Warren G, Smith LG, Lescoe MK, Kane M, Earabino C, Lipford J, Lindblom A, Tannergard P, Bollag RJ, Godwin AR, Ward DC, Nordenskjold M, Fishel R, Kolodner R, Liskay RM. 1994. Mutation in the DNA mismatch repair gene homologue *hMLH1* is associated with hereditary non-polyposis colon cancer. **Nature 368**:258–261.
9. Busque L, Gilliland DG. 1993. Clonal evolution in acute myeloid leukemia. **Blood 82**:337–342.
10. Raimondi SC. 1993. Current status of cytogenetic research in childhood acute lymphoblastic leukemia. **Blood 81**:2237–51.
11. Raimondi SC, Williams DL, Callihan T, Peiper S, Rivera GK, Murphy SB. 1986. Nonrandom involvement of the 12p12 breakpoint in chromosome abnormalities of childhood acute lymphoblastic leukemia. **Blood 68**:69–75.
12. Golub TR, Barker GF, Lovett M, Gilliland DG. 1994. Fusion of PDGF receptor beta to a novel ets-like gene, tel, in chronic myelomonocytic leukemia with t(5;12) chromosomal translocation. **Cell 77**:307–316.
13. Golub TR, Barker GF, Bohlander SK, Hiebert SW, Ward DC, Bray-Ward P, Morgan E, Raimondi SC, Rowley JD, D.G. G. 1995. Fusion of the TEL gene on 12p13 to the AML1 gene on 21q22 in acute lymphoblastic leukemia. **Proc Natl Acad Sci in press**.
14. Stegmaier K, Pendse S, Barker GF, Bray-Ward P, Ward DC, Montgomery KT, Krauter KS, Reynolds C, Sklar J, Donnelly M, Bohlander SK, Rowley JD, Sallan SE, Gilliland DG, Golub TR. 1995. Frequent loss of heterozygosity at the *TEL* gene locus in acute lymphoblastic leukemia of childhood. **Blood 86**:38–44.
15. Sato Y, Suto Y, Pietenpol J, Golub T, Gilliland DG. in press. *TEL* and *KIP1* define the smallest region of deletions on 12p13 in hematopoietic malignancies. **Blood** . .
16. Buijs A, Sherr S, van Baal S, van Bezouw S, van der Plas D, van Kessel AG, Riegman P, Deprez RL, Zwarthoff E, Hagemeijer A, Grosveld G. 1995. Translocation (12;22)(p13;q11) in myeloproliferative disorders results in fusion of the ETS-like *TEL* gene on 12p13 to the *MN1* gene on 22q11. **Oncogene 10**:1511–1519.
17. Sorensen PHB, Lessnick AL, Lopez-Terrada D, Liu XF, Triche TJ, Denny CT. 1994. A second Ewing's sarcoma translocation, t(21;22), fuses the EWS gene to another ETS-family transcription factor, ERG. **Nature Genetics 6**:146–151.

18. Shimizu K, Ichikawa H, Tojo A, Kaneko Y, Maseki N, Hayashi Y, Ohira M, Asano S, Ohki M. 1993. An *ets*-related gene, *ERG*, is rearranged in human myeloid leukemia with t(16;21) chromosomal translocation. **Proceedings of the National Academy of Science USA 90**:10280–10284.
19. Pendergast AM, Quilliam LA, Cripe LD, Bessing CH, Dai Z, Li N, Der CJ, Sclessinger J, Gishizky ML. 1993. BCR-ABL-induced oncogenesis is mediated by direct interaction with the SH2 domain of the GRB-2 adapter protein. **Cell 75**:175–185.
20. Nucifora G, Begy CR, Erickson P, Drabkin HA, Rowley JD. 1993. The 3;21 translocation in myelodysplasia results in a fusion transcript between the AML1 gene and the gene for ETO, a highly conserved protein associated with the Epstein-Barr virus small RNA EBER 1. **Proc Natl Acad Sci USA 90**:7784–7788.
21. Romana SP, Mauchauffe M, Leconiat M, Chumakov I, Le Paslier D, Berger R, Bernard OA. 1995. The t(12;21) of acute lymphoblastic leukemia results in a tel-AML1 gene fusion. **Blood 85**: 3662–3670.

DISCUSSION

T. Graf: I think an important question in trying to understand how TEL participates in cell transformation is whether it can homodimerize. It would be the first Ets-family factor that I know homodimerizes

G. Gilliland: Yes, we do. It is preliminary evidence, but I think the evidence is reasonably convincing. We can demonstrate homodimeric complexes of the TEL gene that can be dissociated or abrogated by deletion of the HLH domain. These are not very sophisticated mutations they are not point mutations within the HLH domain.

T. Graf: In that case, can you functionally replace HLH domain, for example, with that of Max or Myo-D, and would such a modified TEL fused with the PDGF receptor transform in your assay?

G. Gilliland: We have not done the experiment in the wild type TEL gene. I think the idea of using other dimerization motifs like leucine zippers would be a very interesting experiment. The TPR-MET fusion that Dr. Comoglio described yesterday is another good example of a putative dimerization motif that may serve to constitutively activate the MET receptor tyrosine kinase, so that paradigm of dimerization is shared in several examples of transformation and is mediated by receptor tyrosine kinases. But that would be a good experiment to provide support for that theory.

F. Rauscher: The second allele loss is very strange. You are showing it is a dominant transforming gene when it is translocated, however, when you delete the HLH domain you lose that function. Yet in the leukemias you are losing the other allele. So genetically it says it is a tumor suppress gene. And you cannot invoke transdominance through HLH domain to inactivate it

G. Gilliland: Part of the transdominance may depend on sub-cellular localization, and access to the substrate for which the transdominant effect is supposed to be mediated on. The cell systems that we used to look at these kinds of questions are somewhat artifactual. These experiments are performed using an overdrive promoter to express the fusion protein (e.g., LTR's). However, marked overexpression may lead to the same effect that you would see in cells in which the other TEL allele is deleted.

F. Rauscher: Even just the truncated TEL gene without ABL or the rest of it, will that overexpression of just that HLH domain transform?

G. Gilliland: We do not know that. We are doing that experiment.

F. Rauscher: And have you looked at other loci or micro satellite markers from different chromosomes. It is not generalized marker loss, correct?

G. Gilliland: No, this is very specific. In fact, as you move out telomeric and centromeric from that locus there is no evidence for LOH; it is a very well circumscribed one mega base region that contains both TEL and p27 it is not a generalized genomic instability phenomenon.

M. Fried: Is there any specificity in TEL being on in different cell types?

G. Gilliland: TEL is ubiquously expressed. As best we can tell it is expressed in all tissue types.

P. Comoglio: I may have missed the point, but, you showed in the slide that during your deletion experiments you lose cytoskeletal association and transformation. What about dimerization; I mean, the mutant that failed to associate to the cytoskeleton do they dimerize?

G. Gilliland: We do not have direct evidence for dimerization of the TEL-ABL construct, we have examined the TEL wild type cDNA and we would like to extrapolate those findings. So we do not have evidence that dimerization is relevant and we do not know whether in those cells, it exists as a monomer or as a dimer. But that is a good experiment to do.

D. Livingston: What are the characteristics of the MN-1 TEL fusion?

G. Gilliland: To my knowledge, the MN1-TEL fusion has not been characterized except to say that it is associated with the (12;22) translocation and it is expressed, and that is where things stand as far as Gerard Grosveld work goes. If one extrapolates it is quite similar. MN1 has structural features that are similar to the EWS fusion with the fli1 gene, that does contact DNA and binds ets consensus sequences. But what the role of TEL in transcriptional activation is, or how that is different in the MN1-TEL fusion has not been well characterized.

D. Livingston: And in the child's leukemia there is no LOH and on one chromosome there appears to be, at least repeatedly, a big deletion. What is the story with the other chromosome?

G. Gilliland: The other chromosome appears to be perfectly normal from a micro-satellite perspective, and presumably large deletions on that chromosome would be lethal events. So we are in the process of sequencing p27 which is an easy gene to sequence as it has just two exons, to look for mutations. We have actually gone through most of the patients we have so far, and do not have evidence for mutation of p27. TEL has a more complicated genomic structure that spans about 150 kb and we are still working through that, but we do not yet have evidence of mutations in the TEL gene either.

D. Livingston: Is there wild type TEL RNA in those leukemia cells?

G. Gilliland: There are paired samples from Steve Sallen's collection, which are DNA only. We do not have access to RNA, but that is a critical question that could save us a lot of time, if we knew whether TEL was expressed.

D. Livingston: Because the question that comes to mind is whether half a copy is a real problem as in some cases of L-Fraumeni, for example.

G. Gilliland: Yes. It may be. I think you have to go the extra mile to prove that hemizygosity is relevant to disease or not. You would have to exclude involvement of any of the other transcription units in that region.

D. Livingston: So why do you call it LOH?

G. Gilliland: It is loss of heterozygosity for the micro satellite markers than flank these genes. So you are loosing genetic material in the region.

D. Livingston: But there is no reduction to homozygosity yet?

G. Gilliland: No, and I would actually say, also in response to Frank's comments, that this may not be a tumor suppressor gene. It may simply be that deletion of the other TEL allele is permissive for the expression of the dominant activity of a TEL related fusion. So, I think it is important to distinguish loss of function from tumor suppressor activity.

D. Livingston: Although there is no evidence for fusion on the other copy right?

G. Gilliland: No.

D. Livingston: How about regulation of expression?

G. Gilliland: We do not know anything about the regulation expression of the gene. We have not cloned the TEL promoter yet.

M. Oren: Perhaps a philosophical question: Would you care to speculate about the coincidence of losing TEL and p27 together? Have you looked whether TEL expression has anything to do with cell cycle? Does it oscillate in any way?

G. Gilliland: No, we are very attracted by that possibility, by the similarities in structure to yan/pok, by the very elegant work that demonstrated that Elk-1 is a downstream effector for Mad-kinase - maybe its not just a coincidence that it is there, and may be it is not just a coincidence that TEL and PDGF co-segregate. I think the more likely outcome will be that if we look at one thousand kids with ALL we will be able to find some in which the deletion involves only one gene or the other, but we will have to sort through that.

T. Taniguchi: Does wild type TEL expression, for example, suppress colony formation of TEL-ABL induced colony formation or any growth inhibitor effect of that?

G. Gilliland: That is a good experiment, we have not done it.

F. Rauscher: Presumably all of these cell lines you are using for transformation have lost endogenous p27? So, maybe that is really what you are looking at in terms of transforming ability in these transformed cell lines already - the loss of endogenous p27?

G. Gilliland: I do not know what the CDK inhibitors do and. whether they are present or what their function is like, but it is probably an important question to look at.

14

CHARACTERIZATION OF THE TCLI GENE AND ITS INVOLVEMENT IN T-CELL MALIGNANCIES

Laura Virgilio,[1] Gian Domenico Russo,[2] and Carlo M. Croce[1]

[1] Jefferson Cancer Institute
Jefferson Cancer Center and
Department of Microbiology and Immunology
Jefferson Medical College of Thomas Jefferson University
Philadelphia, Pennsylvania 19107
[2] RaggioItalgene
Pomezia, Italy 00040

INTRODUCTION

Most human leukemias and lymphomas exhibit non-random chromosomal alterations. Translocations are the most common form of alteration in hematopoetic malignancies, leading to oncogenic activation either by the formation of chimeric transforming genes or by deregulation of transcription (Croce, 1987; Rabbitts, 1994). Gene fusion is observed in the majority of the myeloid tumors and in soft tissue sarcomas, and less frequently in B and T cell leukemias and lymphomas: good examples of these alterations are the t(9;22) translocation of chronic myelogenous leukemia (CML) and Ph chromosome positive acute lymphocytic leukemia (Ph+ALL) and the t(1;19), t(15;17), t(6;9) and t(4;11) chromosomal translocations observed in pre-B, myeloid and mixed lineage leukemias, all of which generate chimeric transcripts (Nourse et al., 1990, Kamps et al., 1990, and Gu et al. 1992). Deregulation of oncogene transcription is observed in most B and T cell leukemias and lymphomas, in these alterations the immunonoglobulin (Ig) or the T-cell-receptor (TCR) loci become juxtaposed to cellular protoncogenes such as c-MYC, BCL-2, TCL-2, BCL-1, TCL-3 (for a review see Croce, 1987; Rabbitts, 1994). In this latter case the gene justaxposed to the Ig or the TCR locus can be quite close (within 10–30 kb) from the genomic breakpoint, as for BCL-2 on chromosome 18q21, BCL-3 on chromosome 19q13.1, c-MYC on 8q24 in sporadic cases of Burkitt Lymphomas (BLs),or far (up to few hundreds kilobases) as for BCL-1 on chromosome 11q13, and c-MYC, in the endemic cases of BLs. These translocations are belived to be due to errors during the physiological process of the Ig and TCR gene rearrangements, and result in the activation of oncogenes by their juxtaposition to regulatory elements (enhancers) of the Ig or TCR loci .

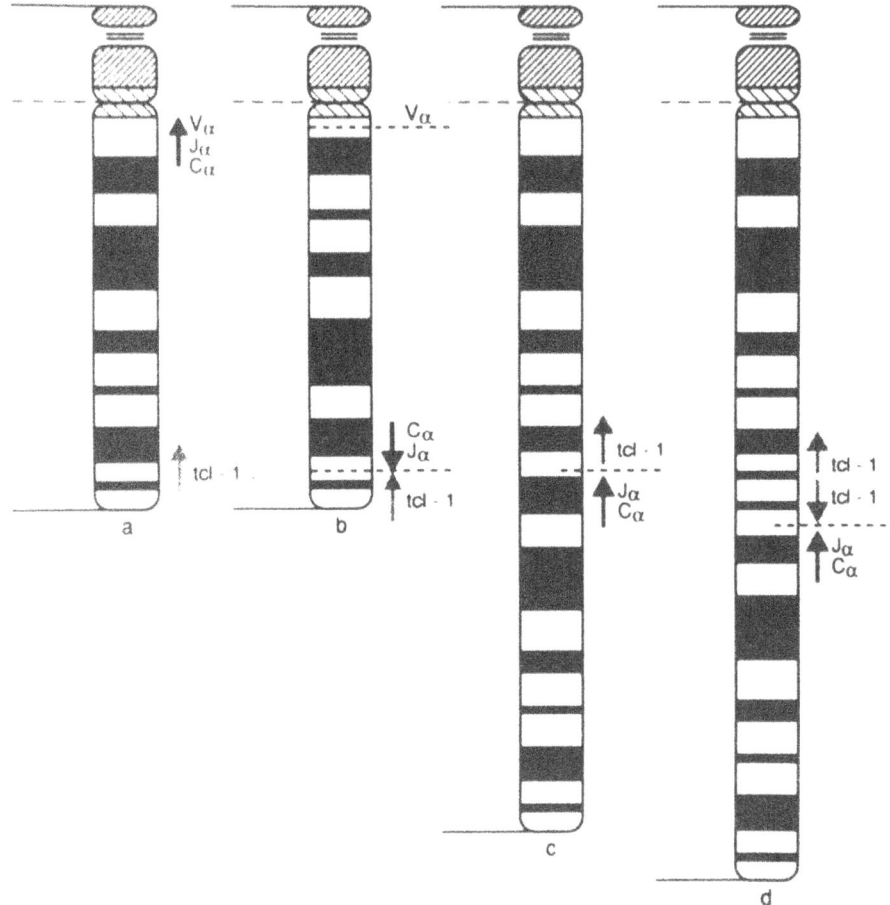

Figure 1. Schematic representation of the chromosomal rearrangements involving the TCL1 locus on chromosome 14q32.1 and the TCRa-chain locus at chromosome 14q11.2. The filled arrow represent the orientation of TCRa, and the open arrow represent the orientation of TCL1 transcription. (a) Normal chromosome 14, (b) An inv(14) chromosomal inversion, (c) A t(14;14)(q11;q32.1) classical chromosomal translocation. (d) A t(14;14)(q11;q32.1) chromosomal translocation with an inverted duplication of 14q32.1–14qter. V_α, J_α, and C_α represent variable, joining, and costant gene segments of TCRα.

The *TCL1* locus is located at chromosome band 14q32.1 and it is predominantly involved in rearrangements with the TCRα/δ locus at 14q11 and seldom with the TCRβ locus at 7q35 in T-cell lymphocytic leukemia (T-CLL) (Russo et al., 1988). Rearrangements at the *TCL1* locus can either be inversions, inv(14)(q11;q32), or simple balanced translocations t(14;14)(q11;q32), or translocations with inverted duplication (see Fig.1.) (Virgilio et al., 1993). In every case the control elements of the Jα/δ segment at 14q11 are juxtaposed to the TCL1 gene either in a head to tail configuration as in the case of inversions and translocations with inverted duplication, or in head to head configuration as in the case of simple translocations (Fig.1).

TCL1 rearrangements are observed in most T-cell chronic lymphocytic leukemia (T-CLL), in 75% of T-prolymphocytic leukemias (T-PLL), a post-thymic type of leukemia, and are particularly common in leukemias developing in patients with Ataxia Telangiectasia (AT), an autosomal recessive immunodeficiency syndrome associated with genomic instabilitiy, defective DNA repair, cerebellar ataxia, and oculocutaneous telangiectasia (Brito-Babapulle and Catovsky, 1991; Virgilio et al., 1993). Patients with AT, because of their underlying defect are prone to cancer especially of the hematopoetic lineage, and unlike non-AT patients where B-cell leukemias are predominant, they more frequently develop leukemia of T-cell origin (Gatti et al., 1994). These T cell leukemias predominantly carry rearrangements involving the *TCL1* locus at 14q32.1 and more rarely the *MTCP1/c6.1B* locus at Xq28(Russo et al., 1989; Brito-Babapulle and Catovsky, 1991; Stern et al., 1993; Kirsch, 1994; Sherrington et al., 1994). Chromosomal alterations involving chromosome band 14q32 have also been reported in 30% of adult T-cell leukemia (ATL), associated with HTLVI infection; ATL as T-PLL represent a post-thymic type of leukemia (Virgilio et al., 1994).

CLONING AND STRUCTURAL CHARACTERIZATION OF THE TCL1 GENE

The *TCL1* locus was cloned through chromosome walking using both a P1 phage and a cosmid human DNA library. It spans a region of about 350Kb as defined by the mapping of all the cloned breakpoints (Fig.2) (Virgilio et al., 1993). The breakpoints form two clusters: a more centromeric cluster containing all the breakpoints derived from inversions or translocations with inverted duplications and a more telomeric cluster containing all the breakpoints from balanced translocations (Virgilio et al., 1993). It became evident to us that the *TCL1* gene to be activated by both kind of alterations had to be positioned between the two sets of breakpoints. In the case of inversions the breaks are centromeric to *TCL1*, the chromosome 14 portion between q11 and q32 inverts and the the Jα/δ region at 14q11 becomes juxtaposed to the gene; in the case of simple translocations the breaks are telomeric to *TCL1* and join with the Jα/δ region of the reciprocal chromosome 14 (Fig.1). Indeed, careful screening of the region by exon trapping and Northern blot hybridization with probes derived from GC rich regions determined the presence of transcribed sequences. The TCL1 cDNA, 1.3Kb in length, was cloned and its sequence revealed the presence of an open reading frame of 342 nucleotides to encode for a protein of 14 kD (Fig.1) (Virgilio et al., 1994). Antibodies raised against recombinant *TCL1* specifically recognized a protein of 14kD, which was later localized to the microsomal fraction of the cell(Fu et al., 1994).

The *TCL1* amino acid sequence did not show any homology with known proteins or the presence of known sequence motives to indicate a possible function of the protein. However, it showed high amino acid homology with the putative protein encoded by one of the open reading frame of the *MTCP1/c6.1B* gene; this gene located at Xq28 is involved in translocations t(X;14) (q28;q11) rarely observed in cases of T-cell lymphoproliferative disorders and T-PLLs (Stern et al., 1993; Sherrington et al., 1994). It is quite striking that two similar genes are both involved in chromosomal translocations and lead to the development of the same type of leukemia.

TCL1 EXPRESSION IN NORMAL AND MALIGNANT CELLS

TCL1 expression is lymphoid specific and it is normally expressed at specific stages during B and T cells differentiation. Analysis of RNA by reverse transcriptase-PCR (RT-

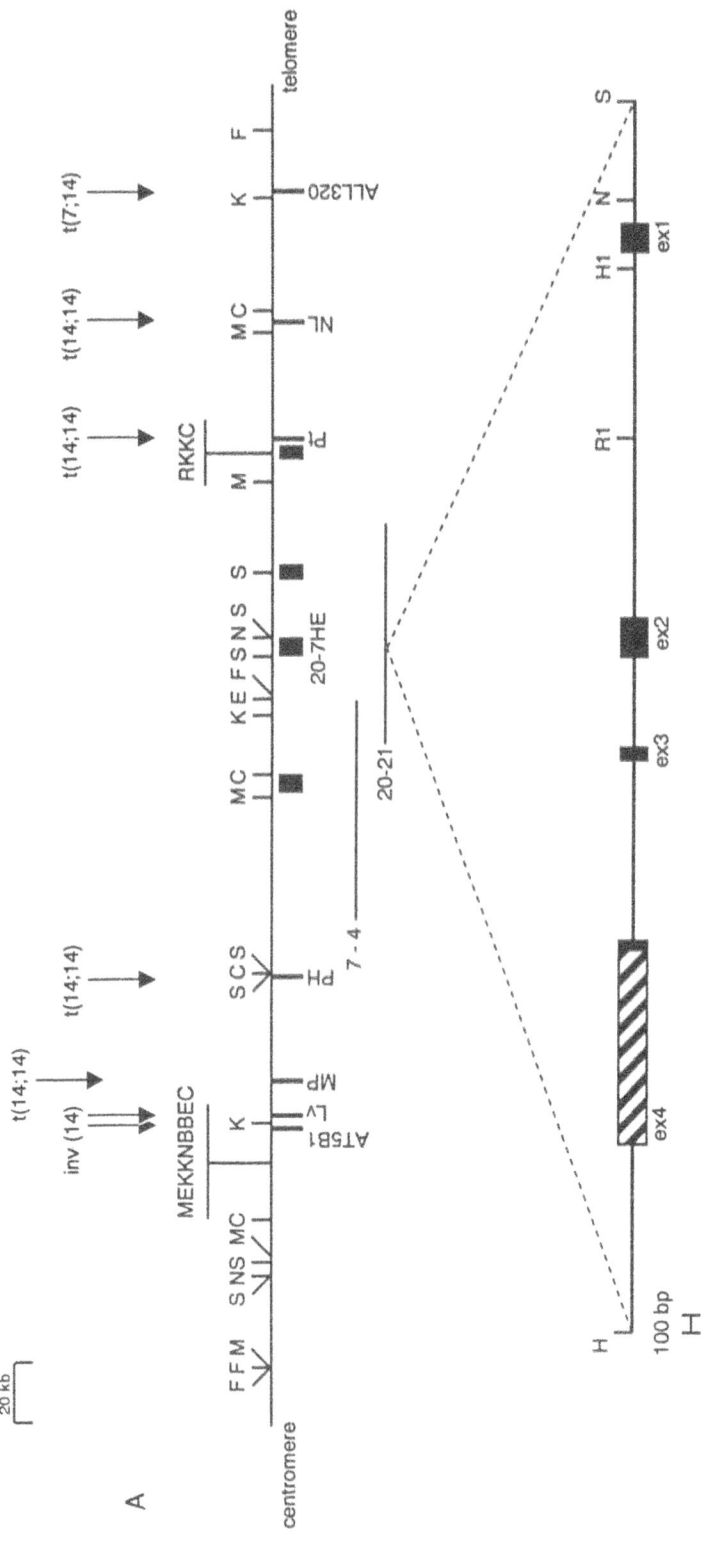

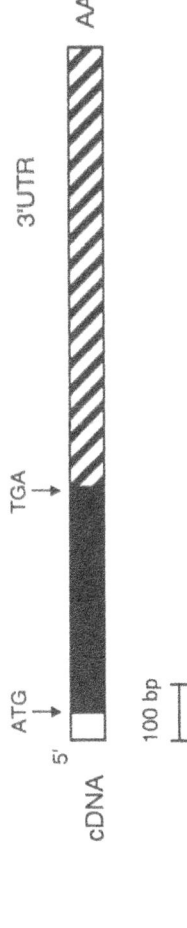

Figure 2. Genomic and cDNA organization of the TCL-1 gene A. Genomic organization of the TCL-1 locus on chromosome 14q32.1. Vertical bars refers to cloned breakpoints in the literature (see Virgilio et al. 1993 for references). Restriction sites are given for BssH II (B), Cla I (C), Eag I (E), Ksp I (K), Mlu I (M), Sfi (F),Not I (N), Nru I (R), Sal I (S), EcoR I (R1), HindIII (H) and BamH I (H1). P1 clones 7–4 and 20–21, covering the 140kb region between the two cluster of breakpoints, are shown by horizontal bars. Solid boxes represent probes used for RNA screening. Enlarged is shown a SalI- HindIII genomic fragment with the organization of the four exons of the TCL-1 gene, and the 3′ untranslated region is shown in diagonal stripes. (B) TCL1 cDNA structure. An open box represent the 5′ untranslated region; a solid box represent the encoding sequence, and the hatched box represent the 3′ untranslated region.

PCR) from cell sorted populations of fetal bone marrow cells, showed that *TCL1* expression is absent in pro-B cells, it is upregulated in pre-B and in B cells expressing IgM surface antigens (Virgilio et al., 1994). In T cells, *TCL1* expression is observed only in very immature CD4⁻CD8⁻ thymocytes, and not in the more mature double positive cells; peripheral T cells will express *TCL1* only when stimulated with phytohemagglutinin (Fig.3). These data were confirmed by analysis of *TCL1* expression in established cell lines, the results of which are summarized in Table 1, and clearly indicate *TCL1* expression is high in cells at the pre-B stage i.e. ALL1, BV173 and cell lines established from patients with endemic Burkitt, but it is absent in cells at the pro-B stage as the MV(4;11) and RS(4;11) and in myeloma and lymphoblastoid cell lines such as the RPMI8866 and the GM1500 respectively. *TCL1* expression is absent in T cell lines established from T-cell leukemias not carrying rearrangements of the TCL1 locus i.e. MOLT4, CEM, and Jurkat (Fig.3)(Virgilio et al., 1994).

We also examined RNA derived from the peripheral T lymphocytes of two patients with T-PLL both carrying an inversions inv(14)(11;q32.1). These two samples showed high levels of *TCL1* expression, indicating that the *TCL1* gene is specifically activated by the rearrangements . Furthemore TCL1 activation was also observed in the T cell line SupT11, which presents a t(14;14) translocation (Fig.3).

Patients with AT represent an excellent model to study tumor progression. Because of their high cancer susceptibility, their lymphocytes can be closely monitored by cytoge-

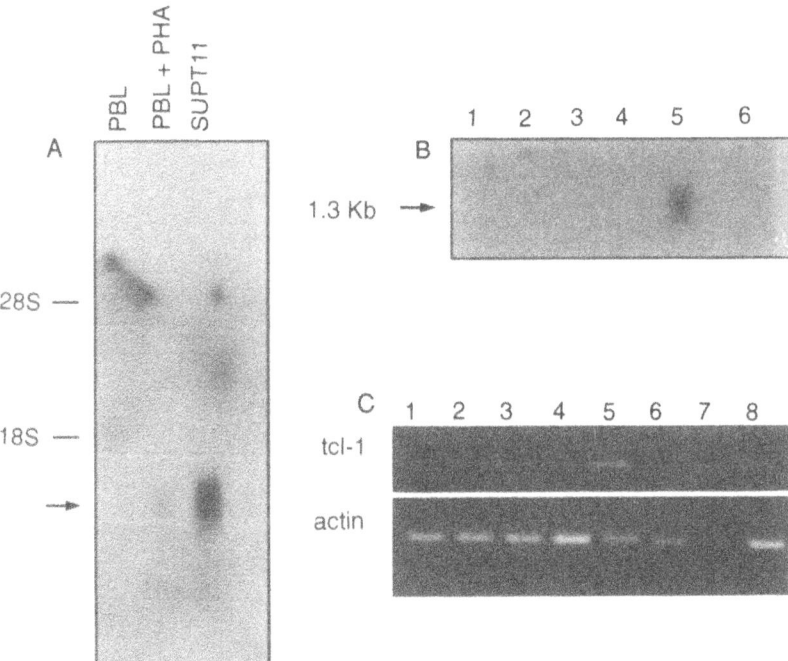

Figure 3. Expression of TCL1 in various T-cells. (A) Northern blot hybridization of stimulated and nonstimulated peripheral blood lymphocytes (PBL) with a TCL1 probe, p697; 11ug of RNA were loaded per lane. (B) Northern blot of RNA from cell lines. Lanes: 1, CEM; 2, MOLT-4; 3, HUT78; 4, SupT1; 5, SupT11; 6, Jurkat. (C) RT-PCRwith TCL1 primers, and with actin specifc primers. Lanes 1, CEM; 2, HUT78; 3, MOLT-4; 4, SupT1; 5, SupT11; 6, PBLs; 7, PHA-activated PBLs; and 8, fetal thymus cells.

Table 1. Expression of *TCL-1* mRNA in cell lines

Cell line	Tumor	Translocation	RNA
RS(4;11)	ALL	t (4;11)	-
MV (4;11)	ALL	t (4;11)	-
B1	ALL	t (4;11)	-
ALL380	ALL	t(8;14), t(14;18)	+
ALL-1	ALL	t (9;22)	+
BV173	ALL	t (9;22)	+
RPMI 8866	B-lymphoblastoid	N/A	-
GM1500	B-lymphoblastoid	Normal	-
RPMI 8226	Myeloma	Multiple Rearrangements	-
U266	Myeloma	Multiple Rearrangements	-
P3HR-1	Endemic Burkitt	t (8;14)	+
AKUA	Endemic Burkitt	t (8;14)	+
Daudi	Endemic Burkitt	t (8;14)	+
SKDHL	Sporadic Burkitt	t (8;14)	-
BL 2	Sporadic Burkitt	t (8;22)	-
RS 11846	High grade B- cell lymphoma	t (14;18), t(8;22)	+
K562	CML	t (9;22)	-
PEER	T-ALL	Multiple Rearrangements	-
Jurkat	T-ALL	Multiple Rearrangements	-
Molt 4	T-ALL	t (7;7), 6q-	-
CEM	T-ALL	Multiple Rearrangments	-
Sup T1	T-ALL	inv (14) (q11;q32.3)	-
SupT11	T-ALL	t (14;14)(q11;q32.1)	+
HUT 78	T-Sezary Syndrome	N/A	-

N/A = not done.
The cell lines with multiple rearrangments do not have translocations or rearrangments at 14q32.1.

netic analysis for the occurrence of aberrations. Two types of translocations are observed in T-cells from AT patients. In one case the rearrangements involve the different TCR loci giving origin to chimeric T cell receptor genes; however cells presenting these rearrangements do not become neoplastic. In the other case the rearrangements are between a TCR locus and the TCL1 locus. These alterations are observed in T cell clonal expansions, that over the course of several years develop into full blown leukemias`(Russo et al., 1989; Brito-Babapulle and Catovsky, 1991; Kirsch, 1994). Therefore it was of interest to determine at which stage of the disease the expression of the *TCL1* gene was activated. We studied T cells from an AT patient with a large T cell clonal expansion carrying a translocation t(14;14) for the expression of *TCL1* , and we observed that *TCL1* expression was elevated before the onset of leukemia (Narducci et al., 1995). This observation indicates that *TCL1* activation is a very early step in the leukemogenic process, and that secondary genetic events must occur before the onset of full blown leukemia.

CONCLUSIONS

The *TCL1* gene is involved in most T-CLL, and in at least 75% of T-PLL. Since the difficulty of T-PLL diagnosis, this number may actually be higher, and rearrangements at chromosome 14q32 have also been observed in 30% of ATL (Brito-Babapulle and Ca-tovsky, 1991; Virgilio et al., 1993). The *TCL1* locus spans a region of 350 kb, and the *TCL1* gene, bracketed between two clusters of breakpoints, can be activated by either in-versions or translocations; in the first case TCR-Jα/δ elements are positioned 3' to the gene and in the second case 5' to it, in a situation resembling that of the *BCL2* gene. The *TCL1* protein has very high similarity with the protein encoded by the *MTCP1* gene, a gene also involved in T cell proliferative disorders (Stern et al., 1993; Fu et al., 1994; Sherrington et al., 1994). The function of *TCL1* and *MTCP1* proteins has not been defined as yet, and they clearly represent of a novel gene family.

The activation of *TCL1* in T-cell clonal expansions, suggests a role of this protein in the initiation of the neoplastic process. *TCL1* expression may confer to the cell either a proliferative or a survival advantage that only over the course of many years and with the accumulation of secondary genetic events will lead to neoplastic transformation. The much lower incidence of *MTCP1* rearrangments could be due either to a lower incidence of the translocation itself or it could suggest that even though the two proteins are very similar, *MTCP1* activation might confer to the cell less of a selective advantage.

Because *TCL1* is involved in the intiation of leukemia with a very slow progression, it is reasonable to postulate that the *TCL1* protein may belong to that class of oncoproteins in-volved in the regulation of programmed cell death as the BCL2 protein in follicular lym-phomas. However further studies expecially involving animal models, such as transgenic mice and null mice, will elucidate the consequences of overexpression or lack of expression of this protein and its role in the lymphoid development and lymphocyte differentiation.

REFERENCES

Brito-Babapulle, V. and Catovsky, D. (1991). Inversion and tandem duplication involving chromosome 14q11 and 14q32 in T-prolymphocytic leukemia in patients with ataxia-telangectasia. Cancer Genet. Cytogenet. *55*, 1–9.

Croce, C. M. (1987). Role of chromosome translocations in human neoplasia. Cell *49*, 155–156.

Fu, T., Virgilio, L., Narducci, M. G., Facchiano, A., Russo, G. and Croce, C. M. (1994). Characterization and lo-calization of the *TCL-1* oncogene product. Cancer Res. *54*, 6297–6301.

Gatti, R. A., Mc Conville, C. M. and Taylor, A. M. R. (1994). Sixth International Workshop on Ataxia Telangiecta-sia. Cancer Res. *54*, 6007-.

Gu, Y., Nakamura, T., Alder, H., Prasad, R., Canaani, O., Cimino, G., Croce, C.M. and Canaani, E. (1992). The t(4;11) chromosome translocation of human acute leukemias fuses the ALL-1 gene, to the Drosophila trithorax, to the AF-4 gene. Cell *71*, 1–20

Kamps, M.P., Murre, C., Sun, X. and Baltimore, D. (1990). A new homeobox gene contributes the DNA binding domain of the t(1;19) translocation protein in pre-B ALL. Cell *60*,547–555

Kirsch, I. R. (1994). V (D) J recombination and ataxia telangiectasia: A review. Int. J. Radiat. Biol. *66*, S97-S108.

Narducci, M. G., Virgilio, L., Isobe, M., Stoppacciaro, A., Elli, R., Fiorilli, M., Carbonari, M., Antonelli, A., Chessa, L., Croce, C. M. and Russo, G. (1995). TCL1 oncogene activation in preleukemic T cells from a case of ataxia-telangiectasia. Blood *86*, 2358–2364.

Nourse, J., Mellentin, J. D., Galili, N., Wilkinson, J., Stanbridge, E., Smith, S.D. and Cleary, M.L. (1990). Chro-mosomal translocation t(1;19) results in the synthesis of a homeobox fusion mRNA that codes for a poten-tial transcription factor. Cell *60*, 535–545

Rabbitts, T. H. (1994). Chromosomal translocation in human cancer. Nature *372*, 143–149.

Russo, G., Isobe, M., Gatti, R., Finan, J., Batuman, O., Huebner, K., Nowell, P. C. and Croce, C. M. (1989). Mo-lecular analysis of a t(14;14) translocation in leukemic T-cells of an ataxia telangiectasia patient. Proc. Natl. Acad. Sci. USA *86*, 602–606.

Russo, G., Isobe, .M., Pegoraro, L., Finan, J., Nowell, P. C. and Croce, C. M. (1988). Molecular analysis of a t(7;14)(q35;q32) chromosome translocation in a T-cell leukemia of a patient with ataxia telangiectasia. Cell *53*, 137–144.

Sherrington, P. D., Fish, P., Taylor, A. M. R. and Rabbitts, T. H. (1994). Clonal evolution of malignant and non-malignant T cells carrying t(14;14) and t(X;14) in patient with ataxia telangectasia. Oncogene 9, 2377–2381.

Stern, M. H., Soulier, J., Rosenzwaig, M., Nakahara, K., Canki-Klain, N., Aurias, A., Sigaux, F. and Kirsh, I. R. (1993). MTCP-1 gene: A novel gene on the human chromosome Xq28 translocated to the T cell receptor a/b locus in mature T cell proliferation. Oncogene 8, 2475-.

Virgilio, L., Isobe, M., Narducci, M. G., Carotenuto, P., Camerini. B., Kurosawa, N., ar-Rushdi, A., Croce, C. M. and Russo, G. (1993). Chromosome walking on the TCL1 locus involved in T-cell neoplasia. Proc. Natl. Acad. Sci. USA 90, 9275–9279.

Virgilio, L., Narducci, M. G., Isobe, M., Bilips, L., Cooper, M., Croce, C. M. and Russo, G. (1994). Identification of the TCL-1 gene involved in T-cell malignances. Proc. Natl. Acad. Sci. USA 91, 12530–12534.

DISCUSSION

F. Rauscher: What happens if you just overexpress full-length ALL-1 in the differentiation system?

C. Croce: We do not know yet. We tried to do that experiment in transgenic mice and we had a difficult time in getting the normal ALL-1 in transgenic mice expressed, probably because of the site. We got a lot of mice having part of the gene in, but never got expression. We also had a problem of the expression of the normal ALL-1 product *in-vitro*. Again, because of the site; only recently it seems that we are succeeding, but I do not know the answer to your question yet.

F. Rauscher: TCL-1: have you looked for direct interactions between BCL-2 protein and TCL-1?

C. Croce: They do not interact, unfortunately. That was the first experiment that we had done in fact.

G. Gilliland: What is the problem of expression of TCL-1 in hematopoietic cells of the wild type gene with reference to your dominant negative hypothesis for the activity of the cell fusion?

C. Croce: TCL-1, I told you, is lymphoid specific. Are you are talking about TCL-1?

G. Gilliland: No, for the ALL-1 gene.

C. Croce: ALL-1 is expressed essentially everywhere. In fact, we did not find a single cell line of any sort which is not expressing ALL-1. I strongly think that ALL-1 action might not be hematopoietic specific, but might occur in a lot of different tissues. It is a very large protein and we know that is processes; it is also involved, or at least a participant, in solid tumor pathogenesis. We have already evidence for that. Now we do not have conclusive evidence concerning the mechanism's mutation of the gene that could be involved in a fraction of solid tumor - the self fusion of the ALL-1, I mentioned to you, we found in gastric cancer. So, clearly, a protein that might have something to do with a hematopoietic differentiation might also have a variety of other actions.

G. Gilliland: So the prediction of your model of dominant negative activity of ALL-1 self fusion or of other ALL-1 fusions would be that overexpression in a hematopoietic cell would lead to a transformed phenotype. Is there evidence for transforming activity?

C. Croce: My idea is that we knock-out the expression of ALL-1 in a hematopoietic cell we will get an acute leukemia.

G. Gilliland: But in leukemic cells in which this has occurred, presumably there is expression of a dominant negative ALL-1.

C. Croce: In all the leukemia we have looked at, we have had also the expression of the normal allele.

G. Gilliland: Could you demonstrate transformation in cultured hematopoietic cells by overexpression of the putative dominant negative ALL-1 mutant?

C. Croce: That is exactly what we are trying to do now.

D. Livingston: If that hypothesis were correct, to follow up on Gary's question, one prediction would be that the wild type allele would be normal. If it was a single dominant negative, then is the wild type allele?

C. Croce: Yes. We did not sequence yet, but if we look at the mRNA, it has the normal size.

D. Livingston: That should be wild type.

C. Croce: It is wild type. So we see always the aberrant transcript coming from the fusion gene and the normal. In all leukemias carrying ALL-1 rearrangement we looked at, there is expression of normal ALL-1. The only places where we did not see ALL-1 normal expression were those gastric cancers having cell fusion of ALL-1.

D. Livingston: In fibroblast, for example, can you see the protein?

C. Croce: We can see the proteins, yes.

D. Livingston: So have you looked in any of the leukemias to see whether there is an off-sized ban other than the fusion protein?

C. Croce: In the leukemia we find the aberrant band and the normal band.

D. Livingston: The normal band - no other band?

C. Croce: No.

D. Livingston: Is it a nuclear protein?

C. Croce: I cannot give you an answer. One of the processed peptides derived from ALL-1 is nuclear. The protein is over 400,000 molecular weight.

D. Livingston: Do you know when during embryogenesis the embryo dies?

C. Croce: Very, very early.

A. Matter: Going back to the Bcl-2 phosphorylation state; would you speculate that carcinogenic action of okadaic acid is mediated by Bcl-2 under phosphorylation.

C. Croce: That could be it. Okadaic acid could have many other effects, we really cannot say that, but in every situation we looked at, there is a pretty good correlation between induction to die and phosphorylation of the BCL-2 protein. I did not mention several cell lines, I mentioned only the pro B-cell leukemias that expresses the phosphorylated form and in fact they are about 20% of cell death all the time. Now we found in other cell line, a lymphoblastoid cell line that is called GM-1500 - in which the treatment with okadaic acid does not induce phosphorylation of BCL-2; those cells are very resistant to okadaic acid. This is consistent with that interpretation. By the way, it was just published a week or two ago in PNAS.

15

TARGETING UBIQUITIN-MEDIATED DEGRADATION FOR PROLIFERATION INHIBITORS

Michele Pagano, Peggy Beer-Romero, Susan Glass, Sun Tam,
Ann Theodoras, Mark Rolfe and Giulio Draetta

Mitotix, Inc.
One Kendall Square, Bldg. 600
Cambridge, Massachusetts 02139

INTRODUCTION

The possibility of developing small molecule cancer chemotherapeutics using mechanism-based drug design has only recently been considered. The anti-cancer drugs presently available to the clinic were initially discovered as substances that inhibit the proliferation of tumors in animal models and/or of cultured cells (see [1,2] for reviews). The field of cancer chemotherapy started with the serendipitous discovery that mustard gas agents used in chemical warfare induced lymphoid hypoplasia, leading the way to their use in the treatment of Hodgkin's and lymphocytic lymphoma. The availability of transplantable tumor models in laboratory animals was also of utmost importance to allow testing of novel chemical agents. The establishment of a mass screening effort at the US National Cancer Institute (NCI) to identify substances that inhibit the proliferation of cultured tumor cells, then led to the discovery of agents that have been useful to treat and cure certain tumors, including leukemias and lymphomas. The NCI approach has primarily focused on the identification of chemical entities that inhibit the proliferation of one or the other histological cell type. With the discovery of the multiple drug resistance (MDR-1) gene and its amplification in tumors, some cell lines that show MDR-1 amplification in addition to their parental lines were introduced into the screen, but still, to this date most of the NCI screening efforts have focused on the identification of novel compounds that inhibit cell proliferation with a distinctive pattern. The identification of the molecular targets of the available anti-cancer drugs, together with the explosion in the discovery of genetic and biochemical abnormalities in cancer cells have suggested the possibility of taking a molecular mechanism-based approach for the development of cancer therapeutics (see[3], for review). The identification of a molecular lesion does indeed allow for the possibility of specifically targeting that defect, using both cell-based and molecular mechanism-based approaches. Both cell-based screens and molecular screens are worth carrying

Cancer Genes, edited by Mihich and Housman
Plenum Press, New York, 1996

to discover specific inhibitors of a certain molecular target. One can indeed screen for inhibition of proliferation of cell lines which carry a certain defect, using as a control wild-type cell lines, as well as molecular screens, in which inhibition of the biochemical activity of the target molecule (generally a protein) is assessed. Molecular screens allow the optimization of the identified inhibitor (i.e. enhancing potency and selectivity) against the target itself, without the need to worry about permeability and metabolic effects, which complicate cell-based screens.

Once the decision is made to develop a molecular approach for the discovery of anti-proliferatives, how should the choice of which target to focus upon be made? Several criteria in our opinion should be obeyed to in deciding which regulatory molecules to target for cancer:

1. there should be evidence of deregulation of the target in a given cancer;
2. the target molecule should have a role in the development of the tumor phenotype, and most importantly should continue to be required for tumor growth;
3. there should be a differential sensitivity between normally proliferating cells and cancer cells to the inhibition of that particular target;
4. the selected molecular target should preferably be an enzyme, since enzyme active sites are traditionally amenable to the development of small molecule inhibitors.

It is indeed difficult to target a molecule that is only present in cancer but not in normal cells. With the notable exceptions of molecules that arise as a result of chromosomal translocations, such as the Bcr-Abl and APL-RARα fusion proteins [45], which due to the genetic rearrangement, represent unique molecules that are not present in normal cells, the same regulatory molecules will be present in all cells of the body. One therefore has to rely on the likelihood that tumor cells which carry a deregulated expression of a certain gene product, might have developed epigenetic changes that make them exquisitely sensitive to inhibition of that function. This is the case for inhibitors of Ras farnesylation which inhibit proliferation of cultured cells and animal tumors carrying mutant Ras, but not of normal cells and non-Ras driven tumors (see [6], for review).

The relative higher responsiveness of some tumors to traditional chemotherapeutics could be attributed to the fact that tumor cells are hypersensitive to perturbations of cell cycle control, given that much of their control mechanisms have been altered. The very same principles that make tumor cells immortal, i.e. insensitive to growth controlling mechanisms, make them more susceptible to die, due to their inability to sense the perturbations caused by chemotherapeutic agents, or by ionizing radiation. It has been suggested to even try to take advantage of these "checkpoint" defects of tumors cells by giving "activators" of cell cycle transitions, hoping that the deregulated cancer cells be killed, under conditions in which normal cells remain unaffected[7]. This checkpoint inhibition approach might be very effective in treating cancers that are insensitive to traditional chemotherapeutics, such as the ones that carry p53 inactivation.

We at Mitotix are working on the identification of inhibitors of cyclin-dependent kinases and Cdc25 phosphatases, as well as inhibitors of the ubiquitin-mediated degradation pathway, in the context of the role that these molecules play in regulating cell proliferation. As opposed to growth factors and signal transduction molecules such as Ras, MAP kinases, protein kinase C etc. which play a role in multiple signal transduction cascades, the molecular pathways we study are only activated in proliferating cells, and are specifically involved in the development of cancer.

CELL CYCLE REGULATION

The induction of eukaryotic cell proliferation in response to growth-stimulatory signals, and conversely the induction of quiescence in response to lack of growth factors, to cell-cell contact, or to cellular damage etc., are mediated by signal transduction cascades that control the activation of cyclin-dependent kinases (Cdks). Multiple molecular controls have evolved to ensure the tight regulation of Cdk activation. These include the regulated synthesis and assembly of cyclin and Cdk subunits; the phosphorylation by a Cdk-activating kinase (Cak); the phosphorylation by a Cdk-inactivating kinase (Wee1); the activating dephosphorylation by a Cdc25-type phosphatase; the regulated accumulation of Cdk inhibitors (Ckis), including p16, p21, p27 and related proteins; the regulated destruction of cyclin and Cki subunits (see [8, 9, 10], for reviews).

While certain of these events mainly occur as part of the normal progression through each cell cycle, others occur in response to cellular damage, and others yet, in response to differentiative stimuli. It is now well established that lack of negative regulation of Cdks plays a determining role in oncogenesis (Fig. 1). Deregulated expression of D and E cyclins, as a consequence of gene amplification or DNA rearrangements, point mutations/deletions in the p16 gene, Cdk4 mutations and pRb mutations all result in the inactivation of the pathway that modulates the G1 to S-phase transition [1112]. The retinoblastoma protein, which is the sole known substrate of cyclin D1 kinase. appears to be a critical factor for the release of cells into S-phase. Recently, it has also been shown that the Cdc25-A and B phosphatases, which likely dephosphorylate Cdk2 and Cdk4[13, 14, 15], are linked to the Ras-Raf signal transduction pathway[16], and that the Cdc25-A and B mRNA are overexpressed in many human tumors[17]. Cdc25 overexpression could affect the ability of the cells to inactivate the Cdk4 and 2 subunits in response to DNA damage[15].

The pRb and p53 tumor suppressor proteins are inactivated at high frequency in human tumors. The demonstration that pRb is the product of a tumor suppressor gene, is in complete agreement with the idea that lack of pRb function plays a fundamental role in the cells becoming unresponsive to growth control mechanisms. On the other hand, the inactivation of p53, or of other elements of its pathway, increases the susceptibility of a tumor cell to DNA damage, creating that phenotype of genetic instability which is characteristic of tumor cells (Fig. 2).

As part of our effort to discover of specific inhibitors of cell proliferation which might be used as anti-proliferative drugs, we have initiated a research investigation on the mechanisms that control the regulated degradation of proteins which play a critical role in cell proliferation. We will summarize here our results on the characterization of the mechanisms responsible for p53 and p27 degradation.

INHIBITION OF p53 DEGRADATION IN HPV INFECTED CELLS

Studies started in P. Howley's laboratory demonstrated that the inactivation of p53 function subsequent to infection of human epithelial cells with human oncogenic papillomaviruses of the 16 and 18 serotypes, is achieved through the induction of p53 degradation in the cell [18]. Their in vitro studies demonstrated that upon addition of p53 to a rabbit reticulocyte lysate, in the presence of added E6 protein p53 was multiubiquitinated and degraded by the proteasome, a multi-subunit complex that is responsible for the degradation of ubiquitinated proteins (see[19], for a review).

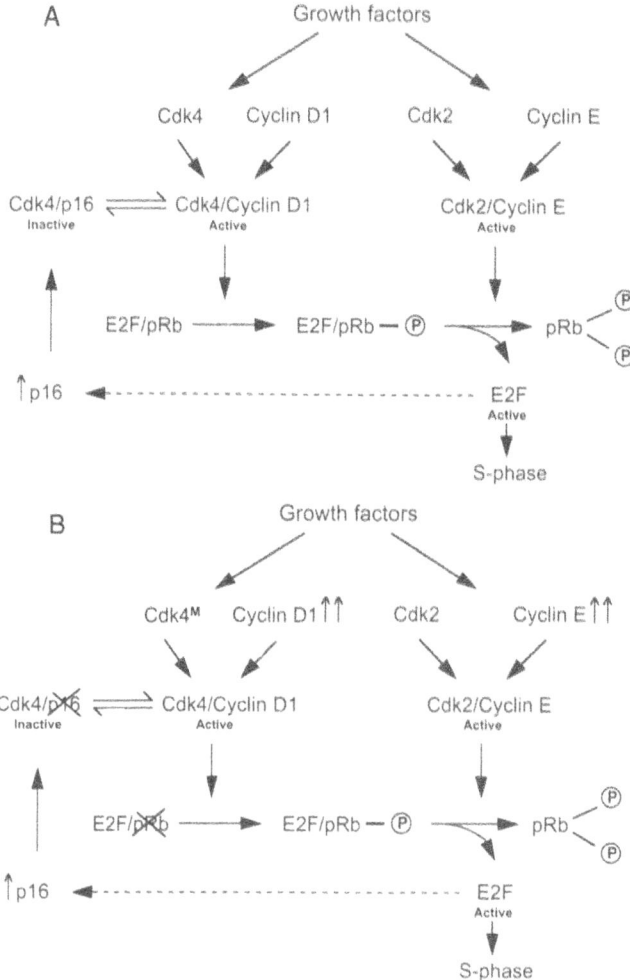

Figure 1. Regulation of cell cycle progression in G1 by the cyclin D and E -dependent kinases. (A) The activation of the G1/S transition in cells stimulated to reenter the cell cycle is achieved though the formation of cyclin D and E kinase complexes. Upon phosphorylation of pRb by D and E cyclins, E2F complexes are released and induce the transcription of genes required for S-phase. (B) In cancer cells, deregulated expression of D-cyclins, mutations in Cdk4 that render it insensitive to p16-type inhibitors, p16 or pRb inactivation all result in the failure of the cell to arrest in response to lack of growth stimuli.

The conjugation of ubiquitin to proteins acts as a signal for their degradation by the proteasome, and it is generated through a biochemical cascade that requires at least three distinct protein components, in addition to ubiquitin [20]. First, an enzyme called ubiquitin - activating enzyme or E1, in the presence of ATP, is linked to ubiquitin via a cysteine in its active site. The formed high energy thioester then transfers its ubiquitin to a ubiquitin-conjugating enzyme, or E2. A further component, a ubiquitin-ligase or E3, which itself might bind covalently ubiquitin through a thioester bonds then releases the ubiquitin to the target substrate by forming a covalent isopeptide bond between the C-terminus of ubiquitin and the ε-amino group of a lysine residue of the target protein. Additional

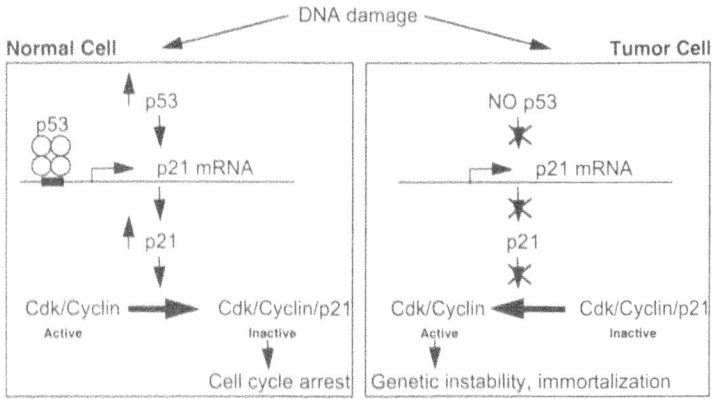

Figure 2. The role of p53 in mediating cell cycle arrest in response to DNA damage. In response to DNA damage, p53 accumulates in cells, binds to specific sites on DNA and induces the transcription of genes including the gene encoding p21, a Cdk inhibitor. The consequent cell cycle arrest allows cells to repair their DNA and possibly reenter the cell cycle. The inactivation of p53 in tumor cells results in a failure for those cells to respond to DNA damage with cell cycle arrest and DNA repair, leading to genetic instability.

ubiquitin molecule are added to the ubiquitin bound to the target protein, creating an ubiquitin tree, that is recognized by the proteasome and rapidly degraded.

As of the component required for p53 degradation in HPV infected cells, Howley et al. identified a factor named E6AP (E6-associated protein) which is required for p53 degradation in the presence of E6 [21]. The identity of other components required for p53 degradation and present in cell lysate, was not known at that time.

We had previously observed that upon injection of p53 expression plasmids in HPV-infected cervical carcinoma cells, these cells did enter apoptosis (M. Pagano et al., unpublished). We thought therefore that specific inhibitors of p53 degradation, could induce apoptosis by elevating the abundance of p53 in HPV-infected cells, while leaving normal cells unharmed. We decided therefore to attempt the identification of the specific ubiquitin-conjugating enzyme(s) responsible for p53 degradation in HPV-infected cells. We cloned a number of human cDNAs encoding human ubiquitin-conjugating enzymes and tested them for the ability to induce p53 ubiquitination in a purified in vitro system containing E6, E6AP, E1, Ub and ATP. One of these enzymes, which we call Ubc4, was in fact a powerful inducer of p53 ubiquitination in vitro[22]. In assessing the order of events in the reactions that lead to p53 ubiquitination, we have found that E6AP is an important intermediary in the reaction, since it receives ubiquitin from Ubc4 and donates it, only if E6 is present, to p53 (Fig. 3). Scheffner et al. have also identified an E2 that is able to induce the ubiquitination of p53 in vitro[23]. They have also recently shown that E6AP is ubiquitinated and have identified a critical Cys residue, that when mutated completely inactivates E6AP [24].

To prove that in fact E6AP and Ubc4 are involved in regulating p53 in living cells as well, we resorted to microinjection of antibodies, antisense or of plasmids encoding proteins carrying a replacement of the active site cysteine with a serine. These proteins fail to be ubiquitinated but still retain the ability to bind their substrates, and therefore behave as dominant interfering mutants. Upon microinjection into living cells, we found that inhibition of Ubc4 or E6AP function prevents the disappearance of p53 caused by HPV-E6 expression (Fig. 4). Furthermore, microinjection of anti-Ubc4 or E6AP antibodies in

HPV-infected cells, but not of anti-Ubc2 antibodies, results in cell death (P. Beer-Romero and M. Rolfe, in preparation).

We predict that if we were able to raise the abundance of p53 in pRb⁻ cells these cells would enter apoptosis. Despite the fact that there is evidence for the involvement of the ubiquitin conjugation pathway in the degradation of p53 in normal cells, and that p53 accumulation upon DNA damage involves stabilization of the protein, we and others have failed to date to generate ubiquitinated p53 in cell extracts which lack HPV-E6. Further-

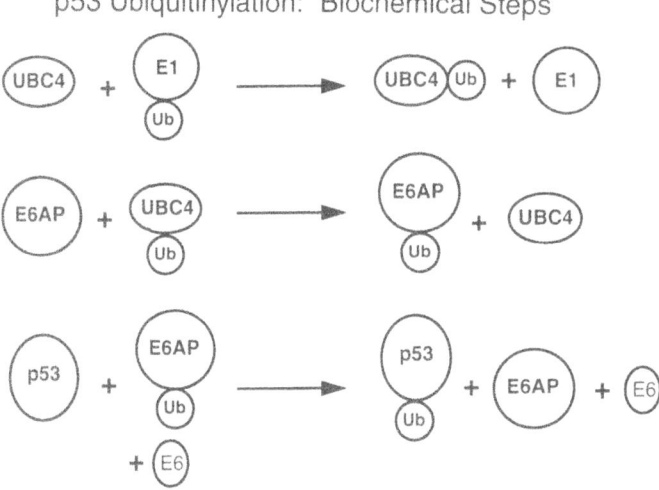

Figure 3. Biochemical pathway responsible for p53 degradation in HPV 18 infected human cells. The E1 enzyme releases its ubiquitin to the UBC4, ubiquitin-conjugating enzyme, which then donates its ubiquitin to E6-AP. In the presence of the viral oncoprotein HPV18-E6, pre is ubiquitinated by UBC4, leading to the activation of p53 destruction through the proteasome.

more, inhibition of E6AP or Ubc4 function in normal cells, did not result in an increased accumulation of p53 (P. Beer-Romero and M. Rolfe, in preparation). It is likely that additional components need to be identified to reconstitute this system in vitro, and that these components are distinct from E6AP and Ubc4. Evidence in favor of a role of the ubiquitin-mediated proteolysis in the degradation of p53, in normal cells, include the fact that cells carrying a temperature-sensitive allele of Ub-E1, at the restrictive temperature show an increased accumulation of p53 [25], and that the addition of proteasome inhibitors to growing cells will induce the accumulation of p53 (P. Beer-Romero and M. Rolfe, in preparation).

INACTIVATION OF THE p27 CDK INHIBITOR BY UBIQUITIN-MEDIATED PROTEOLYSIS

p27 was discovered as a protein that accumulates in cells that have undergone cell cycle arrest in response to transforming-growth factor β and contact inhibition [26,27]. It was

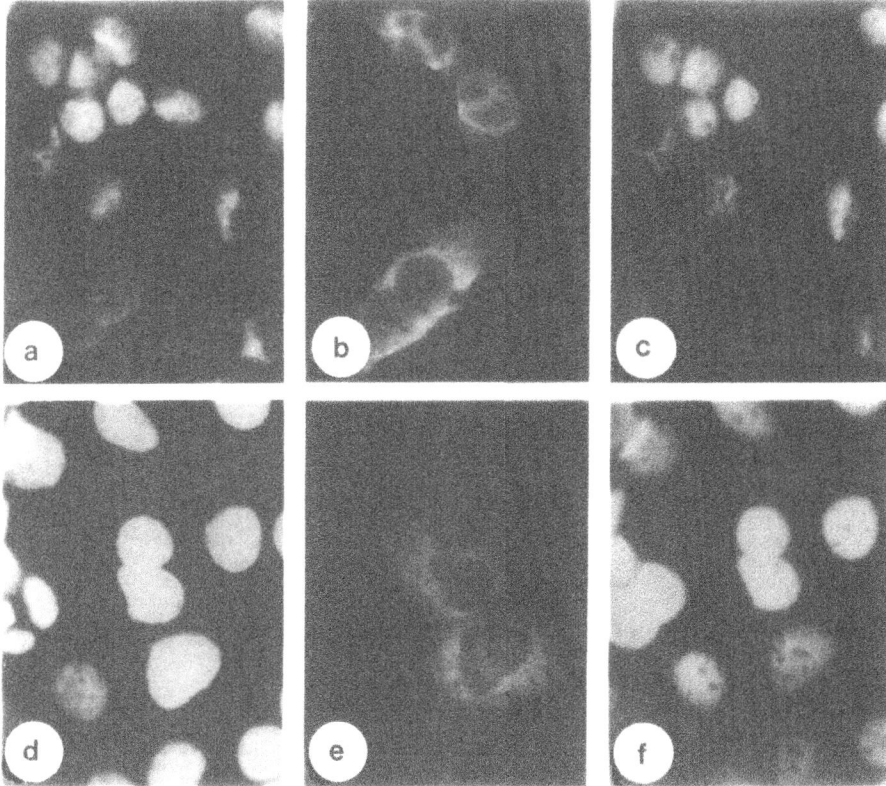

Figure 4. Role of UBC4 in p53 degradation Inhibition of E6-stimulated protein degradation by mutant UBC4 in human cells. Immunofluorescence analysis of microinjected cells. (a-c) cells injected with a plasmid encoding the HPV-18 E6 protein. (d-f): cells injected with both an E6-encoding plasmid and with a plasmid encoding a UBC4 Cys-to-Ser mutant. (a, d) Hoechst staining; (b-e): staining of injected cells; (c-f): p53 staining. (reproduced from [22], with permission).

also cloned using the yeast two hybrid system, as an interactor of Cdk4/Cyclin D1 [28]. It is a powerful inhibitor of Cdk4/2 kinase complexes [26, 29]. The p27 levels are elevated in serum starved osteosarcoma cells (Fig. 5) and in fibroblasts and resting primary T-lymphocytes, compared to growing cells. In T-cells treated with rapamycin or cAMP, p27 levels remain elevated upon growth factor stimulation [29, 30]. Interestingly, the levels of p27 mRNA and the rate of p27 protein synthesis are not significantly different between quiescent and growing cells. In fact, substantial differences are only seen when comparing the half-life of p27 between growing and quiescent cells. In quiescent cells the p27 half-life is 6–8 times higher compared to actively growing cells [31]. This can account for the differences in p27 abundance seen between quiescent and proliferating cells.

We sought to investigate the mechanisms that control p27 degradation [31]. Using an inhibitor of the chymotryptic activity of the proteasome, N-acetyl-leucinyl-leucinyl-norleucinal-H (LLnL) added to growing human osteosarcoma cells MG-63, or normal fibroblasts, we found that p27 levels dramatically increase and slowly migrating p27 bands appear on SDS-PAGE. We were able to demonstrate that those high-molecular weight bands are caused by p27 ubiquitination, since they are recognized by specific antibodies to

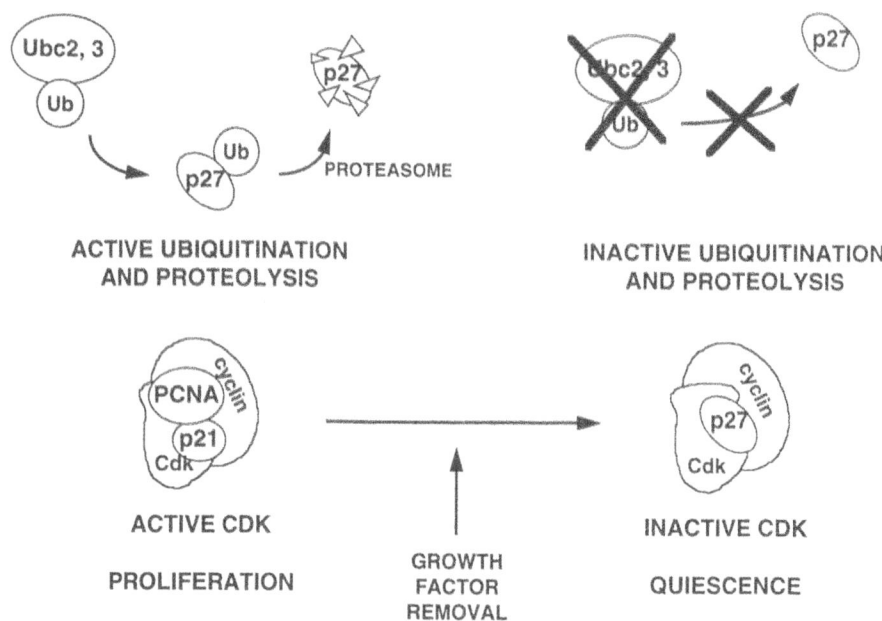

ACTIVE UBIQUITINATION AND PROTEOLYSIS

INACTIVE UBIQUITINATION AND PROTEOLYSIS

ACTIVE CDK

PROLIFERATION

GROWTH FACTOR REMOVAL

INACTIVE CDK

QUIESCENCE

Figure 5. Cell cycle oscillation of p27 protein levels and phosphorylation. Human osteosarcoma MG-63 cells synchronized in G1 by serum deprivation. Arrested cells were stimulated by serum readdition. By 18 hrs 50% of the cells were in S phase and by 24 hrs about 80% of the cells had incorporated BrdU. At different time points cell lysates were analyzed by immunoblotting with antibodies to p27 and to p21. The overall abundance of p27 protein gradually decreased after serum readdition, and by 18 hours reached the lowest level (approx. 6 to 8 fold less protein than in quiescent cells). The state of p27 phosphorylation was determined by labeling cells with pulse of 32P-phosphate (Fig. 1C). p27 was poorly phosphorylated in quiescent cells. Three hours after serum readdition the incorporation of 32P dramatically increased reaching a peak between 6 and 9 hours. This result suggests that p27 phosphorylation may have a role in its degradation. (A) Flow cytometry profiles of serum-deprived MG-63 cells (left) and MG-63 cells 18 hours after serum reactivation (right). Open and closed triangles mark 2N and 4N DNA content, respectively. (B) Immunoblotting with anti-p27 or anti-p21 antibodies, 50 μg protein extract/lane. Lane 1, asynchronous cells (AS); Lanes 2 -6, serum deprived cells reactivated by serum addition and sampled at the indicated intervals (hours). (C) Immunoprecipitations with anti p27 antibodies. Serum deprived cells reactivated by serum addition were labeled for one hour with 32P-orthophosphate and sampled at the indicated intervals (hours).

ubiquitin [31]. Upon addition of proteasome inhibitor to quiescent cells, followed by addition of serum, p27 failed to disappear and remained localized to the nucleus (A. Theodoras and M. Pagano, unpublished results).

p27 is in fact also ubiquitinated in vitro. Using a rabbit reticulocyte lysate system, a good source of ubiquitinating enzymes and proteasome subunits, we could show that p27 was poly-ubiquitinated and degraded in vitro [31]. This reactions, as similar ubiquitination reactions, required ATP and were inhibited by the addition of proteasome inhibitors. We could also show that the ubiquitination and degradation of p27 was enhanced by the addition of either human UBC2 or UBC3 protein. Furthermore, we found that the ubiquitination and degradation of p27 could be prevented by the addition of mutant UBC2 or UBC3 in which the catalytic cysteine had been replaced with a serine, suggesting that these enzymes were competing with the endogenous enzymes for conjugation of Ub to p27.

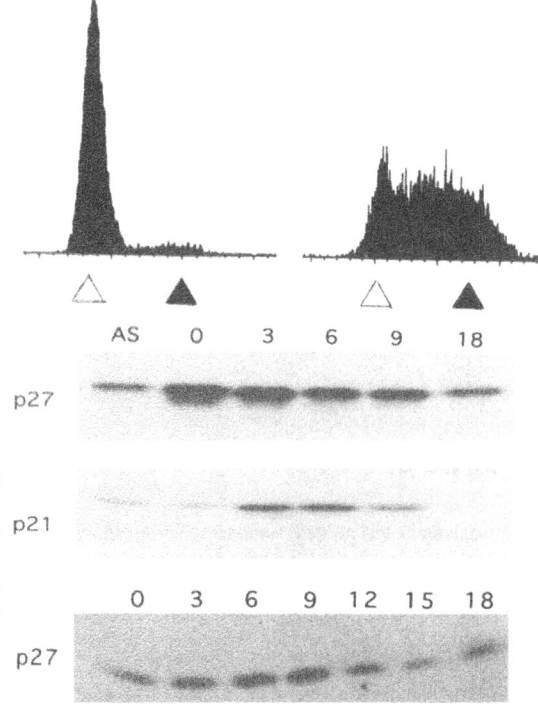

Figure 6. Regulation of p27 degradation in quiescent and growing cells. In quiescent cells, p27 is present at high levels due to an increase in its half-life. UBC2 and 3, the enzymes that are responsible for p27 ubiquitination, and likely a yet to be discovered E3, are inactive in quiescent cells, while they get activated in cells stimulated to reenter the cell cycle with growth factors

In an in vitro reaction with purified components , we noticed that in the presence of E1, ATP, ubiquitin and either UBC2 or UBC3, only a mono-ubiquitinated p27 species was generated. The addition of a cellular extract was indeed necessary to generate the multiple ubiquitinated forms of p27 that are necessary to stimulate degradation. We suspect therefore that an additional component is required to generate the multiubiquitinated forms of p27 and are presently attempting at the purification of this component(s).

The key question about p27 ubiquitination in living cells, is how is it regulated (Fig. 6). We find that extracts from quiescent cells are poor sources of p27 ubiquitination activities compared to proliferating cells, despite the fact that quiescent cells contain similar amounts of UBC2 and UBC3 compared to proliferating cells. We believe that either a change in abundance of a third component, the putative E3 enzyme, or post-translational modifications of p27 and/or of the ubiquitinating enzymes, or both, are responsible for the observed differences. While mutations in the gene encoding p27 have not been detected in tumors [32, 33], we have preliminary evidence that the p27 protein is reduced in abundance in certain tumors (M. Pagano, M. Loda et al., in progress), suggesting that this might have occurred as a result of alterations in the p27 degradation rate. As these studies continue, the identification of the mechanisms involved will allow the development of molecular screen for the discovery of small molecule inhibitors of p27 degradation that might profoundly affect tumor cell proliferation.

TARGETING PROTEIN DEGRADATION FOR SMALL MOLECULE INHIBITORS

What confers specificity to protein degradation reactions that involve ubiquitin? In the reaction cascade that requires components such as E1, an E2, an E3, ubiquitin, ATP, a target substrate and the proteasome complex, it seems likely that the targeting of a given protein for degradation in response to specific signals, is brought about by the activation of E2 and E3 enzymes, rather than by E1, for which only one enzyme per cell has been found, or by the proteasome complex which seems to recognize any ubiquitinated protein and degrade it. Using mechanism-based approaches as well as high through-put screening of chemical libraries, we will be able to identify compounds that inhibit the function of E2's and E3's. We already have evidence for additional levels of regulation of this system, including the evidence that p27 is phosphorylated in living cells (Fig. 5), which we will continue to explore to potentially target further biochemical reactions in the pathway.

In summary, we believe that regulated protein degradation plays a fundamental role in cell cycle control (see also[34], for review) and that by targeting protein degradation with small molecular weight inhibitors, we will be able to block selectively certain cellular processes.

REFERENCES

1. Calabresi, P., and B. Chabner. 1990. Antineoplastic Agents, p. 1209–1263. *In* A. Gilman, T. Rall, A. Nies and P. Taylor (ed.), The Pharmacological Basis of Therapeutics. Pergamon Press, New York.
2. DeVita, V. 1993. Principles of Chemotherapy, p. 276–292. *In* V. DeVita, S. Hellman and S. Rosenberg (ed.), Cancer: Principals and Practice of Oncology, vol. 1. J.B. Lippincott Company, Philadelphia.
3. Karp, J. E., and S. Broder. Molecular foundations of cancer: new targets for intervention. *Nature Medicine* 1:309–320 (1995)
4. Grignani, F., M. Fagioli, M. Alcalay, L. Longo, P. P. Pandolfi, E. Donti, A. Biondi, F. L. Coco, and P. G. Pelicci. Acute promyelocytic leukemia: from genetics to treatment. *Blood* 83:10–25 (1994)
5. Tauchi, T., and H. E. Broxmeyer. BCR/ABL signla transduction. *Int. J. Hematol* 61:105–112 (1995)
6. Gibbs, J. B., and A. Oliff. Pharmaceutical research in molecular oncology. *Cell* 79:193–198 (1994)
7. Hartwell, L. H., and M. B. Kastan. Cell cycle control and cancer. *Science* 266:1821–1828 (1994)
8. Draetta, G. F. cdc2 activation: the interplay of cyclin binding and thr161 phosphorylation. *Trends in Cell Biology* 3:287–289 (1993)
9. Sherr, C., and J. Roberts. Inhibitors of mammalian G1 cyclin-dependent kinases. *Genes& dev.* 9:1149–1163 (1995)
10. Sherr, C. G1 phase progression: cycling on cue. *Cell* 79:551–555 (1994)
11. Draetta. Mammalian G1 cyclins. *Curr. Opin. Cell Biol.* 6:842–846 (1994)
12. Hunter, T., and J. Pines. Cyclins and Cancer II: cyclin D and Cdk inhibitors come of age. *Cell* 79:573–582 (1994)
13. Hoffmann, I., G. Draetta, and E. Karsenti. Activation of the phosphatase activity of human Cdc25 by a cdk-cyclin E dependent phosphorylation at the G1/S transition. *EMBO J.* 13:4302–4310 (1994)
14. Jinno, S., K. Suto, A. Nagata, M. Igarashi, Y. Kanaoka, H. Nojima, and H. Okayama. Cdc25A is a novel phosphatase functioning early in the cell cycle. *EMBO J.* 13:1549–1556 (1994)
15. Terada, Y., M. Tatsuka, S. Jinno, and H. Okayama. Requirement for tyrosine phosphorylation of Cdk4 in G1 arrest induced by ultraviolet irradiation. *Nature* 376:358–362 (1995)
16. Galaktionov, K., C. Jessus, and D. Beach. Raf1 interaction with cdc25 phosphatase ties mitogenic signal transduction to cell cycle activation. *Genes & Develop.* 9:1046–1058 (1995)
17. Galaktionov, K., A. Lee, J. Eckstain, G. Draetta, J. Meckler, M. Loda, and D. Beach. Cdc25 phosphatase as potential human oncogene. *Science* in press:(1995)
18. Scheffner, M., B. Werness, J. Huibregtse, A. Levine, and P. Howley. The E6 Oncoprotein Encoded by Human Papillomavirus Types 16 and 18 Promotes the Degradation of p53. *Cell* 63:1129–1136 (1990)
19. Goldberg, A. L. Functions of the proteasome: the lysis at the end of the tunnel. *Science* 268:522–523 (1995)
20. Ciechanover, A. The Ubiquitin-Proteasome Proteolytic Pathway. *Cell* 79:13–21 (1994)
21. Huibregtse, J., M. Scheffner, and P. Howley. A cellular protein mediates association of p53 with the E6 oncoprotein of human papillomavirus types 16 or 18. *EMBO J.* 10:4129–4135 (1991)
22. Rolfe, M., P. Romero, S. Glass, J. Eckstein, I. Berdo, A. Theodoras, M. Pagano, and G. Draetta. Reconstitution of p53-ubiquitinylation reaction from purified components: the role of human UBC4 and E6AP. *Proc. Natl. Acad. Sci. USA* 92:3264–3268 (1995)

23. Scheffner, M., J. Huibregtse, and P. Howley. Identification of a human ubiquitin-conjugating enzyme that mediates the E6-AP-dependent ubiquitination of p53. *Proc. Natl. Acad. Sci. USA* 91:8797–8801 (1994)
24. Scheffner, M., U. Nuber, and J. Huibregtse. Protein ubiquitination involving an E1-E2-E3 enzyme ubiquitin thioester cascade. *Nature* 373:81–83 (1995)
25. Chowdary, D., J. Dermody, K. Jha, and H. Ozer. Accumulation of p53 in a mutant cell line defective in the ubiquitin pathway. *Mol. Cell. Biol.* 14:1997–2003 (1994)
26. Polyak, K., M. Kato, M. J. Solomon, C. J. Sherr, J. Massague, J. M. Roberts, and A. Koff. p27^{Kip1} and Cyclin D-Cdk4 are interacting regulators of Cdk2, and link TGF-β and contact inhibition to cell cycle arrest. *Genes & Dev.* 8:9–22 (1994)
27. Polyak, K., M. Lee, H. Erdjement-Bromage, A. Koff, J. Roberts, P. Tempst, and J. Massague. Cloning of p27kip1, a cyclin-dependent kinase inhibitor and a potential mediator of extracellular antimitogenic signals. *Cell* 79:59–66 (1994)
28. Toyoshima, and T. Hunter. p27, a novel inhibitor of G1-cyclin-cdk protein kinase activity, is related to p21. *Cell* 78:67–74 (1994)
29. Nourse, J., E. Firpo, M. Flanagan, S. Coats, C. Polyak, M. Lee, J. Massague, G. Crabtree, and J. Roberts. Interleukin-2-mediated elimination of p27Kip1 cyclin-dependent kinase inhibitor prevented by rapamycin. *Nature* 372:570–573 (1994)
30. Kato, J., M. Matsuoka, K. Polyak, J. Massague, and C. J. Sherr. Cyclic AMP-induced G1 phase arrest mediated by an inhibitor (p27^{kip1}) of cyclin-dependent kinase-4 activation. *Cell* 79:487–496 (1994)
31. Pagano, M., S. W. Tam, A. M. Theodoras, P. Romero-Beer, G. Del Sal, V. Chau, R. Yew, G. Draetta, and M. Rolfe. Role of the Ubiquitin-Proteasome pathway in regulating aboundance of the Cyclin-dependent kinase inhibitor p27. *Science* 269:682–685 (1995)
32. Pietenpol, J., S. Bohlander, Y. Sato, N. Papadopoulos, B. Liu, C. Friedman, B. Trask, J. Roberts, K. Kinzler, J. Rowley, and B. Vogelstein. Assignment of the Human *p27^{Kip1}* Gene to 12p13 and Its Analysis in Leukemias. *Cancer Research* 55:1206–1210 (1995)
33. Ponce-Castañeda, V., M. Lee, E. Latres, K. Polyak, L. Lacombe, K. Montgomery, S. Mathew, K. Krauter, J. Sheinfeld, J. Massague, and C. Cordon-Cardo. *p27^{Kip1}*: Chromosomal Mapping to 12p12–12p13.1 and Absence of Mutations in Human Tumors. *Cancer Research* 55:1211–1214 (1995)
34. Barinaga, M. A new twist to the cell cycle. *Science* 269:631–632 (1995)

DISCUSSION

M. Oren: How do you explain the role of E6-AP in transferring ubiquitin to p53?

G. Draetta: Although in our studies we used proteins expressed in recombinant systems such as E. coli or insert cells and purified to homogeneity, we cannot exclude that some contaminating component was present in our assays. On the other hand, our results are supported by a parallel study performed by Martin Scheffner's group in Heidelberg, who demonstrated that a mutation in a conserved cysteine in E6-AP, inhibits p53 ubiquitination. They also found that E6-AP is ubiquitinated *in vitro*. I do really believe therefore that E6-AP is responsible for transferring ubiquitin to p53 in papillomavirus infected cells. Whether or not all E3 enzymes will work as ubiquitin-transferases, I do not know at present. There are four additional sequences known that have sequence similarities to E6-AP, and they all have a cysteine residue in the same consensus. But no similarity to E6-AP is detectable in a yeast E3 enzyme. It is possible therefore that some E3 will have an E6-AP like function, some others will have different functions.

D. Livingston: Is your strategy for elevating the concentration of p53 effective only in Rb$^{+/+}$ cells?

G. Draetta: The strategy would only be effective in a cell that lacks retinoblastoma function.

D. Livingston: What if there were intact Rb protein present if you are thinking death?

G. Draetta: We are thinking death.

D. Livingston: In that case, would you require intact Rb protein?

G. Draetta: That is right. Well, I mean, from that point of view you would think that. Our focus has been to select biochemical pathways that show alterations in human tumors, for the development of proliferation inhibitors. It is possible that the proliferation of normal cells will also be inhibited in response to such inhibitors. On the other hand, we believe that a mechanism-based approach that targets genetic alterations in cancer is the way to go. The recent results obtained by scientists at Merck with ras farnesyl transferase inhibitors, show that despite the involvement of ras in many signaling pathways, tumor cells are exquisitely sensitive to these inhibitors, while normal cells do not seem to be affected much. I think time will tell whether inhibitors of cyclin-dependent kinases will have potent and selective effects on tumor growth.

Y. Xiong: A couple of things that were not clear, and I noticed on your slide, you put an E2F as p16 activator--is that speculation or actually an experimental result?

G. Draetta: Speculation, based on the fact that we see an increase in p16 abundance as soon as cells enter S-phase.

Y: Xiong: You mentioned that in Go cells p27 accumulates and, if I understand it correctly, is that because the activity of the ubiquitin pathway is decreased in the arrested cell?

G. Draetta: That is what we believe.

Y. Xiong: Instead of the increased expression of p27?

G. Draetta: Yes, I did not have time to go through it. But, first of all, several labs have shown that the RNA level is constant in both quiescent and proliferating cells. We looked at p27 rate of synthesis and found there is not much difference between quiescence and proliferating cells. The only difference we see is in the half-life of p27; in a pulse-chase experiment we found that there is a very big difference between quiescent and proliferating cells. The levels of the UBC2 and UBC3 protein are lower in quiescent cells compared to those in proliferating cells. But there is still quite a bit of those proteins in quiescent cells. Therefore, we believe that some additional factor is activated in proliferating cells: This is also because if you incubate simply UBC2 or 3 or UBC2 and 3 with p27 one does not get the polyubiquitination that one gets in the presence of a crude extract. So there must be some other component needed, which we believe is an E3, and we believe that this E3 could be subjected to regulation via phosphorylation or similar mechanisms.

Y. Xiong: Yes, and to follow that up: Steve Reed mentioned that p27 is actually subjected to post-translational control and that in HeLa cells, p27 expression is not increased but appears to be increased in the protein. You think that the decrease in ubiquitous pathway might be one of the mechanisms that accounts for the increase of the p27 protein level? Or is there actually some other kind of mechanism that might be involved?

G. Draetta: All what we can measure is difference in degradation of p27 in other human cells, we tested of course transformed human cells, as well as normal cells, and you see the same thing.

P. Sassone-Corsi: I thought p27 kip was transcriptionally inducible by cAMP; that is how it was described first, right?

G. Draetta: No, it was transcriptionally repressed.

P. Sassone-Corsi: If you treat cells with cAMP p27 transcription goes up at least four or five fold - that is how it was described first, right?

G. Draetta: OK, but if you look at the disappearance of the protein there is an effect on the stability of the protein as well in that case. Also in mouse cells you do not see these kind of effects that we have described. In human cells, in T-lymphocytes you see this accumulation of p27 protein. If you do this in mouse cells you do not often see the huge difference in accumulation of p27.

E. Mihich: I am intrigued by the unknown determinants of whether p53 induces block of proliferation versus apoptosis. And I was wondering whether consideration has been given by those working in this field to the kinetics of the two phenomenon? As you know concentration and time of exposure are important determinants of differential action and I wonder whether some clues could be obtained in discriminating between these two pathways through studies of the kinetic of the effects induced by different concentration of p53 under different conditions.

G. Draetta: I do not think it would depend much on the dosage of p53 in terms of differences in response to p53 elevation between the normal or non-Rb negative and Rb negative cells. I think, as you say, that there is a time difference. I mean, you are going to get apoptosis. I think, and I do not know if Moshe would agree, but it is so relative, you can get apoptosis in a p53 independent manner as well, but it is a matter of dosage - drug dosage and time.

M. Fried: When you use the antisense for UBC4 and E6AP, what cells were those, and did it have any effect on normal cells?

G. Draetta: No significant effect on normal cells in terms of apoptosis.

M. Fried: Were they transformed cells, or infected cells?

G. Draetta: HPV infected cells - again what we are trying to do now is to run experiment in matched cell pairs so we can exclude cell type specific effects and so on. In the normal cells injected with these components we do not see apoptosis.

M. Fried: But with HeLa cells?

G. Draetta: With HeLa cells we see apoptosis.

M. Fried: And what about antisense to E6 itself?

G. Draetta: Not done. The reason why we have not done it is because we cannot detect E6. In the transformed cells E6 is almost impossible to detect, it is at a very, very low abundance. At least with the antibodies we have tested.

M. Fried: But E6 is the foreign gene, whereas, the other ones are host genes. Would not the viral E6 gene be a better target?

G. Draetta: One could target any of those reactions *in vitro* and you might identify compounds that target different reaction mechanisms. One would probably be successful if you were preventing E6 interaction with the other components. A medicinal chemist would say that trying to inhibit protein-protein interaction is much harder than trying to block an enzyme catalytic site.

G. Evan: Can I go back to the cell fate being determined by whether Rb is there or not; whether the cells are going to arrest or die. I mean, sorry to be stupid about this, but where does this idea come from? I know there are examples where this is the case - but there are an enormous amount of examples where cells with wild type Rb e.g., fibroblasts, also die by apoptosis in a p53 dependent manner and if you hit them hard enough in a p53 independent manner. So I just do not see where this sort of idea is really coming from. Clearly, you can modulate apoptosis as David Livingston says, in lots of other ways, completely independently of Rb and p53 as well as Bcl 2 and the other factors. In the case of fibroblasts arrest, in our hands, when we radiate them, principally if you do it in high serum concentration, you have lots of survival factors around which are suppressing cell death. If you actually drop the serum concentration you get a much, much more effective induction of apoptosis and I would not have thought that Rb stasis would be any different, and what is more, the apoptosis is cell cycle dependent.

G. Draetta: I am not assuming that this is a general strategy. In the context of our experiment, what we are trying to do now is actually to have an inducible activation in a cell - in order to show that it does make a difference. Clearly, there are experiments like the Levine experiment and others and, the data presented by Moshe Oren that indicate that in certain cell systems inactivation of Rb, - and induction of p53 result in apoptosis.

M. Oren: I want to partially reiterate what Gerard said and emphasize that there is evidence that overexpressed Rb will protect cells from apoptosis even in the absence of p53. This is a recent study by Mark Israel. Of course, as Gerard mentioned, there are many other cases where p53 can induce apoptosis in cells which have functional Rb as far as one can tell. So probably, what one should expect is not really a yes or a no, but it is likely that if you have the ability to modulate p53 in a cell which has no Rb, that cell will be more susceptible to apoptosis. Perhaps one has to think about it as a magic trigger, which may allow you, when combined with a relatively low dose of chemotherapy radiation, to alter the fate of the cell from no death, into death.

16

SELECTIVE KILLING OF BCR-ABL POSITIVE CELLS WITH A SPECIFIC INHIBITOR OF THE ABL TYROSINE KINASE

Brian J. Druker,[1] Sayuri Ohno,[1] Elisabeth Buchdunger,[2] Shu Tamura,[1] Jürg Zimmermann,[2] and Nicholas B. Lydon[2]

[1] Division of Hematology and Medical Oncology
Oregon Health Sciences University
Portland, Oregon 97201
[2] Ciba Pharmaceuticals Division, Oncology Research Department
Ciba-Geigy Limited
CH-4002, Basel, Switzerland

1. CHRONIC MYELOGENOUS LEUKEMIA

1.1 Clinical Features

Chronic myelogenous leukemia (CML) is a malignancy of the pluripotent hematopoietic stem cell. This disease accounts for 15–20% of all leukemias with an annual incidence of between 1 to 2 cases per 100,000 persons per year. The median age of onset is approximately 50 years of age. Clinically, the disease is characterized by a chronic phase in which the only apparent abnormality is the massive expansion of functionally normal myeloid lineage cells [1]. During this chronic phase, myeloid cells retain the capacity to differentiate normally. Following an average chronic phase duration of about three years, the disease transforms to an accelerated or blast phase in which there is a progressive loss of the capacity for terminal differentiation of myeloid lineage cells along with the accumulation of cytogenetic abnormalities [1].

1.2 Therapy of CML

Allogeneic bone marrow transplantation is currently the only known curative therapy for CML. The cure rate is 70–90% in patients that survive the transplant but the mortality rate from the procedure is 15–25% and increases with the age of the patient and the degree of mismatch [2,3]. However, only 20–25% of patients with CML are eligible for allogeneic bone marrow transplantation due to age or lack of a suitable donor. Patients without a match who are under 50 are eligible for a matched unrelated donor transplant.

Cancer Genes, edited by Mihich and Housman
Plenum Press, New York, 1996

Although the cure rate for survivors is similar, the mortality rate increases to as high as 50%. For patients not eligible for allogeneic bone marrow transplantation, either due to age or lack of a suitable donor, or for patients unwilling to accept the high mortality rate from the procedure, no curative therapy is available.

Standard therapy for patients not undergoing allogeneic bone marrow transplantation is Hydroxyurea or α-Interferon with recent comparative studies of Hydroxyurea versus α-Interferon suggesting a survival advantage for the α-Interferon treated patients [4, 5]. One of the major current focuses in the treatment of CML is autologous bone marrow transplantation. Although no adequate prospective randomized trials have been performed, there is a suggestion that autografting may prolong survival [6, 7].

1.3 The Philadelphia Chromosome and CML

In over 90% of patients with CML, a specific chromosomal translocation known as the Philadelphia (Ph) chromosome is identifiable throughout the course of the disease [8, 9]. The Ph chromosome is a somatic mutation that results from a reciprocal translocation between the long arms of chromosomes 9 and 22 and fuses genetic sequences on chromosome 22 (BCR) with c-ABL sequences translocated from chromosome 9 [9–11] (Figure 1). The Ph chromosome is seen in cells of the erythroid, megakaryoblastic, and myeloid lineages, occasionally B cells, rarely T cells, but never in marrow fibroblasts or other mesenchymal tissues [12]. In the 10% of patients that have clinical features consistent with CML, but are Ph (-), approximately half of these patients can be demonstrated to have BCR-ABL rearrangements [13, 14]. The BCR-ABL fusion gene is transcribed and translated into a 210 kDa chimeric protein in which the first exon of c-ABL has been replaced by sequences from the first and second exons of BCR with or without the third BCR exon [15, 16] (Figure 1).

1.4 Other BCR-ABL Positive Leukemias

Approximately 5% of adults with de novo acute myeloid leukemia are Ph (+) and have the BCR-ABL fusion gene described above [17]. Another 20% of adult patients and 5–10% of pediatric patients with de novo acute lymphocytic leukemia (ALL) will have an identifiable BCR-ABL rearrangement [17, 18]. In at least half of the adult patients the BCR-ABL fusion protein described above is present. However, in the remainder of the adult

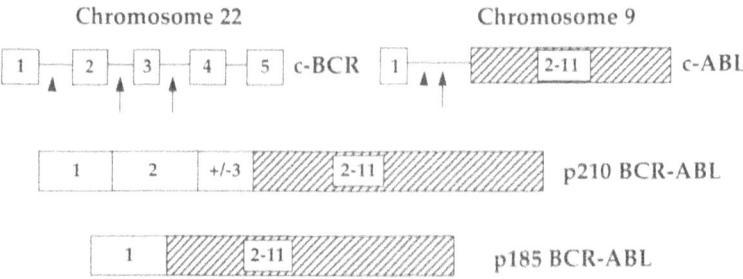

Figure 1. The molecular consequences of the Philadelphia chromosome translocation. A schematic of the ABL and BCR loci on chromosomes 9 and 22 with positions of breakpoints and corresponding chimeric mRNAs and proteins.   BCR encoded exons;   ABL encoded exons;   Introns;   CML Breakpoints;   ALL Breakpoints

cases of ALL and in most pediatric ALL cases, a third BCR-ABL fusion protein of 185 kDa is seen [17]. This fusion protein only contains sequences from BCR exon 1 fused to exons 2–11 of c-ABL [19, 20] (Figure 1).

1.5 BCR-ABL Structure and Function

The fusion protein, p210BCR-ABL, has elevated protein tyrosine kinase activity as compared to c-ABL [21]. It also has been shown to transform immature hematopoietic cells in vitro, and is capable of converting interleukin-3 (IL-3) dependent cell lines to growth factor independence [22–24]. In bone marrow reconstitution studies using bone marrow infected with BCR-ABL, transplanted mice develop a CML-like syndrome along with other leukemias [25, 26]. In mice developing a CML-like syndrome, the disease is capable of being transplanted into sublethally irradiated syngeneic recipients [27].

The portion of BCR that is contained in the BCR-ABL hybrid protein contains several activities, some of which appear to be essential to transformation by BCR-ABL. As ABL proteins with elevated and constitutive tyrosine kinase activity are known to be transforming proteins, it appears that one of the major functions of BCR exon 1 is to activate the tyrosine kinase activity of ABL [28, 29]. Further, the tyrosine kinase activity of the c-ABL portion of this fusion protein is essential to transformation [21, 30]. Therefore, an inhibitor of this tyrosine kinase may be an effective therapy for BCR-ABL positive leukemias. ·

2. A TYROSINE KINASE INHIBITOR WITH SELECTIVE ACTIVITY AGAINST THE ABL TYROSINE KINASE

2.1 Compound Design

CGP 57148 is a compound of the 2-phenylamino pyrimidine class [31]. This class of compounds was designed based on the known structure of the ATP binding site of protein kinases. A series of structurally modified congeners of a base compound of this class were produced and analyzed for their ability to inhibit a series of protein kinases. CGP 57148 (Figure 2) was found to be a potent inhibitor of the ABL tyrosine kinase identified from this screen.

2.2 In Vitro Profiling of CGP 57148

2.2.1 IC50 of Inhibition. Initial studies demonstrated that CGP 57148 was capable of inhibiting substrate phosphorylation by a bacterially expressed v-ABL tyrosine kinase with an IC50 of 0.038 μM, where IC50 represents the concentration of compound required

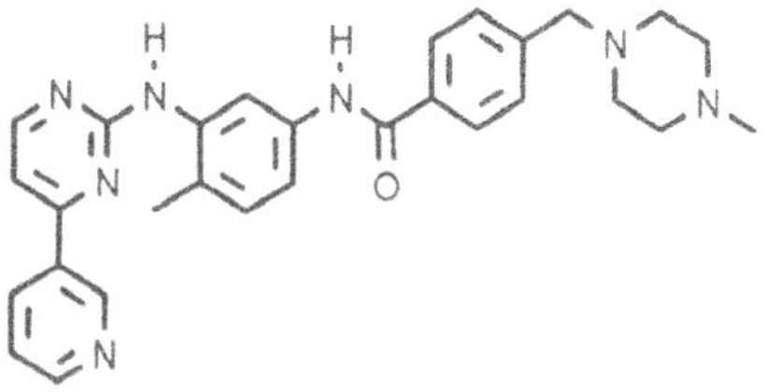

Figure 2. Structure of CGP 57148.

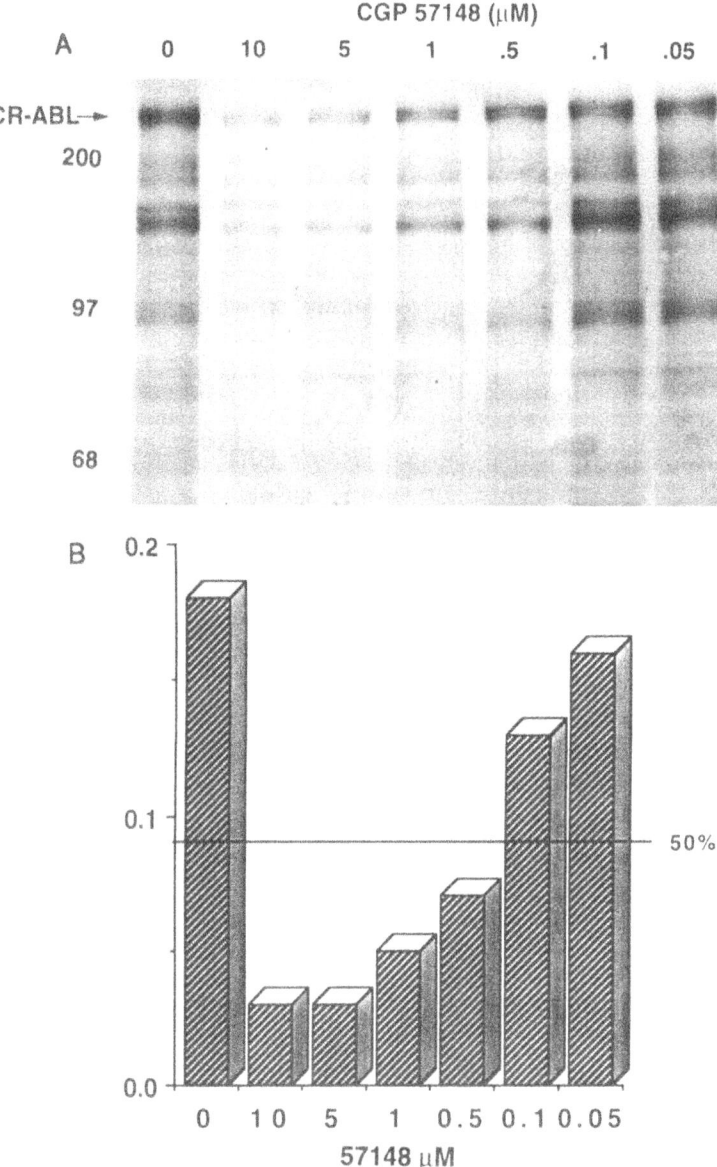

Figure 3. IC50 of inhibition. A. K562 cells were incubated for 1.5 hours with the indicated concentration of inhibitor. Cellular lysates were analyzed by antiphosphotyrosine immunoblotting as described [37] using the monoclonal antiphosphotyrosine antibody 4G10. The migration of BCR-ABL is marked with an arrow and the migration of molecular weight markers is indicated on the left of the panel. B. The BCR-ABL antiphosphotyrosine band was scanned with a laser densitometer and the data from this scan is presented. The IC50 for this assay is defined as a 50% reduction in the intensity of the BCR-ABL phosphotyrosine band.

to achieve a 50% reduction in the phosphorylation of an exogenous substrate [32]. Additional studies were performed using cell based assays for inhibition of autophosphorylation of various protein kinases. Antiphosphotyrosine immunoblots were performed on cellular lysates of BCR-ABL expressing cells incubated for 1.5 hours with various concentrations of inhibitor. No significant differences in the amount of ABL protein were noted on immunoblots using an ABL specific antisera, however, there was a dose dependent decrease in the amount of phosphotyrosine detected in the presence of CGP 57148 (Figure 3a). Densitometric scans of the BCR-ABL phosphotyrosine band (Figure 3b) shows that a 50% reduction in the intensity of the phosphotyrosine staining (IC50) of BCR-ABL using CGP 57148 occurred at a concentration of 0.25 μM.

2.2.2 Specificity of Inhibition. A number of other protein kinases have been examined for inhibition by this compound using either in vitro kinase assays or the cell based assays described above. This includes tyrosine kinases such as the epidermal growth factor receptor, HER2/neu, insulin receptor, insulin like growth factor-1 receptor, platelet derived growth factor receptor, c-and v- fms, c-and v-src, c-fgr, c-lck, c-lyn, and JAK-2. In addition, a variety of protein serine/threonine kinases including protein kinase A, phosphorylase kinase, protein kinase C types α, β1, β2, γ, σ, ε, η, and ζ, cdc2/cyclin, and casein kinases 1 and 2 have been tested for inhibition by this compound. With the exception of the platelet derived growth factor receptor, no inhibitory activity of CGP 57148 was observed at concentrations greater than 100 μM [32]. Thus, CGP 57148 is highly selective for the ABL protein tyrosine kinase.

2.3 Inhibition of Cellular Proliferation by CGP 57148

Although the in vitro profiling of CGP 57148 demonstrated a high degree of specificity, if critical kinases required for cellular growth and proliferation are inhibited by this compound that were not tested above, then inhibition of cellular proliferation would be observed. Similarly, if ABL tyrosine kinase activity is required for cellular proliferation, then treatment of cells with this compound might result in cell death. For these cellular based studies, we used 32Dcl3 cells, a murine myeloid cell line that is dependent on IL-3 for proliferation [33] and MO7e cells, a human megakaryocytic leukemia cell line that requires either GM-CSF, IL-3 or SF for proliferation [34]. Derivatives of these cell lines expressing p210BCR-ABL were created by electroporation with a retrovirus, pGD containing a full length BCR-ABL cDNA as described [35, 36]. 32Dp210 and MO7p210 cells are independent of exogenous growth factor for proliferation.

MTT and viable cell count experiments [30] demonstrated that CGP 57148 at 1 and 10 μM killed BCR-ABL expressing cells but not normal cells (Figure 4). At 100 μM non-specific toxicity has been observed. Interestingly, this compound did not simply revert BCR-ABL expressing cells to growth factor dependence but killed BCR-ABL (+) cells even in the presence of IL-3. This suggests that BCR-ABL is responsible for more than simply growth factor independence in these cells and is required for proliferation or survival of these cells. Other Ph (+) cell lines, including K562 cells are killed by this compound. CGP 57148 had no effect on the proliferation of 32Dcl3 cells expressing v-SRC, c- or v-FMS or IL-3 and GM-CSF dependent cell lines suggesting that the compound's effects are specific for ABL transformed cells.

2.4 Inhibition of Tumor Formation by CGP 57148

32Dcl3 cells expressing p210BCR-ABL or v-SRC are capable of forming tumors in syngeneic C3H/HEJ mice. The ability of CGP 57148 to inhibit tumor formation was tested following inoculation of C3H/HEJ mice with 32Dp210 or 32Dv-Src cells. Tumors typically developed within one week of inoculation of 5×10^6 cells subcutaneously. As shown in Figure 5, there is a dose dependent inhibition of BCR-ABL tumor formation by CGP 57148. No effects of this compound have been seen in animals inoculated with v-SRC expressing cells.

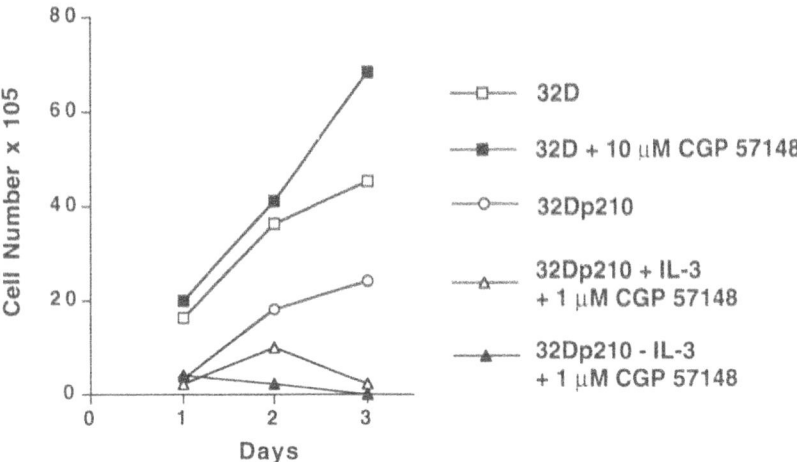

Figure 4. Cell count assay. 32Dcl3 or a factor-independent derivative expressing BCR-ABL (32Dp210) were plated in their regular growth media with or without exogenous growth factor and/or the indicated amount of inhibitor [38]. The number of viable cells were assessed daily by the exclusion of trypan blue.

2.5 Inhibition of Colony Formation of Hematopoietic Cells by CGP 57148

Previous studies have demonstrated that incubation of hematopoietic cells with antisense abl oligonucleotides results in an inhibition of colony formation by committed progenitor cells. Therefore, the effects of the inhibitor on colony formation of samples of normal bone marrow were examined initially. Bone marrow samples from patients undergoing bone marrow transplantation for a variety of non-leukemic disorders were incubated

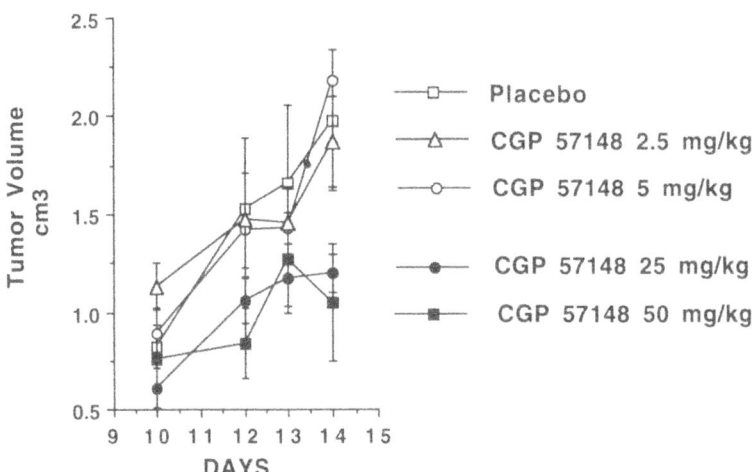

Figure 5. Antitumor activity of CGP 57148. Syngeneic C3H/HEJ mice, four per group, were injected in the left flank with 5 x 10^6 32Dp210 cells. Beginning 10 days later, after palpable tumors had developed, mice were injected daily, intraperitoneally with various amounts of CGP 57148 dissolved in sterile saline. Tumor growth was monitored by daily measurement of perpendicular tumor diameters. Tumor volumes were calculated as described [39] using the formula (π x L x D^2/6).

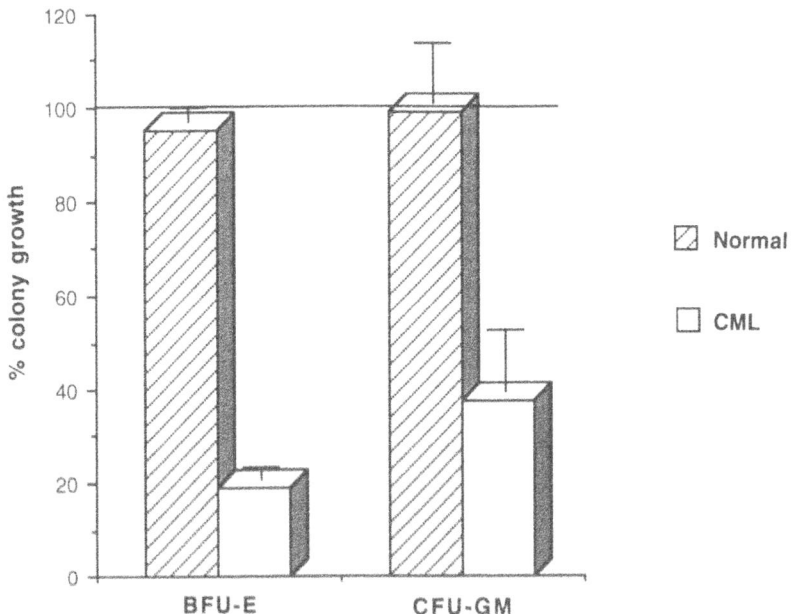

Figure 6. Colony forming assays. Normal bone marrow or CML bone marrow or peripheral blood samples were assayed for colony formation as described [40], either without inhibitor or in the presence of 1 μM CGP 57148. Results are presented as the number of colonies formed with 100% representing the average number of colonies formed without inhibitor. Error bars represent standard deviations.

with 1 μM of CGP 57148. As seen in Figure 6, there was no inhibition of colony formation at this dose. At a dose of 10 μM, colony formation of normal bone marrow was inhibited by approximately 15–20% (data not shown). The difference between our findings and the previous report using an antisense oligonucleotide strategy to target c-Abl could reflect non-specific toxicity of the anti-sense constructs, a kinase independent function of c-Abl in supporting hematopoietic colony formation, or less likely, selectivity of the compound for activated Abl proteins as opposed to endogenous c-Abl. In any case, this data demonstrates that CGP 57148 has little effect on the ability of normal marrow to form colonies at a concentration of up to 10 μM.

In contrast, when peripheral blood or bone marrow was obtained from CML patients known to have the t(9;22) chromosomal translocation, a 60–90% inhibition of colony formation of committed progenitor cells was seen by incubation with CGP 57148 at a concentration of 1 μM 57148 (Figure 6). This data has been updated from our original publication [32] and now includes a total of 12 CML patients, 9 of whom were in the chronic phase of the disease with the other three in accelerated phase or blast crisis. The 60–80% inhibition of colony formation from CML patients remains consistent. When colonies that formed were assayed for the presence of *bcr-abl* transcripts by reverse-transcriptase polymerase chain reaction (RT-PCR), 92–96% of the colonies formed in the absence of inhibitor contained *bcr-abl*. However, of the colonies that formed in the presence of 1 μM CGP 57148, less than 20% of the colonies contained *bcr-abl* transcripts. Combining this data with the 60–90% inhibition of colony formation, there was an overall decrease of *bcr-abl* positive colonies of 92–98%.

CONCLUSIONS

CGP 57148 is a compound that was designed based on the structure of the ATP binding site of protein kinases. It has been shown to be a potent and selective inhibitor of the Abl tyrosine kinase that is capable of selectively killing Bcr-Abl expressing cells in vitro and inhibiting Bcr-Abl induced tumor formation in vivo. Further, this compound is capable of selecting for the growth of benign hematopoietic progenitor cells from CML patients. Thus, this compound may be useful for the in vivo therapy of BCR-ABL positive leukemias and for bone marrow purging in preparation for autologous bone marrow transplantation of these leukemias. This compound serves as an example of a drug that was rationally designed to inhibit the function of a specific protein when the protein's function was known to be involved in the pathogenesis of a specific disease state. It is hoped that by directing therapy toward the underlying disease mechanism, that this will result in more effective and less toxic therapies. Ultimately, clinical trials will be required to determine the potential therapeutic benefit of such compounds.

REFERENCES

1. B. Clarkson, The chronic leukemias. In: J.B. Wyngaarden and L.H. Smiths, Jr. (eds): Cecil Textbook of Medicine, 18th Edition, W. B. Saunders, Philadelphia, p. 988–1001 (1988)
2. H.M. Kantarjian, A.B. Deisseroth, R. Kurzrock, Z. Estrov and M. Talpaz, Chronic myelogenous leukemia: a concise update. *Blood.* 82: 691–703 (1993)
3. J.M. Goldman, Management of chronic myeloid leukaemia. *Blood REv.* 8: 21–29 (1994)
4. The Italian Cooperative Study Group on Chronic Myeloid Leukemia, Interferon alfa-2a as compared with conventional chemotherapy for the treatment of chronic myeloid leukemia. *N Engl J Med.* 330: 820–825 (1994)
5. R. Hehlmann, H. Heimpel, J. Hasford, H.J. Kolb, H. Pralle, D.K. Hossfeld, W. Queisser, H. Loffler, A. Hochhau and B. Heinze, et. al., Randomized comparison of interferon-alpha with busulfan and hydroxyurea in chronic myelogenous leukemia. The German CML Study Group. *Blood.* 84: 4064–4067 (1994)
6. S.G. O'Brien and J.M. Goldman, Autografting in chronic myeloid leukaemia. *Blood Rev.* 8: 63–69 (1994)
7. P.B. McGlave, P. De-Fabritiis, A. Deisseroth, J. Goldman, M. Barnett, J. Reiffers, B. Simonsson, A. Carella and D. Aeppli, Autologous transplants for chronic myelogenous leukaemia: results from eight transplant groups. *Lancet.* 343: 1486–1488 (1994)
8. P.C. Nowell and D.A. Hungerford, A minute chromosome in human chronic granulocytic leukemia. *Science.* 132: 1497–1501 (1960)
9. J.D. Rowley, A new consistent abnormality in chronic myelogenous leukaemia identified by quinacrine, fluorescence and giemsa staining. *Nature.* 243: 290–293 (1973)
10. N. Heisterkamp, J.R. Stephenson, J. Groffen, P.F. Hansen, A. de Klein, C.R. Bartram and G. Grosveld, Localization of the c-abl oncogene adjacent to a translocation break point in chronic myelocytic leukemia. *Nature.* 306: 239–242 (1983)
11. C.R. Bartram, A. de Klein, A. Hagemeijer, T. van Agthoven, A. Geurts von Kessel, D. Bootsma, G. Grosveld, M.A. Ferguson-Smith, T. Davies, M. Stone, N. Heisterkamp, J.R. Stephenson and J. Groffen, Translocation of c-abl correlates with the presence of a Philadelphia chromosome in chronic myelocytic leukemia. *Nature.* 306: 277–280 (1983)
12. M. Nitta, Y. Kato, A. Strife, M. Wachter, J. Fried, A. Perez, S. Jhanwar, R. Duigou-Osterndorf, R.S.K. Chaganti and B. Clarkson, Incidence of involvement of the B and T lymphocyte lineages in chronic myelogenous leukemia. *Blood.* 66: 1053–1061 (1985)
13. C.M. Morris, A.E. Reeve, P.H. Fitzgerald, P.E. Hollings, M.E. Beard and D.C. Heaton, Genomic diversity correlates with clinical variation in Ph'-negative chronic myeloid leukaemia. *Nature.* 320: 281–283 (1986)
14. R. Kurzrock, M.B. Blick, M. Talpaz, W.S. Velasquez, J.M. Trujillo, N.M. Kouttab, W.S. Kloetzer, R.B. Arlinghaus and J.U. Gutterman, Rearrangement in the breakpoint cluster region and the clinical course in Philadelphia-negative chronic myelogenous leukemia. *Ann Intern Med.* 105: 673–679 (1986)

15. E. Shtivelman, B. Lifshitz, R.P. Gale and E. Canaani, Fused transcript of abl and bcr genes in chronic myelogenous leukaemia. *Nature.* 315: 550–554 (1985)
16. Y. Ben-Neriah, G.Q. Daley, A.-M. Mes-Masson, O.N. Witte and D. Baltimore, The chronic myelogenous leukemia-specific P210 protein is the product of the bcr/abl hybrid gene. *Science.* 233: 212–214 (1986)
17. R. Kurzrock, J.U. Gutterman and M. Talpaz, The molecular genetics of Philadelphia chromosome-positive leukemias. *N Engl J Med.* 319: 990–998 (1988)
18. S.A. Cannistra, Chronic myelogenous leukemia as a model for the genetic basis of cancer. *Hematol Oncol Clin North Am.* 4: 337–357 (1990)
19. A. Hermans, N. Heisterkamp, M. von Lindern, S. van Baal, D. Meijer, D. van der Plas, L.M. Wiedemann, J. Groffen, D. Bootsma and G. Grosveld, Unique fusion of bcr and c-abl genes in Philadelphia chromosome positive acute lymphoblastic leukemia. *Cell.* 51: 33–40 (1987)
20. S.S. Clark, J. McLaughlin, M. Timmons, A.M. Pendergast, Y. Ben-Neriah, L.W. Dow, W. Crist, G. Rovera, S.D. Smith and O.N. Witte, Expression of a distinctive BCR-ABL oncogene in Ph1-positive acute lymphocytic leukemia (ALL). *Science.* 775–777 (1988)
21. T.G. Lugo, A.M. Pendergast, A.J. Muller and O.N. Witte, Tyrosine kinase activity and transformation potency of bcr-abl oncogene products. *Science.* 247: 1079–1082 (1990)
22. G.Q. Daley and D. Baltimore, Transformation of an interleukin 3-dependent hematopoietic cell line by the chronic myelogenous leukemia-specific P210bcr/abl protein. *Proc Natl Acad Sci USA.* 85: 9312–9316 (1988)
23. J.B. Konopka, S.M. Watanabe and O.N. Witte, An alteration of the human c-abl protein in K562 unmasks associated tyrosine kinase activity. *Cell.* 37: 1035–1042 (1984)
24. J. McLaughlin, E. Chianese and O.N. Witte, In vitro transformation of immature hematopoietic cells by the P210 BCR/ABL oncogene product of the Philadelphia chromosome. *Proc Natl Acad Sci USA.* 84: 6558–6562 (1987)
25. G.Q. Daley, R.A. Van Etten and D. Baltimore, Induction of chronic myelogenous leukemia in mice by the P210bcr/abl gene of the Philadelphia chromosome. *Science.* 247: 824–830 (1990)
26. M.A. Kelliher, J. McLaughlin, O.N. Witte and N. Rosenberg, Induction of a chronic myelogenous leukemia-like syndrome in mice with v-abl and BCR/ABL. *Proc Natl Acad Sci USA.* 87: 6649–6653 (1990)
27. M.L. Gishizky, J. Johnson-White and O.N. Witte, Efficient transplantation of BCR-ABL-induced chronic myelogenous leukemia-like syndrome in mice. *Proc Natl Acad Sci USA.* 90: 3755–3759 (1993)
28. J.R. McWhirter and J.Y.J. Wang, Activation of tyrosine kinase and microfilament-binding functions of c-abl by bcr sequences in bcr/abl fusion proteins. *Mol Cell Biol.* 11: 1553–1565 (1991)
29. A.J. Muller, J.C. Young, A.M. Pendergast, M. Pondel, N.R. Landau, D.R. Littman and O.N. Witte, BCR first exon sequences specifically activate the BCR/ABL tyrosine kinase oncogene of Philadelphia chromosome-positive human leukemias. *Mol Cell Biol.* 11: 1785–1792 (1991)
30. T. Oda, S. Tamura and B.J. Druker, The SH2 domain of Abl is not required for factor independent growth induced by Bcr-Abl in a murine myeloid cell line. *Leukemia.* 9: 295–301 (1995)
31. E. Buchdunger, J. Zimmermann, H. Mett, T. Meyer, M. Muller, U. Regenass and N.B. Lydon, Selective inhibition of the platelet-derived growth factor signal transduction pathway by a protein-tyrosine kinase inhibitor of the 2-phenylaminopyrimidine class. *Proc Natl Acad Sci USA.* 92: 2558–2562 (1995)
32. B.J. Druker, S. Tamura, E. Buchdunger, S. Ohno, G.M. Segal, J. Zimmermann and N.B. Lydon, Effects of a selective inhibitor of the ABL tyrosine kinase on the growth of BCR-ABL positive cells. *Submitted* (1995)
33. J.S. Greenberger, M.A. Sakakeeny, R.K. Humphries, C.J. Eaves and R.J. Eckner, Demonstration of permanent factor-dependent multipotential (erythroid/neutrophil/basophil) hematopoietic progenitor cell lines. *Proc Natl Acad Sci USA.* 80: 2391–2395 (1983)
34. G.C. Avanzi, P. Lista, B. Giovinazzo, R. Miniero, G. Saglio, G. Benetton, R. Coda, G. Cattoretti and L. Pegoraro, Selective growth response to IL-3 of a human leukaemic cell line with megakaryoblastic features. *Br J Haematol.* 69: 359–366 (1988)
35. T. Matsuguchi, R. Salgia, M. Hallek, M. Eder, B. Druker, T. Ernst and J.D. Griffin, SHC phosphorylation in myeloid cells is regulated by GM-CSF, IL-3, and steel factor and is constitutively increased by p210BCR-ABL. *J Biol Chem.* 269: 5016–5021. (1994)
36. U. Matulonis, R. Salgia, K. Okuda, B. Druker and J.D. Griffin, IL-3 and p210BCR/ABL activate both unique and overlapping pathways of signal transduction in a factor-dependent myeloid cell line. *Exp Hematol.* 21: 1460–1466 (1993)
37. Y. Kanakura, B. Druker, S.A. Cannistra, Y. Furukawa, Y. Torimoto and J.D. Griffin, Signal transduction of the human granulocyte-macrophage colony-stimulating factor and interleukin-3 receptors involves a common set of cytoplasmic proteins. *Blood.* 76: 706–715 (1990)
38. S. Tamura, S. Ohno, E. Buchdunger, J. Zimmermann, N.B. Lydon and B.J. Druker, A selective ABL protein tyrosine kinase inhibitor with potent activity against BCR-ABL positive cells. *Submitted* (1995)

39. B.D. Evans, I.E. Smith, A.J. Shorthouse and J.L. Millar, A comparison of the response of human lung carci-
     noma xenografts to vindesine and vincristine. *Br J Cancer.* 45: 466–468 (1982)
40. G.M. Segal, R.E. Magenis, M. Brown, W. Keeble, T.D. Smith, M.C. Heinrich and G.C. Bagby, Repression
     of Fanconi anemia gene (FACC) expression inhibits growth of hematopoietic progenitor cells. *J Clin In-
     vest.* 94: 846–852 (1994)

DISCUSSION

M. Kulesz-Martin: Why is the inhibitor of the tyrosine kinase activity affecting the transcript levels in the colony forming assays?

B. Druker: We assume that the inhibitor does not affect BCR-ABL transcript levels directly but is working at the protein level. In the colony forming assays using CML patient
samples, we assume that this sample contains a mixture of normal and BCR-ABL expressing hematopoietic progenitors. By picking individual colonies, we are analyzing individual progenitors that could be either BCR-ABL positive or negative. In the absence of
inhibitor, the majority, but not all of the colonies are positive for BCR-ABL. As seen, in
the presence of inhibitor, the majority of colonies no longer contain BCR-ABL. We believe this is due to selective killing of the BCR-ABL expressing progenitors with preser-
vation of the normal progenitors.

T. Taniguchi: When you express BCR-ABL, do the cells become factor independent?

B. Druker: Yes. We have typically used 32Dcl3, a murine myeloid cell line that is IL-3
dependent and MO7e, a human megakaryocytic leukemia cell line that requires IL-3 or
GM-CSF for growth. Expression of BCR-ABL in these cell lines renders the cells independent of these growth factors.

T Taniguchi: And when you add this drug, do they grow?

B. Druker: Yes, that is right. We initially were a bit surprised by this finding. The effect
is more striking in the MO7e cells expressing BCR-ABL than in the 32D cells as the 32D
cells expressing BCR-ABL retain a low level of proliferative capacity as compared to the
MO7e cells that are completely killed by this compound. However, the 32Dp210 cell line
has been passaged in culture for quite some time while the MO7p210 cell line is a relatively recently derived cell line. Similar data to our inhibitor data has also been obtained
using antisense oligonucleotides to the BCR-ABL junction. That is, the cells do not simply revert to factor independent growth but die in the presence of the antisense oligonucleotides. My explanation for these results is that the cells have somehow become
dependent on BCR-ABL for their proliferation as well as their survival and this is dependent on ABL kinase activity. In other words, you do not simply have a cell plus BCR-ABL,
but you have a cell plus BCR-ABL plus all of the changes induced by BCR-ABL expression. When the ABL kinase activity is inhibited, the cells cannot simply revert as they
have been altered by BCR-ABL.

M. Fried: Why do you think the cell is now dependent on BCR-ABL?

B. Druker: This is the focus of my laboratory and a number of other laboratories. We are
trying to figure out which signaling pathways are used by BCR-ABL. The usual cast of

characters for an activated tyrosine kinase seem to be utilized, including SHC, GRB-2, and rasGAP in the ras pathway, PI-3 kinase, and many others. The specific role of these proteins in inducing growth factor independence is currently being investigated.

M. Fried: Is there any toxicity in the mice?

B. Druker: We have not seen any. Ciba-Geigy has performed a fourteen day toxicity study in rats and preliminary results have shown little toxicity with additional toxicity studies in progress.

D. Livingston: Have you tried to detect activity of this compound in the transplantable murine model of CML as reported by the Baltimore and Witte laboratories.

B. Druker: We have not yet tried these experiments. We initially wanted to determine whether the compound would show any in vivo activity. Therefore, we used the simplest test we could perform which was subcutaneous injection of v-ABL or BCR-ABL expressing cells in syngeneic or nude mice. Now that we have seen some activity, we would certainly consider setting up the murine CML model or collaborating with a laboratory that has this model up and running.

D. Livingston: What about testing this compound against the viral Abelson disease in a mouse? That would be a really interesting test. You could compare animals shortly after viral infection, to others in the midst of disease evolution, to animals with full blown disease. This would be a rapid test and a very powerful one if remissions were achieved in this setting.

B. Druker: Yes, I agree that this would be a much simpler model.

W. Cowens: What do you think the relationship of the expression of BCR-ABL is to the progression of the disease as patients go from stable phase to accelerated phase, to blast crisis?

B. Druker: It appears that BCR-ABL is capable of inducing chromosomal instability. What happens with disease progression form the stable phase to blast crisis is that additional chromosomal, in addition to the t(9:22) Philadelphia chromosome, appear. As a result of these additional chromosomal abnormalities, a block to differentiation develops and an acute leukemia develops. There are even a few reported cases where the Philadelphia chromosome and BCR-ABL expression are lost within blast crisis, however, the majority retain BCR-ABL. One of the issues that your question is getting at is whether this inhibitor will only work in the chronic phase of the disease when BCR-ABl is the only demonstrable abnormality as opposed to blast crisis where there might be other abnormalities driving cellular proliferation. In our colony forming assay, we have analyzed six stable phase patients and four patients in accelerated or blast crisis. Our data suggests that the compound is more effective at eliminating BCR-ABL positive cells in the stable phase patient samples, however, the compound was capable of eliminating 50–75% of the BCR-ABL positive cells from the blast crisis samples. Thus, the compound may be less useful in blast crisis but it still appears to have some effects.

G. Evan: I wanted to check on this business of factor independence of BCR-ABL expressing cells. Do they grow and survive in serum-free medium?

B. Druker: Actually, they do not survive in the presence of low serum conditions. So, the MO7p210 and 32Dp210 cells are grown in 10% fetal bovine serum with no additional growth factors. There was a recent report from Jean Wang's laboratory where BCR-ABL expression in fibroblasts abrogated anchorage independent growth but these cells will not proliferate in low serum conditions.

G. Evan: So, in my terms, they are not factor independent.

B. Druker: Yes, that is correct. When I have used the term factor independent, I have meant it in the context of additional growth factors, such as IL-3 that are required in addition to the factors required from serum.

G. Evan: Have you tried growing these cells in plasma?

B. Druker: No, we have not.

F. Rauscher: What kind of cell death occurs? Apoptotic cell death?

B. Druker: We have preliminary data that these cells do undergo programmed cell death when treated with the inhibitor. This experiment is at the top of our list to confirm.

F. Rauscher: Is this drug affected by MDR?

B. Druker: We have not looked at this issue. However, leukemic cells from CML patients, particularly in blast crisis, have been shown to overexpress MDR. It would be interesting to see whether we could correlate a difference in levels of MDR expression with differing sensitivity to the inhibitor.

G. Gilliland: Along those lines, do you know if there are any qualitative or quantitative differences between the 10–15% of colonies that survive treatment with the inhibitor?

B. Druker: We have not performed analyses beyond BCR-ABL expression in the colony forming assays.

G. Gilliland: There is some literature that suggests that progenitors exist that contain the Philadelphia chromosome by do not express BCR-ABL message or protein and that these cells would escape strategies directed at either RNA or protein. Do you think this will have an impact on clinical applications of this compound?

B. Druker: This is a very important point as to whether there are BCR-ABL negative cells that are Philadelphia chromosome positive. That is, positive at the DNA level for the rearrangement but negative at the RNA or protein level for BCR-ABL expression. There initially was a report that suggested that this scenario could occur. However, on more careful examination, the feeling is that the existence of these cells was quite rare, if it occurred at all. However, this allows for two possible models of CML. One is that the genetic rearrangement occurs in a very early progenitor cell, but the protein is not expressed until a later level of hematopoietic development and induces expansion of this later compartment of cells. The second possibility is that the DNA rearrangement and protein expression occur in all cells. I think that DNA or protein based therapy could be successful in either scenario, however these therapies would not be capable of eliminating the earliest diseased progenitor if the first scenario is correct. At this point, I do not think that it is possible to distinguish between these two possibilities, but we may be able to learn more as RNA and protein based therapies begin to be used in this disease.

E. Mihich: I am following up on the question that Dr. Rauscher asked, but in a different way. Has anybody tried, either in your laboratory, at Ciba-Geigy, or in other laboratories, to develop a cell line that is resistant to this or similar tyrosine kinase inhibitors. The usual approach would be to use your BCR-ABL transfected cell line and incubate with extremely low, then increasing doses of the compound in an attempt to select or induce mutations that would rescue the cells from this compound. I think that this would be helpful in verifying the site of action of this compound. The fact that you have a specific inhibitor of the ABL tyrosine kinase is very convincing, but not as convincing as if you were able to demonstrate it in cells that are resistant to this compound.

B. Druker: We have not done these experiments, but I agree that it would be very interesting and convincing.

A. Nordheim: Could you comment on the substrates of ABL?

B. Druker: Endogenous c-ABL is not particularly active as a kinase. It is found both in the cytoplasm and in the nucleus and with overexpression of this kinase being toxic to cells. As far as substrates, a few in vitro substrates have been identified, including the adapter protein CRK and RNA polymerase II. c-ABL has also been shown to bind to the retinoblastoma protein and to F-actin. As far as the oncogenic versions of ABL, they are almost exclusively cytoplasmic or cytoskeletal. A variety of substrates and associated proteins have been identified, including GRB-2, SHC, p120rasGAp and it associated proteins - p190 and p62, BCR, PI-3 kinase, SYP, paxillin, FES, CRKL, a member of the CRK family of adapter proteins and others. The CRKL story is rather interesting as we and other have identified CRKL as the major tyrosine phosphorylated protein in CML patient samples. Although the list of substrates is quite long and continues to grow, what is really required is a detailed analysis of which of these proteins binds directly to BCR-ABL, mapping the binding sites, and determining which of these proteins are required for BCR-ABL function. We have shown, for example, that CRKL binds directly to ABL and have mapped and mutated the binding site, The biological effects of this mutant are currently being examined.

C. Schneider: Do you know anything about the status of p53 in the cells that you are looking at, especially regarding the effects that you have pointed out?

B. Druker: I do not know the status of p53 in the cell lines that we have used. In the disease, CML, it is unusual to see alterations in p53 in the stable phase, however, there is some literature that suggests that p53 mutations are quite rare with disease progression with other reports showing a higher frequency.

17

UNEXPECTED FUNCTIONS OF GRANULOCYTE-MACROPHAGE COLONY STIMULATING FACTOR

Glenn Dranoff[1] and Richard C. Mulligan[2]

[1] Dana-Farber Cancer Institute and
Harvard Medical School, Boston, Massachusetts
[2] Whitehead Institute for Biomedical Research and
Department of Biology
Massachusetts Institute of Technology

INTRODUCTION

Cytokines are small glycoproteins which play critical roles in hematopoiesis, immunity, and inflammation[1]. Two major themes underlying current understanding of cytokine biology are the redundancy and pleiotropy of cytokine functions. Numerous in vitro systems suggest that many cytokines demonstrate overlapping activities, and that any individual cytokine demonstrates multiple activities. These findings, considered together with the complex circuitry of cytokine expression in vivo, render problematic delineating the central and distinctive properties of any given molecule. The limited understanding of cytokine physiology in turn has hindered the most effective application of these proteins to the treatment of clinically important human disorders, including cancer, bone marrow failure, autoimmunity, and infectious disease.

The colony stimulating factors are a subgroup of cytokines originally discovered by virtue of their ability to induce the proliferation in semisolid culture of hematopoietic progenitors into a variety of mature blood cells[2]. Granulocyte-macrophage colony stimulating factor (GM-CSF) was initially identified as an activity present in lung conditioned medium from endotoxin treated animals which supported the growth of neutrophils and monocyte/macrophages from hemopoietic precursors[3]. More detailed studies of this molecule revealed its additional abilities to induce the production from hemopoietic progenitors of erythrocytes, eosinophils, and dendritic cells[4–7]. Adminstration of the recombinant protein to several laboratory animals and humans confirmed the activity of this molecule in stimulating hematopoiesis in vivo as well, with the most pronounced effects evident on monocyte/macrophages, neutrophils, and eosinophils[8–10]. In addition to the ability of GM-CSF to function as a hematopoietic growth factor, a large number of investigations also have illustrated that this molecule can modulate the functions of several mature blood cells. The major described effects include enhancement of antigen presentation[11,12], improved chemotaxis and adhesion[13,14], more efficient antimicrobial killing[15-17], and increased phagocytosis of opsonized material[18,19]. Smaller numbers of studies suggest that this molecule may also exert effects on endothelial cells and the placenta[20,21].

The multiplicity of functions attributed to GM-CSF highlights the uncertainty regarding the physiologic role of this molecule. This finding is likely relevant to the current limited usefulness of GM-CSF as a therapeutic agent. While GM-CSF sometimes is administered to accelerate bone marrow recovery following radiation or chemotherapy, its application is associated with far greater toxicity than that of the more efficacious granulocyte-colony stimulating factor (G-CSF)[22]. Interestingly, mice which have been engineered by gene targeting techniques to lack G-CSF demonstrate a marked reduction in steady state neutrophil production[23]. This suggests that the pharmacologic superiority of G-CSF derives, at least in part, from its normal physiologic function. This finding also raises important questions regarding the role of GM-CSF in hematopoiesis.

We have used gene transfer and gene knockout technologies in order to generate new insights into the functions of GM-CSF in vivo and to reveal new applications of this molecule for the treatment of human disease. We have discovered the surprisingly potent ability of GM-CSF to stimulate specific and long lasting anti-tumor immunity[24] and uncovered a previously unrecognized critical role of GM-CSF in the maintenance of lung homeostasis[25].

STUDIES WITH GENETICALLY MODIFIED TUMOR CELLS

Increasing evidence from both murine and human systems indicates that the host is able to generate a tumor specific, major histocompatibility complex (MHC) restricted T cell response[26]. Genetic and biochemical techniques have begun to establish the targets of this recognition. While some of the protein antigens identified to date are novel products of unknown function (MAGE family)[27] or apparently normal self proteins (tyrosinase)[28], a subset of the targets includes oncogenic proteins which likely are intimately linked to the malignant phenotype. These include various mutant forms of ras[29-31], p53[32-34], and the epidermal growth factor receptor[35], BCR-Abl[36], PML-RAR[37], neu[38], and the human papillomavirus E7 product[39,40]. While identification of T cell targets with relevance to the transformed state has inspired considerable excitement after nearly fifty years of previously unsuccessful searches for tumor antigens, this finding also has underscored the limited understanding of why such antigens fail to provoke an effective anti-tumor immune response.

One variable which may prove decisive in the generation of a host anti-tumor response is the mixture of cytokines produced locally in the tumor microenvironment[41]. Several cell types at this location are potential sources of cytokine secretion, including stromal cells, endothelial cells, tumor cells, macrophages, and tumor infiltrating lymphocytes. Forni and associates pioneered the modification of the cytokine milieu associated with tumors by the simple inoculation of recombinant proteins into the growing mass[42,43]. These studies clearly illustated that the presence of interleukin-2 could lead to the rejection of murine tumor cells by syngeneic hosts. Histologic examination of the host response revealed a complex mixture of inflammatory cells including lymphocytes, natural killer cells, macrophages, neutrophils, and eosinophils.

The experiments of Forni and colleagues stimulated a large number of subsequent investigations which used gene transfer techniques to engineer tumor cells to express a variety of cytokines and other immunomodulators[41]. These studies demonstrated that although a large number of cytokines exerted no appreciable effect on the in vitro growth of several murine tumor cell lines, they nonetheless stimulated a powerful anti-tumor effect in vivo which led to the rejection of the genetically modified tumor cells. The characteristics of the elicited host response varied with the particular molecule introduced, but included infiltrations by most of the formed myeloid and lymphoid cell populations. An intriguing finding from these initial studies was that the inoculation of tumor cells secreting particular molecules sometimes led to the generation of systemic anti-tumor immunity. In particular, animals rejecting tumor cells expressing IL-2, IL-4, γ-interferon, or tumor necrosis factor α in some cases were able to eliminate subsequent challenges of parental tumor, and even small burdens of pre-exisiting tumor[44–49].

While these studies clearly indicated that gene transfer techniques could exert a powerful effect on the host anti-tumor response, they also suggested that it was critically important to understand what properties of particular tumor cells might impact on the anti-tumor response, and to determine whether particular molecules might be relatively more effective at inducing these responses. In order to address these issues, we generated a large panel of high titer, replication defective retroviruses expressing numerous cytokines, adhesion molecules. and other potential immunomodulators[24]. The MFG retroviral backbone used for these studies employs the Moloney murine leukemia virus long terminal repeat to drive expression of both the full length viral transcript which is packaged into viral particles and the spliced transcript from which the inserted gene is translated. This system consistently achieves high levels of gene transfer and gene expression without the requirement for selection of transduced cells. The latter property represents a significant technical advance over most other gene transfer systems used in these investigations, as it permits the study of populations rather than clones of tumor cells. Since there is considerable evidence for antigenic heterogeneity in murine model tumor systems[50], studies employing populations of tumor cells are more representative of the full antigenic repertoire.

In our initial studies examining the effects of ten different immuno-modulators in the B16 melanoma model system, only interleukin-2 expressing tumor cells were rejected by syngeneic C57Bl/6 mice[24]. Several other molecules including IL-4, IL-6, γ-interferon, and tumor necrosis factor-α (TNF-α) exerted modest anti-tumor activity, resulting in significant delays in tumor development. The implantation of cytokine secreting tumor cells in other cases produced distinctive systemic syndromes resembling those found in transgenic mouse systems. Interleukin-5 expressing cells induced dramatic increases in circulating and tissue eosinophil numbers. Interleukin-6 secreting cells induced inflammation of the kidneys and enlargement of the liver and spleen associated with increased plasma cells. TNF-α expressing cells caused systemic wasting and death. Tumor cells synthesizing GM-CSF stimulated profound increases in circulating monocytes, neutrophils, and eosinophils, enlargement of the liver and spleen, and pulmonary hemorrhage.

Since IL-2 expressing cells were rejected by the C57Bl/6 hosts, this allowed testing for the potential development of systemic immunity. In contrast to what previously had been reported in other tumor model systems, no appreciable protection against subsequent challenge with wild type B16 tumor was evident. Over the course of one month following the rejection of IL-2 expressing cells, all mice succumbed to secondary challenges with unmodified B16 cells[24]. The effects of coexpression of IL-2 and a second gene product were then evaluated by superinfecting the IL-2 transduced cells with a second retrovirus. As no packaging functions are transferred to the target cells with the MFG vector and CRIP packaging cell lines[51], there is no resistance to multiple infections of the target cells. Surprisingly, B16 cells coexpressing IL-2 and GM-CSF not only were rejected by the

C57Bl/6 hosts, but also stimulated potent protection against subsequent tumor challenge. All other combinations evaluated generated either weak or no vaccination activity. To explore the hypothesis that the major function of IL-2 in the vaccination response was to induce the rejection of GM-CSF expressing cells, we next tested the activity of gamma-irradiated tumor cells. The classic experiments of Prehn and Main in the 1950s had established that a subset of murine tumors could effectively induce protection against subsequent tumor challenge following the injection of irradiated tumor cells[52]. Irradiation of the infected B16 melanoma cells did not lead to detectable decreases in cytokine production. Irradiated B16 tumor cells expressing only GM-CSF generated potent protection against tumor challenge, in contrast to irradiated wild type B16 cells which stimulated little if any systemic immunity[24]. A reexamination of the vaccination potential of all transduced tumor B16 cells following irradiation demostrated the clear superiority of GM-CSF expressing cells, although weaker activity was detectable in the cases of IL-4 and IL-6 expressing cells.

The superior ability of GM-CSF to elicit systemic anti-tumor immunity was unexpected, given the historical perspective emphasing this molecule's role as a hematopoitic growth factor[2]. To generate some insight into the mechanism of immunostimulation, a detailed pathologic analysis of vaccination and challenge sites was performed[24]. Although irradiated B16 cells did induce a mild influx of lymphocytes, irradiated GM-CSF expressing cells stimulated a dramatic influx of macrophages, eosinophils, and lymphocytes. While the draining lymph node of animals vaccinated with irradiated wild type cells revealed little alteration from naive animals, there was extensive lymphoid hyperplasia in the GM-CSF case, particularly in the paracortical T cell areas, with lesser degrees of germinal center formation. At the challenge sites following vaccination, although only a weak lymphocytic infiltrate was apparent with irradiated wild type cells, a vigorous reaction was evident in the GM-CSF case, characterized by abundant eosinophils, macrophages, and lymphocytes.

The identification of lymphocytes at each stage of the vaccination response suggested that their participation might be crucial. In support of this idea, tumor vaccination could be demonstrated to involve specificity (no cross protection against syngeneic, but irrelevant tumors) and memory (efficient protection maintained months after vaccination), the defining features of immunologic responses. To formally demonstrate the dependence on lymphocytes, a series of mice were depleted of various T cell subsets using monoclonal antibodies. These studies revealed the essential roles of both CD4 and CD8 positive T lymphocytes at both priming and effector phases of the response, whereas natural killer cells proved dispensable at each stage[24]. These results were supported by in vitro assays which demonstrated the generation of tumor specific CD8 blockable lysis by splenocytes and tumor induced proliferation of CD4 positive T cells from the draining lymph node.

Since the B16 melanoma line used in these studies was MHC class II negative and uninducible following gamma interferon exposure, the critical requirement for CD4 positive T cells supports the idea that the tumor cells are not likely to function as the antigen presenting cells initiating the immune response. Rather, host professional antigen presenting cells which are recruited to the site of the tumor vaccine are more likely to function in this capacity. In this context, it is important to note that the macrophages and dendritic cells present at the vaccination site are highly efficient stimulators of T cell activation. Additionally, GM-CSF has been reported to both increase the production of these cell types from hematopoietic progenitors and to enhance their function in antigen presentation[53–55]. A plausible model suggested by these findings is that irradiated tumor cells are recognized, internalized, and processed by stimulated macrophages and dendritic cells, which in turn migrate to the draining lymph node where they efficiently activate T cells which in turn circulate systemically. The presence of eosinophils at both the priming and effector phases of the response also suggest that these cells likely are also playing critical roles, both in tumor destruction and in the shaping of the T cell response.

The activity of GM-CSF expressing cells was not limited to the B16 melanoma model, but was also evident in several other systems, including the Lewis lung carcinoma, RENCA renal cell carcinoma, CT-26 colon carcinoma, CMS-5 fibrosarcoma, WP-4 fibrosarcoma, Dunning prostate carcinoma, MBT-2 bladder carcinoma, and S91 melanoma[24,56-58]. We demonstrated that some of these models (CT-26, CMS-5, RENCA, and WP-4), unlike the B16 system, could be shown to be inherently immunogenic as revealed by vaccination studies with irradiated parental tumor[24]. This inherent immunogenicity complicates the interpretation of the immunostimulatory properties attributed to IL-2, IL-4, TNF, and γ-IFN in these studies. Since these molecules were either inactive or weakly active in the B16 model, perhaps the immunostimulation associated with these molecules is largely dependent on properties intrinsic to the tumor cells. Additional experiments will be necessary to resolve this issue.

The broad activity of irradiated, GM-CSF expressing tumor cells together with the ability to transduce efficiently primary human tumor explants with MFG retroviral vectors[59] has led to the development of three current FDA approved Phase I clinical studies[60]. In these trials, patients with advanced melanoma or renal cell carcinoma are being vaccinated subcutaneously and intradermally with irradiated, autologous tumor cells engineered to secrete human GM-CSF. In addition to determining potential toxicities associated with these vaccinations, these trials will begin to assess whether tumor specific CD4 and CD8 positive T cell responses can be enhanced in patients with metastatic disease by virtue of tumor cell vaccination.

GM-CSF DEFICIENT MICE

The unexpected superiority of GM-CSF in enhancing anti-tumor immunity underscored the need to understand more about the physiologic function of this molecule. Towards this end, we generated GM-CSF deficient mice using gene targeting techniques in embryonic stem cells[25]. The pPNT targeting vector[61] employed in these experiments utilizes the murine phosphoglycerate kinase promoter and polyadenylation sequences to drive expression of the neomycin resistance gene and the Herpes simplex virus thymidine kinase gene. Targeted clones could be obtained by using positive-negative selection with G418 and ganciclovir[62]. The GM-CSF knockout construct deleted exons three and four, which previous in vitro mutagenesis experiments had demonstrated would result in a null allele[63]. D3 embryonic stem cell clones undergoing homologous recombination were identified by Southern analysis, injected into recipient blastocysts, and germ line chimeras obtained. Heterozygous mutant mice were intercrossed to obtain homozygous GM-CSF deficient animals.

Mutant mice are clinically healthy and are fertile. No distortion in the expected Mendelian frequencies have been observed. Analysis of steady state hematopoiesis surprisingly revealed no obvious deficiencies. Examination of peripheral blood cells disclosed no abnormalities in either numbers or morphology of all lineages[25]. Tissue hematopoietic populations are unperturbed, including splenic dendritic cells. This last finding is surprising, given several studies which previously had suggested the critical need for GM-CSF in the production of this cell type from hematopoietic progenitors[53,54].

Analysis of the lymphoid compartment also failed to reveal any significant defect in T or B cell development or secondary lymphoid organ organization.

The normal steady state hematopoiesis is not due to any major alterations in bone marrow progenitor dynamics[25]. No evidence of extramedullary hematopoiesis in liver or spleen has been found. Quantitative assessment of hemopoietic precursors in the marrow and spleen by methycellulose colony formation assay failed to reveal significant differences between mutant and wild type animals. Examination of the response of mutant bone marrow to a severe stress was performed by transplanting mutant bone marrow into lethally irradiated mutant recipients. Although there may have been a small delay in the time to recovery of blood counts in comparison to wild type marrow transplanted into lethally irradiated wild type recipioents, all mutant animals successfully reconstituted. Collectively, these findings indicate that GM-CSF is not essential for steady state hematopoiesis and suggest that the historical view of the requirement for this molecule in blood cell formation needs to be revised[2]. Whether the absence of a more severe defect in hematopoiesis is due to functional redundancy[64] will require additional experiments. Interleukin-3 is an attractive candidate in this regard, and we are currently generating mice doubly deficient in GM-CSF and IL-3.

In contrast to the absence of a clear hematopoietic defect, GM-CSF deficient mice demonstrate an unexpected alteration in lung homeostasis[25]. The animals develop the progressive accumulation of surfactant in the alveolar air space, the pathologic feature characteristic of the idiopathic human disorder pulomonary alveolar proteinosis[65]. Surfactant is a complex mixture of charged phospholipids (predominantly dipalmitoyl phosphatidycholine) and at least four proteins (surfactant proteins A, B, C, and D) which functions in the air space primarily to reduce surface tension and thus prevent lung collapse at exhalation[66]. Its absence in premature infants (synthesis of surfactant is not initiated until the last trimester) is associated with severe respiratory compromise. The accumulation of surfactant that is clinically observed in alveolar proteinosis is also associated with respiratory compromise, although whole lung lavage to remove the excess surfactant is highly therapeutic[67]. We currently are studying patients with this disease to determine whether any carry mutations in the GM-CSF gene.

Surfactant proteins and lipids are synthesized constitutively by specialized type II cells in the respiratory epithelium which secrete the material into the airspace[66]. Surfactant turnover in the alveolus occurs predominantly via uptake by the type II cells which recycle and, to a lesser extent, catabolize the material. Alveolar macrophages also contribute to surfactant clearance, although quantitatively to a lesser extent, through a process involving specific uptake and intracellular digestion. In addition to the surfactant accumuluation, lungs from mutant animals also reveal an extensive lymphoid hyperplasia around both airways and veins[25]. Immunohisto-chemistry indicates that the hyperplasia consists of CD4 and CD8 positive T cells, B cells, and macrophages. Extensive search for various infectious agents has failed to reveal any pathogens. While the etiology of the hyperplasia remains to be determined, a primary disturbance of mucosal immunity is an attractive working model.

To determine the mechanism underlying the surfactant accumulation, we performed S1 nuclease analysis of surfactant protein transcripts in whole lung preparations from wild type and mutant littermates[25]. No evidence for alteration in the levels of these transcripts was found. Further, immunohistochemistry failed to disclose significant increases in surfactant levels in respiratory epithelial type II cells These findings suggest that surfactant production is not likely to be altered, although additional experiments using radioactive precursor labeling of surfactant in whole animals is underway to definitively address this issue. In contrast to the apparently normal surfactant production, examination of alveolar macrophages harvested from the lungs of mutant animals revealed a dramatic intracellular accumulation of surfactant. Since recent studies have indicated that the respiratory epithelium, including type II cells, constitutively synthesizes GM-CSF[68], it is tempting to speculate that GM-CSF is critical to the ability of alveolar macrophages to internalize and degrade surfactant. As surfactant proteins structurally are related to members of the collectin family (conglutinin, mannose binding protein, and C1q) whose function involves the opsonization of particulate material[69], the surfactant accumuluation in our mutant mice may provide a model to study processes potentially relevant to macrophage antigen processing at the vaccination site of irradiated, GM-CSF secreting tumor cells.

REFERENCES

1. Arai K-I, Lee F, Miyajima A, Miyatake S, Arai N, Yokota T. Cytokines: coordinators of immune and inflammatory responses. Annu. Rev. Biochem. 1990;59:783–836.
2. Metcalf D. The Molecular Control of Blood Cells.Cambridge, Massachusetts: Harvard University Press. 1988
3. Burgess A, Camarkis J, Metcalf D. Purification and properties of colony-stimulating factor from mouse lung-conditioned medium. J. Biol. Chem. 1977;252:1998–2003.
4. Johnson G, Metcalf D. Detection of a new type of mouse eosinophil colony by luxol fast blue staining. Exp. Hematol. 1980;8:549–561.
5. Metcalf D. Clonal analysis of proliferation and differentiation of paired daughter cells: Actions of granulocyte-macrophage colony-stimulating factor on granulocyte-macrophage precursors. Proc. Natl. Acad. Sci. U.S.A. 1980;77:5327–5330.
6. Metcalf D, Burgess A, Johnson G, et al. In vitro actions on hemopoietic cells of recombinant murine GM-CSF purified after production in *Escherichia coli*: comparison with purified native GM-CSF. J. Cell. Physiol. 1986;128:421–431.
7. Inaba K, Inaba M, Deguchi M, et al. Granulocytes, macrophages, and dendritic cells arise from a common major histocompatibility complex class II-negative progenitor in mouse bone marrow. Proc. Natl. Acad. Sci. U.S.A. 1993;90:3038–3042.
8. Metcalf D, Begley C, Williamson D, et al. Hemopoietic responses in mice injected with purified recombinant murine GM-CSF. Exp. Hematol. 1987;15:1–9.
9. Donahue R, Wang E, Stone D, et al. Stimulation of haematopoiesis in primates by continuous infusion of recombinant human GM-CSF. Nature 1986;321:872–875.
10. Groopman J, Mitsuyasu R, DeLeo M, Oette D, Golde D. Effect of recombinant granulocyte-macrophage colony-stimulating factor on myelopoiesis in the acquired immunodeficiency syndrome. N. Engl. J. Med. 1987;317:593–598.
11. Morrissey P, Bressler L, Park L, Alpert A, Gillis S. Granulocyte-macrophage colony-stimulating factor augments the primary antibody response by enhancing the function of antigen-presenting cells. J. Immunol. 1987;139:1113–1119.
12. Witmer-Pack M, Olivier W, Valinsky J, Schuler G, Steinman R. Granulocyte-macrophage colony-stimulating factor is essential for the viability and function of cultured murine epidermal Langerhans cells. J. Exp. Med. 1987;166:1484–1498.
13. Arnaout M, Wang E, Clark S, Sieff C. Human recombinant granulocyte-macrophage colony-stimulating factor increases cell-to-cell adhesion and surface expression of adhesion-promoting surface glycoproteins on mature granulocytes. J. Clin. Invest. 1986;78:597–601.
14. Weisbart R, Golde D, Gasson J. Biosynthetic human GM-CSF modulates the number and affinity of neutrophil f-Met-Leu-Phe receptors. J. Immunol. 1986;137:3584–3587.
15. Fleischmann J, Golde D, Weisbart R, Gasson J. Granulocyte-macrophage colony-stimulating factor enhances phagocytosis of bacteria by human neutrophils. Blood 1986;68:708–711.
16. Silberstein D, Owen W, Gasson J, et al. Enhancement of human eosinophil cytotoxicity and leukotriene synthesis by biosynthetic (recombinant) granulocyte-macrophage colony-stimulating factor. J. Immunol. 1986;137:3290–3294.

17. Weiser W, Van Niel A, Clark S, David J, Remold H. Recombinant human granulocyte/macrophage colony-stimulating factor activates intracellular killing of *Leishmania donovani* by human monocyte-derived macrophages. J. Exp. Med. 1987;166:1436–1446.

18. Collins H, Bancroft G. Cytokine enhancement of complement-dependent phagocytosis by macrophages: synergy of tumor necrosis factor-α and granulocyte macrophage colony-stimulating factor for phagocytosis of *Cryptococcus neoformans*. Eur. J. Immunol. 1992;22:1447–1454.

19. Weisbart R, Kacena A, Schuh A, Golde D. GM-CSF induces human neutrophil IgA-mediated phagocytosis by an IgA Fc receptor activation mechanism. Nature 1988;332:647–648.

20. Bussolino F, Wang J, Defilippi P, et al. Granulocyte- and granulocyte-macrophage-colony stimulating factors induce human endothelial cells to migrate and proliferate. Nature 1989;337:471–473.

21. Robertson S, Mayrhofer G, Seamark R. Uterine epithelial cells synthesize granulocyte-macrophage colony-stimulating factor (GM-CSF) and interleukin-6 (Il-6) in pregnant and non-pregnant mice. Biol. Reprod. 1992;46:1069–1079.

22. Lieschke GJ, Burgess AW. Granulocyte colony-stimulating factor and granulocyte-macrophage colony-stimulating factor. N. Engl. J. Med. 1992;327:28–35, 99–106.

23. Lieschke GJ, Grail D, Hodgson G, et al. Mice lacking granulocyte colony-stimulating factor have chronic neutropenia, granulocyte and macrophage progenitor cell deficiency and impaired neutrophil mobilization. Blood 1994;84:1737–1746.

24. Dranoff G, Jaffee E, Lazenby A, et al. Vaccination with irradiated tumor cells engineered to secrete murine granulocyte-macrophage colony-stimulating factor stimulates potent, specific, and long-lasting anti-tumor immunity. Proc. Natl. Acad. Sci. U.S.A. 1993;90:3539–3543.

25. Dranoff G, Crawford AD, Sadelain M, et al. Involvement of granulocyte-macrophage colony-stimulating factor in pulmonary homeostasis. Science 1994;264:713–716.

26. Boon T, Cerottini J-C, Van den Eynde B, van der Bruggen P, Van Pel A. Tumor antigens recognized by T lymphocytes. Ann. Rev. Immunol. 1994;12:337–365.

27. van der Bruggen P, Traversari C, Chomez P, et al. A gene encoding an antigen recognized by cytolytic T lymphocytes on a human melanoma. Science 1991;254:1643–1647.

28. Brichard V, Van Pel A, Wolfel T, et al. The tyrosinase gene codes for an antigen recognized by autologous cytolytic T lymphocytes on HLA-A2 melanomas. J. Exp. Med. 1993;178:489–495.

29. Gedde-Dahl TI, Fossum B, Eriksen JA, Thorsby E, Gaudernack G. T cell clones specific for p21 ras-derived peptides: characterization of their fine specificity and HLA restriction. Eur. J. Immunol. 1993;23:754–760.

30. Jung S, Schluesener HJ. Human T lymphocytes recognize a peptide of single point-mutated, oncogenic ras proteins. J. Exp. Med. 1991;173:273–276.

31. Skipper J, Strauss HJ. Identification of two cytotoxic T lymphocyte-recognized epitopes in the Ras protein. J. Exp. Med. 1993;177:1493–1498.

32. Houbiers JGA, Nijman HW, van der Burg SH, et al. In-vitro induction of human cytotoxic T lymphocyte responses against peptides of mutant and wild type p53. Eur. J. Immunol. 1993;23:2072–2077.

33. Stuber G, Leder GH, Storkus WJ, et al. Identification of wild type and mutant p53 peptides binding to HLA-A2 assessed by a peptide loading-deficient cell line assay and a novel major histocompatibility complex class I peptide binding assay. Eur. J. Immunol. 1994;24:765–768.

34. Yanuck M, Carbone DP, Pendleton CD, et al. A mutant p53 tumor suppressor protein is a target for peptide-induced CD8+ cytotoxic T-cells. Cancer Res. 1993;53:3257–3261.

35. Humphrey PA, Wong AJ, Vogelstein B, et al. Anti-synthetic peptide antibody reacting at the fusion junction of deletion-mutant epidermal growth factor receptors in human glioblastoma. Proc. Natl. Acad. Sci. U.S.A. 1990;87:4207–4211.

36. Chen W, Peace DJ, Rovira DK, You S-G, Cheever MA. T-cell immunity to the joining region of p210 BCR-ABL protein. Proc. Natl. Acad. Sci. U.S.A. 1992;89:1468–1472.

37. Gambacorti-Passerini C, Grignani F, Arienti F, Pandlofi PP, Pelicci PG, Parmiani G. Human CD4 lymphocytes specifically recognize a peptide representing the fusion region of the hybrid protein pml/RARα present in acute promyelocytic leukemia cells. Blood 1993;81:1369–1375.

38. Disis ML, Calenoff E, McLaughlin G, et al. Existent T-cell and antibody immunity to HER-2/neu protein in patients with breast cancer. Cancer Res. 1994;54:16–20.

39. Chen L, Thomas EK, Hu S-L, Hellstrom I, Hellstrom KE. Human papillomavirus type 16 nucleoprotein E7 is a tumor rejection antigen. Proc. Natl. Acad. Sci. U.S.A. 1991;88:110–114.

40. Feltcamp MCW, Smits HL, Vierboom MPM, et al. Vaccination with cytotoxic T lymphocyte epitop-containing peptide protects against a tumor induced by Human Papillomavirus type 16-transformed cells. Eur. J. Immunol. 1993;24:605–610.

41. Dranoff G, Mulligan RC. Gene transfer as cancer therapy. Adv. Immunol. 1995;58:417–454.

42. Forni G, Giovarelli M, Santoni A. Lymphokine-activated tumor inhibition in vivo. I The local administration of interleukin-2 triggers nonreactive lymphocytes from tumorbearing mice to inhibit tumor growth in vivo. J. Immunol. 1985;134:1305–1312.

43. Forni G, Fujiwara H, Martino F, et al. Helper strategy in tumor immunology: expansion of helper lymphocytes and utilization of helper lymphokines for experimental and clinical immunotherapy. Cancer and Metast. Rev. 1988;7:289–309.

44. Asher AL, Mule JJ, Kasid A, et al. Murine tumor cells transduced with the gene for tumor necrosis factor-α. J. Immunol. 1991;146:3227–3234.

45. Fearon ER, Pardoll DM, Itaya T, et al. Interleukin-2 production by tumor cells bypasses T helper function in the generation of an antitumor response. Cell 1990;60:397–403.

46. Gansbacher B, Zier K, Daniels B, Kronin K, Bannerji R, Gilboa E. Interleukin-2 gene transfer into tumor cells abrogates tumorigenicity and induces protective immunity. J. Exp. Med. 1990;172:1217–1224.

47. Gansbacher B, Bannerji R, Daniels B, Zier K, Cronin K, Gilboa E. Retroviral vector-mediated γ-interferon gene transfer into tumor cells generates potent and long lasting antitumor immunity. Cancer Res. 1990;50:7820–7825.

48. Golumbek PT, Lazenby AJ, Levitsky HI, et al. Treatment of established renal cancer by tumor cells engineered to secrete interleukin-4. Science 1991;254:713–716.

49. Watanabe Y, Kuribayashi K, Miyatake S, et al. Exogenous expression of mouse interferon γ cDNA in mouse neuroblastoma C1300 cells results in reduced tumorigenicity by augmented anti-tumor immunity. Proc. Natl. Acad. Sci. U.S.A. 1989;86:9456–9460.

50. Basombrio MA. Search for common antigenicity among twenty-five sarcomas induced by methylcholanthrene. Cancer Res. 1970;30:2458–2462.

51. Danos O, Mulligan RC. Safe and efficient generation of recombinant retroviruses with amphotropic and ecotropic host ranges. Proc. Natl. Acad. Sci. U.S.A. 1988;85:6460–6464.

52. Prehn RT, Main JM. Immunity to methylcholanthrene-induced sarcomas. J. Natl. Cancer Inst. 1957;18:769–778.

53. Caux C, Dezutter-Dambuyant C, Schmitt D, Banchereau J. GM-CSF and TNF-α cooperate in the generation of dendritic Langerhans cells. Nature 1992;360:258–261.

54. Inaba K, Inaba M, Romani N, et al. Generation of large numbers of dendritic cells from mouse bone marrow cultures supplemented with granulocyte/macrophage colony-stimulating factor. J. Exp. Med. 1992;176:1693–1702.

55. Steinman RM. The dendritic cell system and its role in immunogenicity. Ann. Rev. Immunol. 1991;9:271–296.

56. Schmidt W, Schweighoffer T, Herbst E, et al. Cancer vaccines: the interleukin 2 dosage effect. Proc. Natl. Acad. Sci. U.S.A. 1995;92:4711–4714.

57. Sanda MG, Ayyagari SR, Jaffee EM, et al. Demonstration of a rational strategy for human prostate cancer gene therapy. J. Urol. 1994;151:622–628.

58. Saito S, Bannerji R, Gansbacher B, et al. Immunotherapy of bladder cancer with cytokine gene-modified tumor vaccines. Cancer Res. 1994;54:3516–3520.

59. Jaffee EM, Dranoff G, Cohen LK, et al. High efficiency gene transfer into primary human tumor explants without cell selection. Cancer Res. 1993;53:2221–2226.

60. Berns AJM, Clift S, Cohen LK, et al. Phase I study of non-replicating autologous tumor cell injections using cells prepared with or without GM-CSF gene transduction in patients with metastatic renal cell carcinoma. Hum. Gene Ther. 1995;6(3):347–368.

61. Tybulewicz V, Crawford C, Jackson P, Bronson R, Mulligan RC. Neonatal lethality and lymphopenia in mice with a homozygous disruption of the c-abl proto-oncogene. Cell 1991;65:1153–1163.

62. Mansour S, Thomas K, Capecchi M. Disruption of the proto-oncogene int-2 in mouse embryo-derived stem cells: a general strategy for targeting mutations to non-selectable genes. Nature 1988;336:348–352.

63. Shanafelt A, Kastelein R. Identification of critical regions in mouse granulocyte-macrophage colony-stimulating factor by scanning deletion analysis. Proc. Natl. Acad. Sci. U.S.A. 1989;86:4872–4876.

64. Metcalf D. Hemopoietic regulators: redundancy or subtlety? Blood 1993;82:3515–3523.

65. Rosen S, Castleman B, Liebow A. Pulmonary alveolar proteinosis. N. Engl. J. Med. 1958;258:1123–1142.

66. Wright J, Dobbs L. Regulation of pulmonary surfactant secretion and clearance. Annu. Rev. Physiol. 1991;53:395–414.

67. Hoffman R, Rogers R. Pulmonary alveolar proteinosis. In: III JPL, DeRemee RA, ed. Immunologically Mediated Pulmonary Disease. Philadelphia: Lippincott, 1991: 449–472.

68. Tazi A. Evidence that granulocyte macrophage-colony-stimulating factor regulates the distribution and differentiated state of dendritic cells/Langerhans cells in human lung and lung cancers. J. Clin. Invest. 1993;91:566–576.

69. Sastry K, Ezekowitz R. Collectins: pattern recognition molecules involved in first line host defense. Curr. Opin. Immunol. 1993;5:59–66.

DISCUSSION

G. Evan: It is a comment really, and I wondered what you thought about this: I am very intrigued by your knockout experiments which indicate, to me, that critical cells - though thought to be, in the main, dependent upon particular survival factors and mitogenic factors, are not. Now is this not good news for cancer treatment in principle because you could make a very good argument that if a cancer cell undergoes some sort of mitogenic or survival lesion then there may not be a lot of selected pressure on it? So tumor cells when they arise may be critically dependent upon a relatively small number of lesions. Where is, what your data shows, and what the other data show, the fact that the IGF-1 knockout is not lethal, IGF-2 knockout and so on: Is it that somatic cells appear to be dependent for survival and proliferation upon an array of survival factors. And they are not critically dependent upon any one? So does that not suggest, as it does to me, that if you could find out why it is that tumor cells are surviving when they should not; there may be very small number of lesions and therefore, very susceptible to correction of those lesions.

G. Dranoff: I think that the interpretation of the phenotypes of growth factor knockouts is still a matter for discussion. In some cases, such knockouts produce obvious defects in hematopoiesis. G-CSF deficient mice demonstrate reductions in the number of neutrophils. M-CSF deficient mice have significant reductions in many macrophage populations. IL-5 knockout mice show fewer numbers of eosinophils. Stem cell factor knockout mice have clear reductions in tissue mast cells. The absence of obvious hematopoietic defects in the GM-CSF deficient mouse could mean either that this factor does not have a major role in hematopoiesis or that there is functional redundancy. How these findings relate to the relative dependence of cancer cells on growth factors is not yet clear.

G. Evan: There is one other point which I guess you could answer with your GM-CSF knockout. Where you put back GM-CSF in particular tissues. Which is that of course the defects that you see are chronic defects where their genes have been ablated throughout development. So the question now is, if you are going to try to treat a tumor by knocking out GM-CSF survival pathway, for example, that is not chronic, that is acute; the question now is even when these things appear essential for a fully functional, healthy, happy mouse, what might be the effects of acute knocking out of these particular survival factor pathways on peripheral cells?

G. Dranoff: The use of conditional targeting would allow that question to be addressed.

D. Livingston: Is one physiologic function of GM to allow macrophages to digest certain objects?

G. Dranoff: Yes, I think that is very clear.

D. Livingston: So, in keeping with the findings of Baltimore's laboratory on NF-KB, are your macrophages defective in phagocytosis?

G. Dranoff: That is an important issue currently under study. The alveolar macrophage are able to phagocytose antibody coated red blood cells and zymosan particles. Peritoneal macrophages are able to ingest thioglycollate. Systemic challenge of the mice with pathogens thought to require intact macrophage function such as Listeria, Candida, and Pseudomonas has not yet revealed any major susceptibility. It may be that the difficulty in handling surfactant is due to a very specific macrophage defect.

D. Livingston: But can they not clear surfactant even though they can eat it?

G. Dranoff: That is correct.

D. Livingston: Second question: Can you re-address macrophages to new locations?

G. Dranoff: That is an intriguing experiment. We have transplanted wild type bone marrow into the GM-CSF mutant mice, but this failed to correct the alveolar proteinosis. Similarly, transplantation of GM-CSF deficient bone marrow into a normal host failed to transmit the disease.

D. Livingston: Do wild type marrow progenitors give rise to macrophages that home to the alveoli?

G. Dranoff: That is a difficult experiment to do without surface marked cells. We did, however, demonstrate by Southern analysis of peripheral blood that the mutant animals were reconstituted with wild type marrow. Experiments reported in the literature have demonstrated that alveolar macrophages derive from bone marrow progenitors.

D. Livingston: Can you demonstrate that this defect is in digesting as opposed to ingesting?

G. Dranoff: Could be either one, if it is ingested in the wrong way.

D. Livingston: So if you take a GM minus animal's alveolar macrophages, are they defective in vitro? That is a prelude to the last question.

G. Dranoff: It has been difficult to demonstrate a specific defect in vitro to date because the normal mouse alveolar macrophage depends on growth factors like GM-CSF to maintain viability in culture.

D. Livingston: Is there autocrine stimulation by GM produced by alveolar macrophages?

G. Dranoff: Other macrophage populations can be maintained in culture with just fetal calf serum. It is interesting that if they are incubated with surfactant, they also become "stuffed" and resemble the alveolar macrophages from the GM-CSF knockout.

E. Mihich: I have three sets of questions: The first has to do with whether we are dealing solely or prominently with a vaccine effect as compared to a regional effect related to the secretion of the cytokine that is being transfected. You have a lot of data that are leaning strongly toward vaccination effect but is it possible to explore the question whether there is an effect perhaps on the tumor related suppression of the response. As you know in most of these systems, including B16 the tumor is suppressing T cell responses, for instance, and you could have both effects - the memory and the T cell responses speak strongly in favor of a vaccine effect. But one should not perhaps take for granted the fact that you might have a molecular event in the tumor itself, that would prevent tumor induced suppression and perhaps put into evidence the innate tumor immunogenicity which then would be reflected in the cross-reactivity that you were showing.

G. Dranoff: That is certainly a possibility. I should highlight the fact that live B16 tumor cells secreting GM-CSF are not rejected by the host, nor do they induce significant systemic anti-tumor immunity. Irradiation appears to be an important ingredient in the mix. Inhibition of tumor suppression is not likely to be the whole story.

E. Mihich: But it could be a component.

G. Dranoff: Certainly.

E. Mihich: In relation to the effect on function - discussed by Livingston and others - you mentioned that there is dependency on T cell function, both CD4 and CD8. Do you see a differential, I could not spot it in the slide - do you see a quantitative differential between CD4 and CD8 positive cells; is the effect more dependent on CD8 than on CD4, or is it sort of equally dependent on CD4 and CD8? I am asking this because, as you know, we have been doing a lot of work on the immunomodulation by adriamycin and IL2 combination for example, and we also see a dependence on CD8 and CD4 but the CD4 dependence is partial, compared to the CD8 dependence.

G. Dranoff: It does appear that if you make the challenge dose less stringent, then you do not need the CD4 cells as much. So that would be consistent with your result.

E. Mihich: And in terms of the macrophages: Can you try to paralyze your RES either systemically or specifically, and would you see an effect? In other words, are you dependent on macrophages?

G. Dranoff: That was actually the motivation to generate the GM-CSF deficient mouse. I have not presented any tumor vaccination experiments in the knockout mice today because we are still backcrossing the mutation onto the C57Bl/6 and Balb/c backgrounds.

E. Mihich: And the last set is: Why is x-ray putting into evidence the immunogenic potential of the transfected cells? What happens? They are still producing the cytokine GM-CSF but you showed us very well that GM-CSF was much less effective than IL2 in the normal cell, but if you irradiate it then you put it back into evidence. What is happening in the cell that puts it into evidence?

G. Dranoff: This matter is under study. One possibility relates to the oxidative damage that irradiation generates; this substrate may be effectively recognized by the host.

A. Matter: The effector cell is actually antibody dependent ADCC or direct killing?

G. Dranoff: We have not detected tumor specific antibodies to date. Protection appears to depend more on cellular than humoral mechanisms.

INDEX

The manufacturer's authorised representative in the EU is Springer
Nature Customer Service Centre GmbH, Europaplatz 3, 69115 Heidelberg,
Germany. If you have any concerns regarding our products, please
contact ProductSafety@springernature.com

Printed and bound by CPI Group (UK) Ltd, Croydon, CR0 4YY
23/04/2026
02095607-0014